INSTRUCTOR'S GUIDE FOR

PHARMACOTHERAPEUTICS:

A NURSING PROCESS APPROACH

2nd edition

Carolyn S. Brown, R.N., M.N., CCRN
Instructor
Louisiana State University, Medical Center
School of Nursing
New Orleans, Louisiana

F. A. Davis Company • Philadelphia

Printed in the United States of America

ISBN 0-8036-5924-5

Key to Codes That Accompany Situation and Review Questions

NP =	Nursing process phase	CL =	Cognitive level
	AS = Assessment		KN = Knowledge
	AN = Analysis		CO = Comprehension
	PL = Planning		AP = Application
	IM = Implementation		AN = Analysis
	EV = Evaluation		

* Indicates correct answer

TABLE OF CONTENTS

Chapter

CHAPTER 1: THE NURSING PROCESS AND FUNDAMENTALS OF DRUG THERAPY

Situation from Text

Situation 1-1

Jim Case is employed as a charge nurse in a skilled nursing facility at a small rural hospital. The following questions relate to typical patient situations he encounters.

1. Jean Coyle, a 79-year-old diabetic, is being admitted to the unit for rehabilitation care following a fracture of the right hip. Which question would be most helpful in eliciting information for an admission nursing assessment?
   a. "You do not have problems with giving yourself insulin, do you?"
   b. "Who told you figs could be included in your diet?"
   *c. "What do you do if you become shaky?"
   d. "Do you take daily laxatives?"

   [NP: AS, CL: AN]

   Rationale: Hypothetical questions are useful in determining patient comprehension of previously learned material.

2. Mrs. Coyle tells Jim that she is allergic to penicillin. Which symptom indicates an allergic reaction to this drug?
   *a. rash
   b. nausea
   c. dizziness
   d. drowsiness

   [NP: AS, CL: CO]

   Rationale: An allergic reaction may be manifested by a rash. The other symptoms are considered undesirable adverse drug effects.

3. Mr. Fell, an 80-year-old asthmatic, has been receiving theophylline (a bronchodilator) to decrease bronchospasm. Which statement by Mr. Fell should alert the nurse that the dosage may have to be altered to be effective?
   *a. "I smoke a pack of cigarettes a day."
   b. "My bowels haven't moved in two days."
   c. "I'm not sleeping well at night."
   d. "I have a bad headache."

   [NP: EV, CL: AN]

   Rationale: Heavy smokers may require higher doses of theophylline in order for it to be effective.

4. Jim is evaluating the effectiveness of barbiturates ordered for Mr. Syms, a 79-year-old patient who is very agitated. Which statement by Mr. Syms indicates that he may be having an idiosyncratic reaction to the drug?
   a. "My stomach feels upset."
   *b. "I just can't sit still."
   c. "There is a rash on my neck."
   d. "It burns when I urinate."

   [NP: EV, CL: AN]

   Rationale: Barbiturates may cause unexpected abnormal reactions, such as restlessness and excitability, in the elderly.

5. Mr. Syms is started on a MAO inhibitor for depression. Jim teaches him to avoid the following food:
   a. fish

b. eggs
c. chicken
*d. red wine

[NP: IM, CL: AP]

Rationale: Alcohol may cause a rapid rise in blood pressure when taken with MAO inhibitors.

6. Eighty-five-year-old Rose Santa has been receiving Warfarin to prevent progression of neurologic deficits. Which of the following statements by Rose indicates that health teaching regarding the medication has been ineffective?
a. "I ate a chocolate candy bar yesterday."
b. "My legs feel heavy."
*c. "I always have a bottle of aspirin with me."
d. "I must be catching a bad cold."

[NP: EV, CL: AN]

Rationale: A drug interaction between Warfarin and aspirin may result in bleeding.

Additional Situation Not Presented in Text

Robert Lems is a 59-year-old patient on a medical surgical floor. He has just been diagnosed as having Parkinson's disease. As the primary nurse, Ms. Adams is concerned with providing comprehensive nursing care.

1. Before giving Mr. Lems any medication, the nurse must first assess all of the following EXCEPT:
a. medication allergies
b. other medical problems
*c. family support
d. condition of his skin

[NP: AS, CL: CO]

Rationale: Answers a, b, and d must first be assessed when medications are to be administered. Family support would be important with respect to patient compliance.

2. Mr. Lems was recently started on levadopa. During health teaching, the following dietary changes would be stressed:
a. Avoid rich, fatty foods.
*b. Limit foods high in protein.
c. Eat small frequent meals.
d. Avoid foods high in sodium.

[NP: IM, CL: CO]

Rationale: High protein intake may interfere with the absorption of levadopa.

3. As Ms. Adams hands Mr. Lems his morning medications, he states, "Just take all those pills away; they are not doing me any good." The nurse's best response would be:
a. "But the pills are helping you, Mr. Lems."
b. "It sounds to me like you are angry."
c. "Where did you get the idea that the pills are not helping?"
*d. "Does it upset you to have to take medication?"

[NP: AS, CL: AN]

Rationale: A mirror response is useful in understanding underlying meanings which are not clearly verbalized. Answer d encourages patient response without being threatening or evaluative.

4. Which statement by Mr. Lems would indicate that health teaching was ineffective?

a. "I have always had trouble taking medicine on time."
b. "My uncle had Parkinson's disease and he lived a long time."
*c. "Missing a pill now and then shouldn't matter."
d. "It's best to take my medication on an empty stomach."

[NP: EV, CL: AN]

Rationale: This statement indicates a lack of understanding about the importance of taking medication as ordered.

5. The following would be an appropriate outcome for Mr. Lems:
The patient will:
*a. state the reasons for taking medicines on time
b. know how to take his medications
c. understand why he must watch for side effects
d. understand his disease process

[NP: PL, CL: AP]

Rationale: This answer is more specific and easily measurable. Verbs such as "understand" and "know" are vague and difficult to measure.

6. It is important for Ms. Adams to gather information about Mr. Lems. All of the following are examples of data gathered during the verbal interchange phase EXCEPT:
a. social interactions
b. perceptions about illness
c. ways of coping
*d. gait disturbances

[NP: AS, CL: CO]

Rationale: The verbal interchange phase elicits information about the patient and significant others. Gait disturbances would be an example of findings related to physical assessment.

Review Questions from Text

1. A major responsibility of the nursing profession is to:
a. discourage the use of over-the-counter medications
*b. teach consumers about the benefits and dangers of medications
c. control the administration of medications in the hospital setting
d. alter the consumer's values and beliefs concerning medication use

[CL: KN]

Rationale: Nursing is primarily responsible for patient teaching and for ensuring that patients are adequately informed about the chosen therapy.

2. What is the first condition which must be met in order for a patient to comply with the medication regime?
a. adequate knowledge about the disease process
b. examination of cultural beliefs which may affect compliance
*c. acceptance of the diagnosis
d. adequate family support

Rationale: Answers a, b, and d are important aspects of compliance; however, the nurse must first ensure that the patient accepts the diagnosis and is willing to comply with the treatment.

3. For the cognitive domain of learning, teaching involves:
a. evaluating feedback from the learner about thoughts and feelings
b. ensuring that the patient can perform a procedure

c. demonstrating activities necessary for learning
*d. giving factual information

[CL: KN]

Rationale: The cognitive domain emphasizes the intellectual aspects associated with learning. Answer a reflects the affective domain, and answers b and c reflect the psychomotor domain.

4. Tasks of the affective teaching domain include all of the following except:
*a. analyzing
b. receiving
c. valuing
d. organizing

[CL: CO]

Rationale: Analyzing involves intellectual or thinking processes and, therefore, is a task of the cognitive domain.

5. Which of the following is an example of a dermatologic toxic reaction?
a. mild rash
b. alopecia
*c. hives
d. skin pigmentation

[CL: CO]

Rationale: Hives represent a toxic dermatologic effect which would require discontinuation of the medication.

6. Symptoms related to anemia and leukopenia are referred to as:
a. idiosyncratic reactions
b. adverse effects
c. allergic reactions
*d. toxic effects

[CL: KN]

Rationale: Anemia and leukopenia can result in harm to the patient and are considered toxic effects.

7. During the planning stage of the nursing process:
a. the patient's actual and potential health problems are identified
b. nursing actions are based on nursing orders
c. objective and subjective data are evaluated
*d. goals are established which become the outcomes of nursing care

[CL: KN]

Rationale: The planning phase of the nursing process involves establishing short-term and long-term goals.

8. Which statement is correct regarding interviewing techniques used by nurses to elicit patient information?
a. Open-ended questions impose limitations on patient responses.
*b. Loaded questions should be avoided in an information-gathering interview.
c. Closed-ended questions allow the greatest freedom of response.
d. Mirror-response questions are evaluative and threatening.

[CL: KN]

Rationale: Avoid loaded questions, as they tend to be stated in emotional terms and suggest the desired patient response.

9. In taking a medication history, the nurse knows the following statement to be true:

a. Heavy smokers may require smaller doses if taking theophylline, a bronchodilator.
b. Alcohol consumption decreases the action of tranquilizers and CNS depressants.
c. Over-the-counter drugs should not be included in a medication history.
*d. Patients allergic to fish may also be allergic to contrast dyes used in radiology.

[CL: KN]

Rationale: Cross allergies may occur in patients who are allergic to both fish and x-ray dyes which contain iodine.

10. All of the following statements are true regarding health teaching <u>except</u>:
a. The primary aim of health teaching is to ensure patient compliance.
b. Patients are likely to change behavior if they understand the need and the benefits.
*c. It is inappropriate for the nurse to solicit and evaluate patient feedback to assess learning.
d. Teaching may involve the cognitive, affective, and psychomotor domains of learning.

[CL: CO]

Rationale: An important aspect of health teaching involves evaluation of patient feedback in order to assess learning.

<u>Additional Review Questions Not Presented in Text</u>

1. Pharmacotherapeutics is defined as:
a. using pharmacists to dispense medications
b. studying drug actions on a living system
*c. treating all aspects of disease with medications
d. using a combination of therapies to treat disease

[CL: KN]

Rationale: Pharmacotherapeutics is an encompassing term denoting medication therapy used to treat, diagnose, or cure disease.

2. A constructive listening technique is:
*a. paying attention to ideas that bind facts together
b. reacting to the patient rather than the message
c. responding on an emotional level to what the patient says
d. hearing only isolated facts and drawing conclusions

[CL: CO]

Rationale: Facts alone are not as important as linking them with whole thoughts and ideas in order to understand what the patient is saying.

3. The purpose of the nursing diagnosis is to:
a. identify only the patient's actual health problems
b. evaluate the patient's response to treatment and medications
*c. focus on patient response to treatment and underlying pathology
d. lead to the development of objectives which are to be implemented

[CL: KN]

Rationale: Nursing diagnoses are developed from the data base and focus on actual or potential problems as the patient responds to symptoms and their pathology.

4. Which statment is not true regarding the intervention stage of the nursing process?
*a. Health teaching is withheld until the patient asks for information about the diagnosis.
b. Health maintenance and disease prevention are aspects of nursing care.

c. Nursing orders evolve from nursing goals and are written in behavioral terms.
d. Nursing care is based on the nursing orders in the nursing care plan.

[CL: CO]

Rationale: The nurse does not wait to perform health teaching until the patient asks for information about the diagnosis. Health teaching is based on patient needs and readiness to learn.

CHAPTER 2: HISTORY, LEGISLATION, AND STANDARDS

Situation from Text

Situation 2-1

Amy Forbes, a new graduate nurse, has been assigned to work on a medical-surgical unit. Many of the patients under her care are receiving controlled drugs. The following questions relate to Amy's knowledge of drug legislation and standards.

1. In administering hydromorphone (Dilaudid), a narcotic, to Jim Nesbit, who has a fractured left femur, the nurse has the responsibility to:
   a. rewrite the prescription on the day of expiration
   b. document and save any remaining medication
   *c. provide health teaching regarding the drug's action
   d. obtain a telephone reorder one day before expiration

   [NP: DM, CL: CO]

   Rationale: One of the nurse's major responsibilities is to provide education regarding drug effectiveness and adverse effects.

2. Sixty-two-year-old James Able is receiving Valium 5 mg T.I.D. for nervousness. Which of the following is true regarding Valium?
   *a. It must be reordered every seven days by the physician.
   b. As a Schedule II drug, it is reordered every 72 hours.
   c. Studies have shown Valium to have a low abuse potential.
   d. It can be dispensed without a prescription in most states.

   [NP: PL, CL: KN]

   Rationale: Hospital orders for Valium are valid for seven days and require a physician's reorder for continuation.

3. Ruth Lee is being prepared for discharge following a laminectomy. The physician has ordered Talwin 50 mg po q 6 hours prn for pain. Amy teaches that Talwin is:
   a. non-addictive if taken only as ordered
   b. a mild tranquilizer which is not subject to regulation
   *c. reordered by the physician every 6 months or after 5 refills
   d. a non-narcotic which can be purchased over-the-counter

   [NP: IM, CL: KN]

   Rationale: Talwin is classified as a Schedule V controlled drug, and a prescription must be rewritten after 6 months or 5 refills.

4. Joseph Starr has been diagnosed as having AIDS. He is being considered for treatment with a new drug. Joseph asks the nurse, "What does the term 'new drug' mean?" All of the following statements regarding new drugs are correct <u>except</u>:
   a. The drugs are initially administered to animals to establish a data base.
   b. The FDA reviews animal study reports on safety and effectiveness.
   c. Clinical Phase I uses healthy volunteers to administer the drug.
   *d. Once the FDA approves the new drug, safety is assured.

   [NP: PL, CL: CO]

   Rationale: Even with FDA approval, medications may be discovered to be toxic or fatal once administered to a large group of individuals.

5. Amy prepares a morphine (narcotic) injection for Mr. Cane as requested. When Amy takes the medication into Mr. Cane's room, he informs her that he has changed his mind and would rather not take the shot. Amy has the legal responsibility to:
   *a. return the drug to the point of origin, such as the hospital pharmacy
   b. discard the drug while another nurse observes and documents her action
   c. save the drug in the syringe in case Mr. Cane requests it later
   d. encourage Mr. Cane to take the medication since it has already been prepared

   [NP: IM, CL: AP]

   Rationale: Narcotics which are drawn up and not used must be returned to the point of origin, usually the hospital pharmacy. The nurse cannot discard the entire dose.

6. Bob Lockhart is receiving Demerol 50 mg IM for postoperative pain. Amy notices that the drug order has expired. She is aware that:
   a. the physician must rewrite the Demerol order every 48 hours
   b. a nurse cannot accept a telephone order for a drug renewal
   *c. the physician must countersign a verbal order within 48 hours
   d. as a Schedule III drug, Demerol is only renewed one time

   [NP: IM, CL: AP]

   Rationale: In obtaining a verbal order for a Schedule II substance, such as Demerol, the physician must countersign the order within 48 hours.

Additional Situation Not Presented in Text

James Meyer is a staff nurse on a neurological unit of a large urban hospital. The following questions relate to standards of medication administration.

1. Kevin Joules, a 76-year-old admitted with a severe head injury and seizures, is on Clonazepam (Clonopin) 1 mg BID. James is aware that this drug:
   a. is a Schedule III narcotic
   b. must be reordered every 48 hours
   *c. is a Schedule IV depressant
   d. represents a high abuse potential

   [NP: PL, CL: KN]

   Rationale: Clonazepam (Clonopin) is a Schedule IV depressant which differs from Schedule III in penalties for legal possession.

2. Mrs. Bell is being treated with a new drug for multiple sclerosis in a Phase 3 Clinical Trial. James teachs Mrs. Bell and her family that Phase 3 Clinical Trials often involve:
   a. observing a group of patients for side effects
   *b. using double-blind studies
   c. refining the drug dosage
   d. comparing data with animal studies

   [NP: IM, CL: CO]

   Rationale: Phase 3 Clinical Trials often use double-blind studies in order to reduce bias.

3. James is preparing discharge instructions for Thomas Corley, who will be taking Lomotil prn for diarrhea. It is important for James to be aware that:
   a. state penalties for illegal possession may differ
   b. the prescription may be refilled only two times
   *c. state regulations may require a prescription
   d. the drug must be reordered every 6 months

[NP: PL, CL: AP]

Rationale: As a Schedule V drug, Lomotil may be dispensed without a prescription unless additional state regulations apply.

4. In order to administer Dilaudid (narcotic) to Laura Norman, a 47-year-old with a spinal tumor, James has the legal responsibility to record all of the following information on the narcotics log <u>except</u>:
 a. date of administration
 b. time of administration
 c. prescriber's name
 *d. copy of the physician's order

[NP: IM, CL: CO]

Rationale: Answers a, b, and c represent information required by law whenever a nurse administers a controlled substance.

5. Before giving medications to any patient, James observes the five rights of medication administration. A sixth right refers to:
 *a. the right to refuse medication
 b. the right to take medication without the nurse present
 c. the right to review the nurse's credentials
 d. the right to withhold personal identity

[NP: IM, CL: KN]

Rationale: The patient has the right to refuse medication; this is often referred to as the sixth right.

6. While giving a patient Flurazepam (Dalmane) for sleep, the pill is accidentally dropped on the floor. James has the responsibility to:
 a. discard the pill in the presence of another nurse and document action
 *b. mark the pill as contaminated and return it to the pharmacy
 c. mark the pill as contaminated and return it to the patient's medication drawer
 d. record the contaminated dose on the pharmacy narcotics log and discard

[NP: IM, CL: AP]

Rationale: If a dose of narcotic or controlled substance is contaminated, it should be labeled and returned to the pharmacy.

<u>Review Questions from Text</u>

1. Early history demonstrates that people of past cultures:
 *a. attempted to treat illness through medical intervention
 b. were successful in curing illness through surgical intervention
 c. had few illnesses related to present day forms
 d. had great insight into the causes of disease and related treatments

[CL: KN]

Rationale: Through the discovery of ancient artifacts and drawings, it is believed that early cultures attempted to treat illness by medical intervention.

2. The following statement is true about the early post-Christian era:
 a. Hippocrates was the most famous physician of this era.
 b. Great strides occurred in medicine and pharmacology.
 *c. The Catholic Church controlled the knowledge of healing and medicine.
 d. Egyptians were the first to employ the use of belladonna and narcotics.

[CL: CO]

Rationale: The role of the Catholic Church was very influential during the early post-Christian era.

3. Contributions of the Arabs to the history of pharmacy include all of the following except:
   a. established hospitals and medical schools
   b. separated pharmacy from the practice of medicine
   c. introduced the use of decimal notation
   *d. popularized the principle of polypharmacy

   [CL: CO]

   Rationale: The Arabian influence in the history began during the eighth century. Answers a, b, and c represent important contribtions. Galen, the Greek physician, popularized the principle of polypharmacy.

4. The empirical stage of therapeutics was characterized by:
   a. a lack of detailed record-keeping
   *b. clinical evidence that a drug was effective
   c. an understanding of drug action
   d. all of the above

   [CL: KN]

   Rationale: Empirical therapeutics is based on evidence that a drug is effective, although the mechanism of action may not be understood.

5. The physician-scientist who advocated the use of specific compounds to treat disease was:
   *a. Paracelsus
   b. Asclepius
   c. Hippocrates
   d. Dioscorides

   [CL: KN]

   Rationale: Individuals such as Paracelsus (1493-1541) questioned superstitious medicinal beliefs and advocated specific compounds to treat disease.

6. The mystical stage of the science of therapeutics employed all of the following forms of therapy except:
   a. prayer
   *b. alchemy
   c. surgery
   d. medication

   [CL: KN]

   Rationale: The mystical stage of therapeutics employed prayers, surgery, and drugs as modes of therapy.

7. Place the following drugs in order of discovery:
   a. colchicine, digitalis, opium, ether
   b. opium, ether, digitalis, colchicine
   c. ether, opium, digitalis, colchicine
   *d. opium, colchicine, ether, digitalis

   [CL: CO]

   Rationale: Opium was discovered in the first century A.D. Colchicine was discovered in the sixth century A.D. Ether was discovered in the sixteenth century A.D., and digitalis was discovered in the eighteenth century A.D.

8. An approved drug label must have all of the following except:
   a. the name and business address of the manufacturer
   b. the suggested dose and frequency of use
   *c. the date of drug manufacture and distribution

d. the kind, quantity, and proportion of ingredients

[CL: KN]

Rationale: The Federal Food, Drug, and Cosmetic Act (FFDCA) of 1938 established requirements for all drug labels. All but answer d are required.

9. Which statement is not true regarding the development of the nurse's role in drug administrations?
   a. As early as 1920, the curriculum for student nurses included two courses dealing with medications.
   *b. By the late 1920's, nurses were given the authority to administer intramuscular injections.
   c. In the late 1930's, health teaching regarding medications became a more defined nursing role.
   d. At the present time, the nursing process is the scientific framework used by the nurse in medication administration.

   [CL: CO]

   Rationale: Nurses became responsible for the administration of intramuscular injections during the 1940's.

10. The Federal Food, Drug, and Cosmetic Act (FFDCA) of 1906 contributed to medication safety by:
   a. empowering state governments to enforce official drug standards
   b. requiring only narcotic drugs to comply with standards set by USP and NF
   c. requiring synthetic drugs to list side effects on the label
   *d. designating the USP and NF as official drug standards

   [CL: CO]

   Rationale: The Federal Food, Drug, and Cosmetic Act of 1906 was the first to designate the USP and NF as the official standards for drugs, thereby providing public protection.

Additional Review Questions Not Presented in Text

1. Schedule I controlled drug classification includes:
   a. all drugs containing opiates
   *b. all drugs used for investigative purposes
   c. drugs that may be reordered only twice
   d. drugs not requiring clearance from the FDA

   [CL: KN]

   Rationale: Drugs classified as Schedule I are legally used for research purposes only.

2. Which drug was discovered in the twentieth century A.D.?
   *a. insulin
   b. ether
   c. digitalis
   d. nitroglycerin

   [CL: CO]

   Rationale: Insulin was discovered by Banting in 1922.

3. A significant event affecting the area of healing occurred in the 1860's. That event was:
   a. St. Thomas Hospital's establishment of nursing "sisters"
   *b. Florence Nightingale's organization of nursing
   c. Paracelsus' study of chemical remedies
   d. Dioscorides' contribution to drug knowledge

   [CL: CO]

   Rationale: Florence Nightingale opened the first school of nursing in the 1860's.

4. Of the following statements, which one is true regarding the Pharmacopeia of the United States (USP) and the National Formulary (NF)?
   *a. In 1880, the NF was established to supplement the USP.
   b. The USP formerly listed drug mixtures rather than single drugs as in the NF.
   c. The USP and NF are revised every ten years.
   d. The USP and NF were first published in 1850.

   [CL: KN]

   Rationale: In 1888, the NF was established as a reference for mixtures and formulas to supplement the USP.

5. Drugs classified in Schedule V are those:
   a. having a high abuse potential
   b. requring a prescription
   *c. sold over the counter
   d. having refill regulations

   [CL: KN]

   Rationale: Drugs classified as Schedule V have a low abuse potential and do not require a prescription.

6. Schedule II controlled drugs:
   a. must be reordered after 6 months or 5 refills
   b. may be sold over the counter
   c. may be refilled without regulation
   *d. have high abuse potential

   [CL: KN]

   Rationale: Schedule II drugs are accepted as therapeutic but possess physical and/or psychological abuse potential.

CHAPTER 3: ADMINISTERING MEDICATIONS WITH SAFETY

Situations from Text

Situation 3-1

The nurse is administering medications to 28-year-old Nina Averton, who is hospitalized with bronchial pneumonia.

1. The nurse will administer several local-acting medications to Nina. All of the following types of drug preparations can produce local therapeutic effects except a:
   a. troche
   b. suppository
   c. gel
   *d. caplet

   [NP: IM, CL: CO]

   Rationale: Local medications produce effects that are confined to one area of the body; a caplet is an oral dosage form that is absorbed systematically.

2. Nina is ordered the expectorant guaifenesin. The nurse will administer this drug:
   *a. with a glass of water
   b. on an empty stomach
   c. through an n/g tube
   d. mixed in applesauce

   [NP: IM, CL: AP]

   Rationale: Administration of water with guaifenesin will ensure entry into the stomach and enhance absorption.

3. One of Nina's respiratory medications is in the form of a sustained-release tablet. The nurse should avoid:
   a. administering the tablet with another medication
   b. mixing the drug with an antacid
   *c. crushing the tablet before administration
   d. administering the tablet with water

   [NP: IM, CL: AP]

   Rationale: Crushing a sustained-release drug will interfere with the timed-release property of the drug preparation.

4. The nurse is preparing to administer antibiotics to Nina. The fastest and most effective route of administration is:
   a. oral
   b. subcutaneous
   *c. intravenous
   d. intramuscular

   [NP: IM, CL: KN]

   Rationale: IV administration places the drug directly into the vasculature, thus bypassing all barriers to drug absorption.

5. Nina is ordered an aspirin rectal suppository as needed for fever. The nurse is aware that the medication is:
   a. administered with its covering intact
   *b. stored in the refrigerator
   c. mixed with a gel before insertion
   d. expelled within a minute after insertion

   [NP: AN, CL: AP]

Rationale: Suppositories are designed to melt at body temperature; thus, they are stored in a cool place.

6. Nina is planning to take an Alaskan cruise during the next month, and her physician prescribes scopolamine disks to prevent motion sickness. The nurse instructs Nina to:
   a. apply the disk to any hairy body surface
   b. wear gloves when applying the disk
   *c. continue to shower while wearing the disk
   d. rub the disk with forceful pressure after application

   [NP: IM, CL: AP]

   Rationale: Transdermal scopolamine disks are applied behind the ear and are not affected by water.

Situation 3-2

Raul Estosa is a patient in the Medical Intensive Care Unit following an automobile accident. He is on multiple drug therapy.

1. Mr. Estosa is ordered the antibiotic Wycillin 600,000 U IM tid. The <u>best</u> schedule for the nurse to follow in administering the Wycillin is:
   a. 10 AM, 2 PM, and 6 PM
   b. 7 AM, 4 PM, and 8 PM
   c. 8 AM, 1 PM, and 6 PM
   *d. 9 AM, 6 PM, and 1 AM

   [NP: PL, CL: CO]

   Rationale: Antibiotics are best given around the clock at regular intervals to maintain therapeutic blood levels.

2. When implementing drug therapy for Mr. Estosa, the nurse's responsibilities include all of the following <u>except</u>:
   a. observing for drug effects
   b. instructing the patient about the drug's use
   c. checking for the correct dose of the drug
   *d. changing the dose if side effects occur

   [NP: IM, CL: CO]

   Rationale: The nurse is responsible for administering the correct dose of the ordered drug. The physician is responsible for changing the dosage if needed.

3. Each of the following is an appropriate nursing diagnosis related to administering medication to Mr. Estosa <u>except</u>:
   a. potential for injury from medication administration
   b. knowledge deficit related to current need for IV therapy
   c. anxiety related to frequent intramuscular injections
   *d. impaired social interaction related to IV therapy

   [NP: AN, CL: AP]

   Rationale: The implementation of IV therapy has no direct effect on social interaction.

4. Before administering medication to Mr. Estosa, the nurse will do all of the following <u>except</u>:
   *a. withhold medication if his pulse is rapid
   b. check his identification band
   c. assess his mental status
   d. honor his right to refuse medication

   [NP: IM, CL: CO]

   Rationale: Answers b, c, and d are all important for the nurse to assess prior to administering medications. A rapid pulse may not be a reason to withhold medication.

5. A heparin lock is placed in order to administer medications to Mr. Estosa. Nursing responsibilities associated with this device include:
   a. preceding and following medication administration with heparin solution
   b. mixing all multiple IV medications before injection
   *c. washing hands prior to administering medication
   d. assessing for dehydration and decreased blood pressure following medication administration

   [NP: IM, CL: AP]

   Rationale: Effective handwashing will decrease the chance of infection.

6. The nurse administers an IV bolus of a bronchodilator to facilitate Mr. Estosa's breathing. A bolus is a:
   a. continuous infusion given over a 24-hour period
   *b. concentrated dose given over a short time period
   c. slow infusion given over one hour
   d. diluted dose given one to six times a day

   [NP: IM, CL: KN]

   Rationale: A concentrated, or bolus, dose is given directly into the vein over a period of at least 1 to 2 minutes.

<u>**Additional Situation Not Presented in Text**</u>

Lynda James, a senior nursing student, is preparing drugs for administration during a clinical experience.

1. Lynda is looking up information on Lanoxin[R]. She realizes that this drug name is termed:

   a. chemical
   b. proprietary
   c. official
   d. generic

   [NP: AS, CL: KN]

   Rationale: A trade, or proprietary, name is created by the manufacturer. It is always capitalized and, if registered, is followed by a trademark symbol.

2. Lynda will be administering several topical medications. Which of the following is <u>not</u> a specific effect of a local medication?
   a. anesthetic
   b. anti-inflammatory
   c. bacteriostatic
   *d. antiarrhythmic

   [NP: PL, CL: CO]

   Rationale: Topical medications do not exert effects on the conduction system of the myocardium.

3. In administering drugs to alcoholic patients taking disulfiram (Antabuse), Lynda will avoid:
   *a. elixirs
   b. magmas
   c. syrups
   d. lozenges

   [NP: PL, CL: AP]

   Rationale: Elixirs are hydroalcoholic liquids that may produce severe reactions in patients receiving Antabuse therapy.

4. Lynda informs her instructor that the advantage of sublingual administration of medication is that the:
   a. first-pass effect occurs more quickly
   b. dosage design allows for slow dissolution
   *c. drug is not damaged by GI secretions
   d. vascular nature of the lingual area is avoided

   [NP: IM, CL: CO]

   Rationale: Through bypassing the oral route, the drug does not come into contact with GI secretions, thereby preventing possible damage.

5. Lynda prepares to administer the following drug order: Garamycin gtt i OS. She will administer the drug in the patient's:
   a. left ear
   b. right ear
   *c. left eye
   d. right eye

   [NP: IM, CL: AN]

   Rationale: OS is the common medical abbreviation for the left eye.

6. Lynda instructs a patient to prepare a tablespoon of liquid medication for administration at home by using a:
   *a. standard measuring spoon
   b. cap from the medication bottle
   c. flatware tablespoon
   d. small water glass

   [NP: IM, CL: AP]

   Rationale: A standard measuring spoon provides the necessary degree of accuracy for a household medication dosage.

<u>**Review Questions from Text**</u>

1. Local medication preparations may be:
   a. applied to the skin for rapid reabsorption
   b. injected into muscle tissue for altered absorption
   *c. injected into a joint cavity
   d. administered safely to all patients

   [CL: KN]

   Rationale: An anti-inflammatory effect is produced as the drug is absorbed into the local vasculature.

2. Which statement is <u>true</u> regarding administration of medications by the oral route?
   a. Gastric upsets rarely occur.
   *b. Inadvertent aspiration may occur in the seriously ill patient.
   c. Water given with the medication retards absorption.
   d. Oral administration is best for all patients.

   [CL: CO]

   Rationale: The seriously ill patient may not have adequate control of muscles used in the act of swallowing.

3. Parenteral administration of medications includes all of the following routes <u>except</u>:
   *a. oral
   b. intra-articular
   c. subcutaneous

d. intrathecal

[CL: KN]

Rationale: Parenteral medications are introduced into the body via a needle.

4. Which of the following nursing actions is incorrect relative to medication administration and patient safety?
 a. checking the five rights of medication administration
 *b. withholding medication if the patient is confused
 c. asking the patient to state his or her name
 d. checking the patient's ID band

[CL: CO]

Rationale: Special care is taken to identify a confused patient, thus properly administering needed medications.

5. In administering a pain-relieving injection, the nurse will implement all of the following actions except:
 a. select a non-excoriated site
 *b. insert and remove the needle slowly
 c. inject the medicine slowly
 d. apply direct pressure to the area afterwards

[CL: CO]

Rationale: Inserting and removing the needle rapidly will decrease the patient's pain sensation.

6. To avoid medication errors, the nurse will:
 a. refuse to interpret illegible handwriting
 *b. question the use of multiple tablets to provide a single dose
 c. use the dropper of one medication to administer another
 d. decline to investigate atypical drug names

[CL: AP]

Rationale: A common cause of medication errors is administering the wrong dose.

7. One characteristic of generic medications is that they are often:
 *a. less expensive than brand name drugs
 b. not as potent as brand name drugs
 c. more difficult to obtain from the pharmacist
 d. less regulated by law with respect to drug purity

[CL: KN]

Rationale: Generic substitutes reduce the cost of medical care by being less expensive than their brand name equivalents.

8. In order to alleviate gastric discomfort associated with taking medication, the nurse should instruct the patient to take the medication:
 *a. with breakfast
 b. in the evening
 c. with an antiemetic
 d. in divided doses

[CL: AP]

Rationale: Administering a medication with meals may decrease a drug's gastrointestinal side effects.

9. Which of the following statements is true regarding a parenteral administration of vitamin B_{12}?

a. It must be injected just under the skin surface.
b. The drug may be destroyed by enzymes in the blood.
c. It must be given by the Z-track method.
*d. It must be administered by specially trained individuals.

[CL: AP]

Rationale: Parenteral drugs are those medications introduced into the body via a needle. This type of drug administration requires specialized training and education.

10. Side effects of a headache associated with nitroglycerin ointment are an example of which type of drug effect?
a. local
b. anaesthetic
*c. systemic
d. first-pass

[CL: AP]

Rationale: A systemic effect such as a headache resulting from vasodilation of cerebral vessels occurs due to absorption of the drug through the skin.

Additional Review Questions Not Presented in Text

1. The physician has written an order to administer Decadron 0.22% gtt i OD daily. The nurse instills:
a. one drop of medication in both eyes daily
b. one drop of medication in the left eye daily
*c. one drop of medication in the right eye daily
d. no medication and verifies the physician's order

[CL: AP]

Rationale: OD is the common medical abbreviation for the right eye.

2. A nursing responsibility associated with medication administration includes:
a. returning unused medication to a stock bottle
b. administering a medication prepared by another nurse
c. leaving the medication at the bedside if the patient is not in the room
*d. signing out narcotics at the time of removal from the narcotic cabinet

[CL: CO]

Rationale: Narcotics are controlled substances; their intended use must be documented, and they must be accounted for prior to their removal from the narcotics cabinet.

3. Assessment of the patient receiving medications includes all of the following nursing actions except:
a. taking a nursing history to establish a data base
b. including an allergy history
c. examining the patient's skin
*d. changing the medication in order to accommodate the patient

[CL: KN]

Rationale: In most cases, the physician is responsible for prescribing the proper medication dosage for the patient.

4. In administering oral medications to patients, the nurse:
a. administers oils and cough medicines first
*b. ensures successful swallowing by administering tablets with water
c. withholds medications if the patient has a nasogastric tube

d. crushes enteric-coated tablets if the patient has difficulty swallowing

[CL: KN]

Rationale: Both large and small tablets should be followed with at least 100 ml of water to ensure successful swallowing.

5. The appropriate needle gauge and length for intramuscular injection would be:
 a. 26 gauge and 3/8 inch
 b. 25 gauge and 1/2 inch
 *c. 22 gauge and 1-1/2 inch
 d. 16 gauge and 1-1/2 inch

[CL: CO]

Rationale: The correct needle gauge for an intramuscular injection is 20-23, length 1-3 inches.

CHAPTER 4: THE PHASES OF DRUG ACTION

Situation from Text

Situation 4-1

Ann Matlock works as a nurse in an out-patient clinic of a small community hospital. The following are situations she frequently encounters while serving in that position.

1. Mr. King has been diagnosed as having pneumonia and ordered on penicillin 250 mg po q 6 hours. When Ann enters the room to administer the first dose, Mr. King states that he was on penicillin four years ago and developed hives. Based on this information, Ann:
   a. administers the drug as ordered and observes for a reaction
   b. combines the drug with an antihistamine to decrease the chance of reaction
   *c. withholds the drug and informs the physician of the patient's allergy
   d. administers the drug intramuscularly to bypass gastric absorption

   [NP: IM, CL: AN]

   Rationale: A prior occurrence of hives following penicillin administration indicates that the patient has developed an allergy to the drug and should not receive penicillin or related preparations again.

2. Mr. Ames is receiving an antibiotic (erythromycin) to treat a respiratory infection. Ann teaches Mr. Ames that taking erythromycin with food will:
   a. increase the rate of absorption
   b. have no effect on therapeutic action
   c. decrease gastric side effects
   *d. delay the rate of absorption

   [NP: IM, CL: AP]

   Rationale: Food decreases the absorption rate of erythromycin.

3. Mr. Downs is receiving aspirin to relieve arthritic pain. Ann administers the first dose with an antacid to:
   *a. increase the absorption rate in the small intestine
   b. reduce the effects of an acidic drug on absorption
   c. provide the drug in a time-release form
   d. provide a lipid base for greater absorption

   [NP: IM, CL: AP]

   Rationale: Aspirin, an acidic drug, is better absorbed in the small intestine if administered with an antacid.

4. John Foley came to the clinic complaining of headache and a stiff neck. Following a diagnosis of meningitis, the physician ordered penicillin G as part of the therapy. One reason for selection of this drug for treatment is that penicillin G is:
   *a. lipid soluble and able to cross the blood brain barrier
   b. utilized by brain cells via an active transport sytem
   c. water soluble and easily absorbed through the blood brain barrier
   d. transported into the central nervous system via facilitated diffusion

   [NP: PL, CL: CO]

   Rationale: Penicillin G is able to cross the blood brain barrier and provide effective treatment for central nervous system pathology.

5. Leo Cordell, a 75-year-old, comes to the clinic with a complaint of shortness of breath. During a nursing assessment, Ann learns that Mr. Cordell is an alcoholic who smokes a pack of cigarettes a day. Ann will assess Mr. Cordell for possible drug toxic effects primarily due to:

a. increased lung capacity
b. spasticity of the colon
*c. diminished liver function
d. ineffective cardiac function

[NP: IM, CL: AN]

Rationale: Elderly patients may have decreased function of the liver enzyme systems needed for drug biotransformation, with resultant toxic drug complications.

6. Mr. Brown, an asthmatic, complains that his bronchial inhaler (Isuprel) does not work as it used to. Ann is aware that this represents an example of:
a. supersensitivity
*b. desensitization
c. receptor agonist effect
d. hypersensitivity

[NP: AS, CL: AP]

Rationale: Desensitization may occur with repeated use of beta-adrenergic bronchodilators, resulting in decreased response to treatment.

Additional Situation Not Presented in Text

Don Hammond is the medication nurse on a medical/oncology unit. This position requires that he be aware of the phases of drug action.

1. Janice Harrell, a 60-year-old with lung cancer, is on an antibiotic (tetracycline). Don teaches Mrs. Harrell that tetracycline should not be taken with milk products or antacids because:
a. protein in the stomach inhibits absorption of the drug
*b. calcium binds with the drug and decreases absorption
c. milk products and antacids increase gastric motility, thereby decreasing absorption
d. milk products and antacids alter the pH of gastric secretions

[NP: IM, CL: CO]

Rationale: Tetracycline is not administered with milk, cheese, or antacids because the calcium binds with the drug and inhibits absorption.

2. Don has been monitoring the nutritional intake of Mr. Simpson, who is on multiple medications for treatment of a lymphoma. Mr. Simpson's lab work reflects hypoalbuminemia. Don is concerned about a low serum protein for all of the following reasons except:
a. Most medications are bound to albumin in the serum.
b. The patient will have difficulty transporting medications.
c. Excess free drug may result in an exaggerated effect.
*d. Decreased free drug may result in reduced therapeutic effect.

[NP: AS, CL: AN]

Rationale: Most medications are bound in the serum to albumin and, if hypoalbuminemia is present, the patient will have difficulty transporting medications. The excess free drug may result in an exaggerated effect.

3. George Prince is receiving an anticancer agent (cisplatin) intravenously. An advantage of giving cisplatin in the evening is that:
*a. the kidneys absorb less cisplatin
b. nausea and vomiting occur less frequently
c. bone marrow is less affected by the drug
d. the drug is less likely to cause alopecia

[NP: PL, CL: AN]

Rationale: Cisplatin is best given in the evening, when the kidneys normally process large quantities of fluid; therefore, less renal toxicity occurs.

4. Mrs. Hamilton is taking an anticoagulant (warfarin) for recurrent thrombophlebitis. She has also been taking aspirin for arthritic pain. Don notifies the physician because he is aware that:
   a. warfarin displaces aspirin from the binding site, creating toxic effects
   *b. aspirin displaces warfarin from the binding site, increasing free warfarin levels
   c. aspirin creates an acidic medium, which inhibits warfarin absorption
   d. warfarin, in the presence of aspirin compounds, causes excessive clotting

   [NP: AS, CL: CO]

   Rationale: Aspirin displaces warfarin from the binding site, thereby increasing free warfarin and causing bleeding.

5. Matthew Thornton is a 60-year-old receiving an anticancer drug (doxorubicin). Don administers this drug early in the morning because:
   a. the endorphin level is at its peak
   b. renal toxicity is less of a threat
   *c. the bone marrow is less vulnerable
   d. cancer cells are dividing quickly at this time

   [NP: IM, CL: KN]

   Rationale: Doxorubicin is best administered in the morning, when the bone marrow is less vulnerable. At this time, the cells are not dividing as quickly.

6. Mrs. Rogers has been on propranolol (Inderal) 1 mg q 12 hours intravenously, but is now able to take the oral form. A dose of 10 mg po quid is ordered. Don is aware that Inderal is not as effective by the oral route, due to:
   a. enterohepatic recirculation
   b. antagonistic effects
   c. Michaelis-Menton kinetics
   *d. hepatic first-pass effect

   [NP: PL, CL: AP]

   Rationale: Inderal taken orally is a drug which is metabolized by the liver on the first pass; therefore, oral doses must be much higher than parenteral doses. This is an example of a hepatic first-pass effect.

Review Questions from Text

1. Which statement is true regarding the pharmacokinetic phase of drug administration?
   a. The immature liver or kidneys of the very young may accelerate drug metabolism and excretion.
   b. Medications enter the body in solid form and change into solution for absorption aand utilization.
   *c. Medication absorption, distribution to tissues, metabolism, and elimination from the body are studied.
   d. A therapeutic effect occurs as the medication reaches the target cell.

   [CL: KN]

   Rationale: The pharmacokinetic phase involves the total process of drug administration from absorption, distribution, and metabolism to elimination from the body.

2. The following statements are concerned with the mechanism of drug absorption. Which statement is false?
   a. Active transport moves substances against a concentration gradient.
   *b. Passive transport provides for one-way drug transport into the cell.
   c. Energy is not required or utilized during passive diffusion.
   d. Protein carriers can only carry specific drugs.

   [CL: CO]

Rationale: Passive transport is a two-way process allowing drug molecules to move into and out of cells without energy expenditure.

3. Which statement is true regarding drug solubility?
   a. Medications in aqueous solutions are absorbed more slowly than oil-based products.
   b. Lipid-soluble substances are too large to cross the blood brain barrier.
   c. Alcohol-based products have a slower absorption rate than oil-based drugs.
   *d. Only nonionized drug forms are available for absorption.

   [CL: KN]

   Rationale: Nonionized drugs are lipid soluble and diffusable; therefore, they are available for absorption.

4. During the phase of drug distribution:
   a. most medications are bound in the serum to hormones
   b. reduced cardiac output increases tissue drug saturation and concentration
   *c. tissues such as the bone and middle ear take longer for drug distribution
   d. substances pass the placental barrier by an active transport system

   [CL: KN]

   Rationale: Bone, middle ear, skin, and fat are areas with minimal blood supply, and the distribution of medication is slower.

5. Which statement is true regarding the half-life of medications?
   a. Doubling the dose will double the medication half-life.
   b. Approximately 6 half-lives are required for a medication to be completely excreted.
   c. Patients with renal or hepatic disease usually have decreased drug half-lives.
   *d. The half-life of a drug determines how often the drug is to be administered.

   [CL: KN]

   Rationale: Drug dosage schedules are determined according to their biological half-life. The half-life of a drug ultimately determines how often a drug is to be given.

6. Which statement is false regarding medication selectivity?
   a. The therapeutic range is the level at which the medication is effective.
   b. The margin of safety is the dose with the most therapeutic results and the fewest toxic effects.
   *c. A medication reference book listing all known adverse and toxic effects is of great use to determine selectivity.
   d. Drug selectivity summarizes the pattern and incidence of adverse side effects produced by the therapeutic dose.

   [CL: CO]

   Rationale: The best reference for drug selectivity lists the most and least common toxic drug effects, not all known adverse effects.

7. All of the following are factors which affect patient response to medication except:
   *a. sex
   b. climate
   c. weight
   d. age

   [CL: CO]

   Rationale: Individual differences occur in response to medications; these include body weight, age, disease, and psychological states, immune and environmental factors, and the time of administration. Sex is not a factor.

8. The majority of acid drugs are better absorbed in the small intestine, due to the:

a. presence of an acidic medium
*b. increased surface area
c. dissociation into ionized forms
d. presence of a basic medium

[CL: CO]

Rationale: Acid drugs return to an ionized form in the small intestine; however, the majority of acidic drugs are absorbed because of increased surface area.

9. Which of the following processes is associated with passive transport?
a. carrier transport
b. pinocytosis
*c. facilitated diffusion
d. one-way transport

[CL: KN]

Rationale: Facilitated diffusion is a process of passive transport in which a carrier is needed to cross the cell membrane. This process differs from active transport in that it does not require energy.

10. The following statements refer to plasma drug concentration. Select the statement which is true.
a. The plasma concentration is the amount of bound drug in plasma.
*b. As the peak concentration is reached, maximal effect usually occurs.
c. The plasma concentration is the amount of free drug in plasma.
d. Peak concentration is reached when all of the drug becomes unbound.

[CL: KN]

Rationale: Peak concentration of a drug is achieved when the maximal amount is absorbed into the target tissue, usually causing the maximal effect.

Additional Review Questions Not Presented in Text

1. Regarding the absorption stage of the pharmacokinetic phase of drug administration:
*a. medications injected directly by the intravenous route are 100 percent absorbed
b. most oral medications are absorbed from the large intestine
c. the convoluted lining of the stomach enhances absorption into the central compartment
d. tetracycline (an antibiotic) is better absorbed if given with an antacid

[CL: CO]

Rationale: Intravenous medications enter directly into the central compartment and are completely absorbed.

2. All of the following statements are true regarding routes of drug absorption except:
a. Parenteral medications are given via the intravenous, intramuscular, or subcutaneous route.
b. Medications can be applied to the mucous membrane of the eye, vagina, urethra, and rectum.
c. Systemic toxicity can occur when excessive medication is absorbed from the skin.
*d. The skin is usually more permeable than other ports of entry.

[CL: KN]

Rationale: The skin is usually less permeable than other ports of entry.

3. Of the following statements, which one is false regarding drug absorption from the stomach?
a. Basic drugs (i.e., morphine) tend to remain ionized and are not absorbed.
*b. In general, an empty stomach slows absorption, whereas food accelerates absorption.
c. Administering an antacid with a basic drug may enhance drug absorption.
d. Acid drugs (i.e., aspirin) tend to remain nonionized and are readily absorbed.

[CL: KN]

Rationale: Usually an empty stomach enhances absorption, while the presence of food delays absorption.

4. The phase of biotransformation:
   *a. converts some medications into a harmless metabolite for excretion
   b. converts most medication to an active form to be absorbed by tissues
   c. occurs primarily in the pancreas through an enzyme-catalyst reaction
   d. occurs through the processes of both active and passive transport

[CL: KN]

Rationale: Biotransformation refers to the enzymatic alteration of a drug molecule, converting some drugs to an inactive metabolite which is then excreted by the kidney.

5. All of the following statements are true regarding drug excretion <u>except</u>:
   a. Medications are eliminated primarily through the renal system.
   b. Cumulation results when excretion decreases and serum drug levels rise.
   *c. As serum drug concentration rises, excretion or clearance decreases.
   d. Effectiveness of excretion is measured by the drug's half-life.

[CL: CO]

Rationale: Normally as drug plasma concentration increases, clearance or excretion also increases.

6. During the pharmacodynamic phase of medication action:
   a. medications are detoxified or broken down by the liver
   b. alterations in cell environment or cell function rarely occur
   *c. the biochemical and physiologic effects of the drug are studied
   d. medications are dissolved into absorbable, nonionized compounds

[CL: KN]

Rationale: The pharmacodynamic drug phase studies the biochemical and physiologic effects of medication which occurs when the drug reaches the target cell.

CHAPTER 5: DRUG INTERACTIONS

Situations from Text

Situation 5-1

Scott Preston is a medication nurse on a medical surgical unit in a large urban hospital. The following questions relate to situations involving drug interactions.

1. Scott checks on a patient admitted with digitalis toxicity. The patient had been taking digoxin and the anti-arrhythmic agent, guinidine, for several months. Scott is aware that the presenting symptoms may be due to:
   a. increased biotransformation of guinidine by digoxin
   *b. displacement of digoxin from its tissue binding sites by guinidine
   c. increased penetration of guinidine into tissue in the presence of digoxin
   d. displacement of guinidine from its binding sites by digoxin

   [NP: AN, CL: AN]

   Rationale: Quinidine is capable of displacing digoxin from its tissue binding sites. When these drugs are given together, digoxin dosage needs to be reduced.

2. Thirty-eight-year-old Emma Smythe is receiving gentamicin, an aminoglycoside antibiotic, and furosemide (Lasix), a loop diuretic, as part of her drug therapy. Which of the following statements by Emma indicates a serious drug interaction resulting from this combination?
   a. "I've been passing my water a lot."
   b. "I didn't move my bowels today."
   c. "My mouth feels so dry."
   *d. "I'm having trouble hearing you."

   [NP: EV, CL: AN]

   Rationale: Ototoxicity is the manifestation of a combined toxicity when an aminoglycoside antibiotic and furosemide is used together in therapy.

3. Following discharge from the hospital, which of these actions is most likely to compromise the patient's drug therapy?
   a. Taking erythromycin on an empty stomach
   b. Using antacids two hours after amphetamines
   c. Combining vitamin C with mineral oil
   *d. Drinking a glass of milk with tetracycline

   [NP: EV, CL: CO]

   Rationale: Calcium, a heavy metal found in milk, forms a complex with tetracycline, thus decreasing absorption of this antibiotic.

4. In administering oral medications to patients receiving cancer chemotherapy, Scott carefully considers the following patient characteristic:
   a. Blood pressure
   *b. Mucosal integrity
   c. Emotional status
   d. Taste sensations

   [NP: PL, CL: AN]

   Rationale: Drug absorption is affected by altering the intestinal mucosa as with antineoplastic therapy.

5. Which of the following patients will Scott expect to experience alterations in drug biotransformation?
   *a. 52-year-old male with cirrhosis

b. 35-year-old female with ulcerative colitis
c. 41-year-old male with cancer of the stomach
d. 60-year-old female with acute renal failure

[NP: AN, CL: AN]

Rationale: Biotransformation, which occurs in the liver, can affect drug concentration at the site of action.

6. When completing a medication history on a patient recently admitted to his unit, Scott notes the following patient statement as being significant to drug therapy while hospitalized:
 a. "I always take Tylenol when I get a headache."
 *b. "I've been taking Tagamet for my ulcer."
 c. "I always take my pills with a glass of water."
 d. "I keep a list of the medications that I take."

[NP: AS, CL: AN]

Rationale: Tagamet alters GI pH and thus may alter oral drug absorption.

Situation 5-2

Hillside Manor, a rural extended-care facility, has a large number of patients on multiple drug therapy. The medication nurse frequently deals with the following patient situations.

1. Sixty-eight-year-old Mary Taggart is experiencing phantom limb pain following a recent amputation. The nurse administers aspirin and codeine together for pain relief. This is an example of which type of effect?
 a. synergistic
 b. antagonistic
 c. potentiated
 *d. additive

[NP: IM, CL: AP]

Rationale: An additive effect occurs when two drugs with the same effect, such as aspirin and codeine, are combined. The result is an enhanced effect.

2. Jake McBride, seventy-two years old, receives furosemide (Lasix), a diuretic, and propranolol (Inderal), a beta-adrenergic blocker, for control of his hypertension. The pharmacodynamic interaction responsible for the therapeutic antihypertensive effect is:
 a. addition
 b. antagonism
 *c. synergism
 d. potentiation

[NP: AN, CL: CO]

Rationale: The two drugs, working to lower the blood pressure by different mechanisms, produce an antihypertensive effect greater than either drug would by itself. This is an example of synergism.

3. Sixty-two-year-old Jane Coleman is taking calcium supplements for hypocalcemia. The nurse should avoid administering the drug with:
 a. ginger ale
 *b. chocolate milk
 c. orange juice
 d. iced tea

[NP: IM, CL: AP]

Rationale: Calcium binds with chocolate, thus reducing the absorption of the drug.

4. Which of the following statements by a visitor to Hillside Manor reflects good insight into a serious food-drug interaction?
   a. "Mom never ate breakfast, but now she takes her digitalis pill every morning with a bowl of bran flakes."
   b. "Mom always takes her penicillin with tomato juice instead of milk in the morning."
   *c. "Mom loves black licorice, but she hasn't had any since she's been taking Lasix."
   d. "Mom's been eating a lot of yogurt since she started on those blood pressure pills."

   [NP: EV, CL: AN]

   Rationale: Licorice promotes potassium excretion, which is also a major adverse effect of diuretics such as Lasix.

5. Seventy-year-old Mildred Rankin is on MAO inhibitor therapy for depression. After appropriate teaching by the nurse, Mildred should avoid the following menu choice:
   a. broiled trout
   b. tomato vegetable soup
   c. baked stuffed flounder
   *d. chicken chow mein

   [NP: EV, CL: AP]

   Rationale: Chinese food often contains large amounts of monosodium glutamate, which can enhance the effects of MAO inhibitors.

6. Betty Thomas, on isoniazid (INH) for a history of tuberculosis, recently ate a large portion of tuna fish casserole for dinner. Betty would be expected to manifest this response:
   *a. severe headaches
   b. constipation
   c. diuresis
   d. no ill effects

   [NP: EV, CL: AP]

   Rationale: Tuna fish contains a high histamine content, which may interact with isoniazid to produce a histamine reaction.

Additional Situation Not Presented in Text

Ella Sanchez and her two children, seventeen-year-old Chad and twelve-year-old Maria, attend a local out-patient clinic. They are discussing their drug therapy with the clinic nurse.

1. In reviewing the medication record of each member of the Sanchez family, the nurse has the responsibility to:
   a. Be aware of all published drug interactions, regardless of significance.
   b. Suggest changes in medication dosages if the desired effect is not achieved.
   *c. Question all orders which could potentially result in an adverse drug interaction.
   d. Continue medication administration according to the physician's original order.

   [NP: IM, CL: KN]

   Rationale: The nurse has a legal responsibility to question drug orders that may adversely affect the patient.

2. Mrs. Sanchez is started on oral iron therapy with Feosol. The nurse will teach her to avoid the following dietary product:
   a. milk
   *b. coffee
   c. bread
   d. tomatoes

   [NP: IM, CL: AP]

Rationale: Concurrent administration of caffeine-containing products results in decreased oral iron effects.

3. Chad is ordered tetracycline for an upper respiratory infection. The nurse instructs Chad to take the medication:
   a. With each meal and at bedtime
   *b. Before each meal and at bedtime
   c. After each meal and at bedtime
   d. Without regard to meals and bedtime

   [NP: IM, CL: AP]

   Rationale: Tetracycline should be taken on an empty stomach for best absorption.

4. Ella is on anticoagulant therapy with Coumadin. Which of the following statements will assure the nurse that Ella has understood the recent patient teaching that she received?
   *a. "I check with the pharmacist before taking any over-the-counter products."
   b. "I take a lot of aspirin for those cramps that I often get."
   c. "My boyfriend and I like to drink a glass of wine with dinner every evening."
   d. "If I forget to take my medication one day, I just take two the next."

   [NP: EV, CL: AN]

   Rationale: Components of OTC products may interfere with blood coagulation and thus may alter the effects of anticoagulant therapy.

5. Maria has been ordered oral griseofulvin for the treatment of a fungal infection. To promote optimum drug absorption, the nurse will instruct Maria to:
   a. Take the drug on an empty stomach
   b. Avoid protein foods when taking the drug
   *c. Take the drug with fatty meals
   d. Avoid acidic foods when taking the drug

   [NP: IM, CL: AP]

   Rationale: Griseofulvin is best absorbed when taken with meals containing fat.

6. Ella was taking Marplan, an MAO inhibitor antidepressant, and was admitted last month to the hospital in an acute hypertensive crisis. She reflects insight into her problem by the following statement:
   a. "I shouldn't have taken that aspirin for my arthritis."
   *b. "I should never have indulged at that wine and cheese party."
   c. "I really learned my lesson -- no more milk and eggs for me."
   d. "Citrus fruits are totally off limits for me now."

   [NP: EV, CL: AN]

   Rationale: Concurrent ingestion of tyramine-containing foods while an MAO inhibitor therapy may result in potentiation of sympathetic cardiovascular effects.

Review Questions from Text

1. A pharmacokinetic drug interaction:
   a. Occurs in the drug preparation phase of drug therapy
   b. Produces the majority of drug incompatibility reactions
   c. May have additive, synergistic, or antagonistic effects
   *d. Affects the absorption, distribution, biotransformation, and excretion of drugs

   [CL: CO]

   Rationale: Pharmacokinetic interactions involve reactions where the absorption, distribution, biotransformation, or excretion of one drug is affected by another drug.

2. A pharmacodynamic drug interaction:
   a. Occurs when liver function is compromised
   b. Refers to a type of drug incompatibility
   *c. May have additive, synergistic, or antagonistic effects
   d. Occurs when plasma protein-binding is modified

   [CL: KN]

   Rationale: Pharmacodynamic interactions result from the combined effects of drugs.

3. An antagonistic drug interaction occurs when:
   a. Drug absorption is decreased by the presence of food in the stomach
   *b. A second drug is added to diminish or eliminate the effect of the first
   c. A second drug is added that possesses the same overt effect as the first
   d. Drug distribution is enhanced by displacement of a protein-bound drug

   [CL: KN]

   Rationale: Antagonism results in a combined effect that is less than either active component alone.

4. Major mechanisms of drug interaction include all of the following classifications except:
   *a. incompatibility effects
   b. protein-binding changes
   c. absorption
   d. biotransformation

   [CL: KN]

   Rationale: Drug incompatibilities are not synonymous with drug interactions, chemical or physical reactions that occur among two or more drugs.

5. Medications that increase or inhibit liver enzyme activity can affect drug action. Which of the following statements is true regarding biotransformation in the liver?
   a. Alcohol inhibits liver enzyme activity, resulting in increased activity of certain drugs.
   *b. Phenobarbital stimulated liver enzyme activity, resulting in increased metabolism of certain drugs.
   c. Cimetidine (Tagamet) stimulates liver enzyme activity, resulting in increased effect of certain drugs.
   d. Rifampin inhibits liver enzyme activity, resulting in decreased metabolism of certain drugs.

   [CL: CO]

   Rationale: Stimulation of microsomal activity in the liver increases the biotransformation of certain drugs, thus decreasing their effect in the body.

6. An example of combined toxicity is:
   a. warfarin and phenylbutazone
   b. quinidine and digoxin
   c. acetazolamine (Diamox) and aspirin
   *d. gentamicin and furosemide (Lasix)

   [CL: CO]

   Rationale: Combined toxicity occurs when two drugs with toxic effects, such as gentamicin and Lasix, are combined for therapy. Both cause ototoxicity.

7. Which statement is true concerning absorption of oral medications?
   a. The faster the drug passes through the intestinal tract, the greater the amount absorbed.
   *b. Drugs such as morphine and codeine prolong emptying time, increasing drug absorption.
   c. Metoclopramide hastens gastric emptying and increases drug absorption in the small intestine.
   d. Anticholinergics decrease gastric emptying time and increase drug absorption.

[CL: KN]

Rationale: The longer a drug remains in the gastrointestinal tract, the greater the amount absorbed. Drugs such as morphine and codeine prolong emptying time and increase drug absorption.

8. Mineral oil inhibits the absorption of fat soluble vitamins. This effect is known as:
   *a. sequestration
   b. antagonism
   c. complexation
   d. potentiation

   [CL: CO]

   Rationale: Sequestration occurs when a drug is surrounded by a lipoid substance, and, therefore, cannot be absorbed.

9. Patients who are taking phenytoin (Dilantin) or phenobarbital must be observed for:
   a. toxic sodium levels
   b. elevated magnesium levels
   *c. decreased calcium levels
   d. decreased phosphorus levels

   [CL: AP]

   Rationale: Phenytoin and phenobarbital can cause malabsorption of calcium and subsequent development of osteomalacia.

10. The correct action for the nurse who suspects that a drug interaction is occurring would be to:
    a. withhold all medications until the physician sees the patient
    b. continue the medication and document all reactions in the nurse's notes
    c. give all medications as ordered and inform the physician
    *d. withhold the suspected medication and inform the physician

    [CL: CO]

    Rationale: The nurse has the legal right to withhold the medication which is suspected to be causing an interaction until the physician evaluates the patient.

Additional Review Questions Not Presented in Text

1. An additive drug interaction results when:
   *a. Two drugs possessing the same overt effect are combined
   b. One of two drugs exerts the action that is made greater by the presence of the second drug
   c. Two drugs, not possessing the same overt effect, are used together to yield a combined effect
   d. Two drugs produce a combined effect that is less than either active component alone

   [CL: KN]

   Rationale: Addition is a type of pharmacodynamic interaction.

2. A synergistic drug interaction occurs when the following drugs are administered together:
   a. aspirin and codeine
   *b. diazepam (Valium) and alcohol
   c. propranolol (Inderal) and epinephrine
   d. Heparin and alcohol

   [CL: CO]

   Rationale: Synergism involves a combined drug effect, the result of which is greater than either active component alone.

3. The absorption of which of the following drugs is delayed or reduced by food?
   *a. Digoxin (Lanoxin)
   b. Chlorothiazide (Diuril)
   c. Propranolol (Inderal)
   d. Griseofulvin (Grisactin)

   [CL: KN]

   Rationale: The absorption of digoxin is delayed by food.

4. Which of the following statements is <u>true</u> regarding drug interactions involving the mechanism of absorption?
   a. Antacids increase digoxin (Lanoxin) absorption.
   b. Iron increases tetracycline absorption.
   *c. Antacids decrease tetracycline absorption.
   d. Cholestyramine (Questran) increases digitalis absorption.

   [CL: CO]

   Rationale: Antacids contain heavy metals that chelate with the tetracycline molecule).

5. An example of a drug altering the urinary excretion of another drug is:
   a. Probenecid (Benemid) increasing tubular excretion of penicillin)
   b. Quinidine increasing tubular excretion of digoxin (Lanoxin)
   *c. Tetracycline decreasing renal excretion of lithium
   d. Allopurinol (Zyloprim) increasing renal excretion of chlorothiazide (Diuril)

   [CL: KN]

   Rationale: Decreased renal excretion of lithium will result in increased lithium toxicity.

CHAPTER 6: DRUG TOXICITY

Situation from Text

Situation 6-1

Helen Andrews is the charge nurse on nights in the emergency room at a large metropolitan hospital. She frequently encounters patients with problems related to drug toxicity.

1. A seven-year-old, Liza Steiner, has a fever (temperature 38^{6}C, 101^{5}F), rash, and enlarged lymph nodes. Helen questions Liza's mother about medications which her daughter has been taking. The mother responds, "All Liza has had is a diptheria-tetanus shot last week." Helen is aware that this reaction represents a:
   a. Type I--anaphylactic
   *b. Type II--serum sickness
   c. type III--auto-immune
   d. Type IV-cel-mediated

   [NP: AS, CL: AP]

   Rationale: Type II allergic reactions are often seen in patients receiving diptheria and tetanus antitoxin. Symptoms include fever, rash, arthralgia, splenomegaly, and lymph node enlargement.

2. Mike Benson arrives in the emergency room in acute respiratory distress. He also has an extensive rash and heart palpitation. A nursing assessment reveals that he recently began taking penicillin for bronchitis. Helen prepares to administer all of the following except:
   a. vasopressors
   b. antihistamines
   c. bronchodilators
   *d. antibiotics

   [AP: PL, CL: AN]

   Rationale: This patient presents signs and symptoms related to an anaphylactic reaction due to penicillin. Emergency treatment includes epinephrine, antihistamines, bronchodilators, and vasopressors.

3. Jason Mills, a seventy-year-old, complains of itching and a rash related to a topical cream containing benzene. The first appropriate action for Helen would be to:
   a. prepare to administer an antihistamine
   b. neutralize the benzene by applying sodium bicarbonate
   *c. wash the product off of the skin
   d. prepare to administer epinephrine

   [NP: IM, CL: CO]

   Rationale: One of the most common drugs which cause a delayed hypersensitivity reaction is benzene. If symptoms of contact dermatitis occur, the product should be completly washed from the skin and not used again.

4. Harry Evans, a 66-year-old with a history of a recent myocardial infarction, comes to the emergency room because of sudden symptoms related to systemic lupus erythematosus. During the assessment, Helen discovers that Mr. Evans began taking Pronestyl a week earlier. Helen is aware that this may represent the following type of reaction:
   *a. idiosyncratic
   b. cell-mediated
   c. anaphylactic
   d. delayed toxicity

   [NP: AN, CL: CO]

Rationale: An idiosyncratic reaction is one that occurs unexpectedly in a small portion of patients. An example of this type of reaction would be symptoms of systemic lupus erythematosus related to Pronestyl. The reaction is due to a deficiency of N-acetyltransferase.

5. Edna Carson has been feeling very tired and presents to the emergency room after noticing a bloody stool. Lab results reveal a low platelet count and hematocrit. Helen investigates the medications that Mrs. Carson takes. Of the following list of drugs, which would most likely be related to Mrs. Carson's symptoms?
   a. digoxin
   *b. quinidine
   c. theophylline
   d. captopril

   [NP: AS, CL: AP]

   Rationale: Quinidine is a drug known to cause thrombocytopenia (reduced platelets).

6. Mr. Graham arrives in a comatose state via an ambulance from a nearby mental hospital. The patient has a history of attempted suicide by drug overdose. Helen will implement the following intervention first:
   a. obtain blood samples for a drug screen
   b. assess neurological function
   c. elevate the legs to increase circulation
   *d. take a set of vital signs

   [NP: AS, CL: AP]

   Rationale: The first action should be to take a set of vital signs as a baseline assessment.

Additional Situation Not Presented in Text

As a community health nurse, Maye Fortam encounters many situations in which knowledge of drug toxicity is vital.

1. When Maye instructs young mothers on safety and poisoning prevention, she stresses that:
   a. medication should be removed from the original container for storage
   b. all empty medication vials should be kept for future use
   c. medication should be referred to as "candy" when administered to children
   *d. medications which are no longer in use should always be discarded

   [NP: IM, CL: CO]

   Rationale: Patients should be taught to discard old medications rather than to save them for another time.

2. Maye discovers that 18-year-old Simon Jones has taken an overdose of amphetamines. She contacts his doctor and is prepared to administer which of the following drugs in order to promote excretion:
   *a. ammonium chloride
   b. mucomyst
   c. sodium nitrate
   d. sodium bicarbonate

   [NP: IM, CL: AP]

   Rationale: The excretion of amphetamines is promoted by acidifying the urine with ammonium chloride administration.

3. Jason Harrell is a six-year-old who has taken an unknown quantity of scopolamine. While Maye waits for the ambulance to arrive, she will pay particular attention to:
   *a. heart rate
   b. abdominal distention
   c. signs of hypoglycemia

d. signs of hyperglycemia

[NP: AS, CL: AP]

Rationale: Management of anticholinergic overdose includes careful cardiac assessment.

4. Mrs. Breaux complains of color vision disturbances since her discharge from the hospital after an episode of congestive heart failure. Which of the following drugs is likely to be related to this effect?
   a. Aldomet
   b. Diuril
   *c. digoxin
   d. quinidine

   [NP: AS, CL: AP]

   Rationale: Patients may complain of color vision disturbances when taking digitalis products.

5. Maye examines the site of a tuberculin skin test, which was administered to Mr. White 48 hours earlier. The area shows reddening and induration of the skin. This type of reaction is an example of:
   a. cell-mediated response
   *b. delayed hypersensitivity
   c. auto-immune reaction
   d. cytotoxic reaction

   [NP: AS, CL: CO]

   Rationale: The tuberculin skin test is an example of delayed hypersensitivity.

6. Mrs. Lopez is taking chlorothiazide (Diuril) for fluid management. When teaching about the possible adverse effects of the drug, Maye stresses that Mrs. Lopez should report the following immediately:
   a. heart rate below 70
   *b. increased bruising
   c. warm, moist skin
   d. increased urine output

   [NP: IM, CL: AN]

   Rationale: This drug is known to cause thrombocytopenia. Patients should report any increase in bruising or bleeding.

<u>Review Questions from Text</u>

1. Toxicology is concerned with all of the following <u>except</u>:
   a. drugs used in therapy
   b. environmental pollution
   c. industrial waste
   *d. safety-related injuries

   [CL: CO]

   Rationale: Toxicology is concerned with drugs used in therapy, as well as with chemicals which are responsible for household, environmental, or industrial intoxication.

2. Which of the following statements is <u>true</u> regarding the adverse effects of drug therapy?
   a. Pharmacologic products should be tested to assure that there are no risks involved.
   *b. Toxic effects will occur in all persons given sufficient dosage.
   c. Drug allergies and hypersensitivity reactions are effects which can be predicted.
   d. Adverse reactions to drugs usually take only minutes to manifest.

   [CL: CO]

Rationale: Toxic effects are dose-related and will occur in all persons who are given a sufficient dosage of a drug.

3. Adverse reactions are more likely to occur in:
   a. male patients
   b. very young patients
   c. patients with nerve damage
   *d. patients with renal dysfunction

   [CL: CO]

   Rationale: Adverse effects are more likely to occur in patients with impaired renal function.

4. An example of a primary drug reaction would be:
   a. excessive drowsiness from antihistamines
   b. impotence from antihypertensives
   *c. excessive lethargy from sedatives
   d. extreme agitation from bronchodilators

   [CL: CO]

   Rationale: Primary reactions are effects that are extensions of the desired action of the drug, such as an overdose.

5. Which of the following statements is <u>true</u> concerning an anaphylactic reaction?
   a. It is a Type III allergic reaction involving the lung and cardiovascular system.
   b. IGE antibodies attach to red blood cells, liberating large amounts of epinephrine.
   *c. When the offending drug is administered, mast cells liberate large doses of histamine.
   d. The resulting effect of substrate release includes bronchodilation and peripheral vasoconstriction.

   [CL: KN]

   Rationale: Anaphylaxis refers to a Type I allergic reaction involving histamine release which causes bronchoconstriction in the lung, peripheral vasodilation, and vascular permeability.

6. The Type II allergic reaction is most often seen in persons receiving:
   a. streptomycin
   *b. penicillin
   c. tetracycline
   d. thiazide diuretics

   [CL: KN]

   Rationale: The Type II allergic reaction or serum sickness is most often seen in patients receiving penicillin or diptheria and tetanus antitoxin.

7. The inflammatory process and tissue destruction associated with an auto-immune reaction is mediated by:
   *a. activation of complement
   b. increased amounts of IGE
   c. complexation with red blood cells
   d. activation of T-lymphocytes

   [CL: KN]

   Rationale: Local ischemia and necrosis associated with Type III allergic auto-immune reaction results as a consequence of complement activation.

8. Hemolytic anemia can result secondarily to:
   a. cell-mediated reaction

b. auto-immune reaction
c. anaphylaxis
*d. serum sickness

[CL: CO]

Rationale: Hemolytic anemia, a blood dyscrasia, can result secondarily to a Type II allergic reaction.

9. Which one of the following statements is true concerning chemical poisoning?
   a. In general, substances which are inhaled have a slower onset of action.
   *b. Poisoning is the fifth most common cause of accidental death in the United States.
   c. The number of cases involving poisoning has increased over several years.
   d. The signs and symptoms of poisoning are very distinctive, facilitating early diagnosis.

   [CL: KN]

   Rationale: Poisoning, a common medical emergency, is th efifth most common cause of accidental death in the United States.

10. Hemodialysis enhances elimination of toxins from the blood. Which one of the following types of toxins is removed by this method?
    a. lipid-bound
    b. protein-bound
    *c. low-molecular-weight
    d. high-molecular-weight

    [CL: KN]

    Rationale: Hemodialysis exposes blood to a semi-permeable membrane to remove low-molecular-weight toxins.

Additional Review Questions Not Presented in Text

1. An example of a secondary drug reaction would be:
   *a. impotence from antihypertensives
   b. increased bleeding tendencies from anticoagulants
   c. hypotension from antihypertensives
   d. drowsiness from hypnotics

   [CL: KN]

   Rationale: Secondary drug reactions are those undesired reactions which are not an extension of the desired action of the drug.

2. The following statement is false regarding drug allergies:
   a. Drugs have no antigenic activity.
   b. Drugs must stimulate antibody production in order to produce a reaction.
   *c. Drug allergies are confined to those of an immediate reaction only.
   d. A drug-protein complex stimulates antibody formation.

   [CL: CO]

   Rationale: Drug allergies may manifest in a wide variety of immediate and delayed reactions.

3. Atopic reactions may result from:
   a. lysis of target cells
   b. IGM antibodies attached to mast cells
   c. contact with lymphokine
   *d. IGA deficiency

   [CL: CO]

Rationale: Atopic reactions may result from IGA deficiency.

4. A drug associated with auto-immune reactions is:
   a. diptheria and tetanus antitoxin
   *b. streptomycin
   c. iodine
   d. sulfonamide

[CL: CO]

Rationale: Streptomycin is capable of causing a Type III or auto-immune reaction.

5. In delayed hypersensitivity reactions, the T cell/antigen reaction releases all of the following substances <u>except</u>:
   a. macrophage inhibitory factor
   b. macrophage activating factor
   *c. necrotying enzymes
   d. chemotactic substances

[CL: CO]

Rationale: The T cell/antigen reaction releases substances which modulate the inflammatory response. These include macrophage migration inhibitory factor (MIF), macrophage activating factor (MAF), and chemotactic factors which attract macrophages into the area.

CHAPTER 7: OVER-THE-COUNTER MEDICATIONS

<u>**Situation from Text**</u>

Situation 7-1

Nora Carter, RN, applies knowledge of over-the-counter medications while managing patients in the office of a physician who specializes in internal medicine.

1. Mr. Schmidt is taking an antihistamine for symptoms associated with a cold. To minimize the side effect of sedation, Nora will teach Mr. Schmidt to:
   *a. take the antihistamine at bedtime
   b. ingest extra coffee during the day
   c. continue to perform his usual activities despite drowsiness
   d. combine the antihistamine with a CNS stimulant

   [NP: IM, CL: AP]

   Rationale: Taking antihistamines at bedtime will reduce the effect of sedation.

2. When antihistamines are recommended for elderly patients, Nora will teach the patients and families to report all of the following <u>except</u>:
   a. dizziness
   b. confusion
   c. hypotension
   *d. reduced rhinorrhea

   [NP: IM, CL: CO]

   Rationale: In elderly patients, antihistamines may cause dizziness, confusion, and hypotension. Reduced rhinorrhea is a desired effect.

3. An antacid is prescribed for Julia Reel, who has a duodenal ulcer. Which of the following antacids would <u>not</u> be indicated for treatment?
   a. sodium bicarbonate
   b. magnesium carbonate
   *c. calcium carbonate
   d. aluminum hydroxide

   [NP: AN, CL: AP]

   Rationale: Calcium carbonate, a calcium-containing antacid, may cause increased gastric secretion and should be avoided when ulcer healing is indicated.

4. Mr. Plunkett, a 67-year-old with narrow-angle glaucoma, calls to find out which medications he should take for cold and flu symptoms. Nora will tell him to <u>avoid</u>:
   *a. antihistamines
   b. antitussives
   c. expectorants
   d. aspirin compounds

   [NP: IM, CL: AP]

   Rationale: Antihistamines are contraindicated for patients with narrow-angle glaucoma.

5. Mrs. Arnold has been taking Sudafed for a cold. She is also taking digoxin daily. Optimally, Mrs. Arnold should discontinue the decongestant due to:
   a. decreased absorption of digoxin
   *b. increased potential for arrhythmias

c. potential for digitalis toxicity
d. decreased effects of both drugs

[NP: AN, CL: CO]

Rationale: Arrhythmias may occur when digitalis preparations are taken with decongestants.

6. Aluminum hydroxide is the antacid recommended for Mr. Farrell, who has chronic renal failure, because it:
   a. has reduced potential for constipation
   *b. prevents absorption of phosphate from the GI tract
   c. blocks absorption of calcium from the GI tract
   d. interferes with nitrogen and protein assimilation

   [NP: PL, CL: AP]

   Rationale: Aluminum hydroxide is used to treat hyperphosphatemia, common in renal failure patients, because it prevents absorption of phosphate from the GI tract.

Additional Situation Not Presented in Text

Rhonda Landry is a public health nurse helping to serve the health needs of a large urban area. The following are situations which require that Rhonda be informed about OTC medications.

1. Mr. Martinez has been using a nasal spray for relief of congestion of a cold. Rhonda teaches Mr. Martinez about the drug. Which of the following is true of topical decongestants?
   a. They reverse nasal congestion by vasodilating the nasal mucosa blood vessels.
   b. The duration of effect of nasal sprays is long acting and potentially addictive.
   *c. The use of topical nasal decongestants should be limited to 3 days.
   d. Frequent application causes a cycle of vasodilation followed by rebound vasoconstriction.

   [NP: IM, CL: KN]

   Rationale: Topical nasal decongestants can become habit forming and should be limited to 3 days and used no more than 4 times a day.

2. Mrs. Helmes prefers to take an antacid in a tablet form. Which of the following responses indicates successful patient teaching with regard to this form of antacid?
   a. "I swallow the tablets with at least two glasses of water."
   b. "I allow the tablets to dissolve completely in my mouth."
   c. "The tablets are better because they are more effective than the liquid form."
   *d. "I chew the tablets completely and drink lots of water."

   [NP: EV, CL: AN]

   Rationale: To exert desired effects, an antacid must be in a liquid form. Tablets must be chewed thoroughly and taken with plenty of water.

3. Josephine Locke takes Metamucil daily as part of her bowel regime. Rhonda teaches Mrs. Locke not to take the psyllium-containing laxative concurrently with her other medications because of:
   a. potential for nausea and vomiting
   *b. potential absorption of the drugs in the stool
   c. risk of inactivation of the drugs by psyllium
   d. excessive cathartic effects

   [NP: IM, CL: CO]

   Rationale: An adverse effect of bulk-forming laxatives such as Metamucil is potential absorption of drugs concurrently administered.

4. When Mr. Tran complains of symptoms related to a cold, Rhonda informs him that he should contact the

physician if he experiences:
a. throat soreness without fever
b. nasal congestion
c. nonproductive cough
*d. symptoms persistent longer than 7 days

[NP: IM, CL: CO]

Rationale: Patients should contact a health care provider if cold symptoms persist longer than one week.

5. Mr. Washington has a productive cough without a fever. Rhonda suggests that he may utilize all of the following <u>except</u>:
a. saline gargles
b. rest
*c. cough suppressants
d. smoking cessation

[NP: PL, CL: AP]

Rationale: Cough suppressants are contraindicated in patients with a productive cough.

6. Joshua Ames is a 77-year-old with hypertension and a history of a hiatus hernia. He has been complaining of constipation and is currently impacted with stool. Rhonda suspects that his symptoms may be associated with the abuse or chronic use of:
a. laxatives
b. antihypertensives
*c. antacids
d. nasal decongestants

[NP: AS, CL: AP]

Rationale: Constipation and impaction in the elderly may be symptoms suggestive of chronic use or misuse of antacids.

<u>Review Questions from Text</u>

1. Over-the-counter drugs are:
a. categorized as legend drugs
b. not required to prove effectiveness
*c. defined as safe for use without medical supervision
d. used for permanent relief of annoying symptoms

[CL: KN]

Rationale: By definition, the FDA has found OTC medications to be safe for use without medical supervision.

2. Which statement is true regarding aspirin?
*a. Gastrointestinal discomfort is the most common adverse effect.
b. Buffered aspirin are therapeutically superior to plain aspirin.
c. Liquid aspirin is preferred for pediatric use.
d. Enteric-coated aspirin should be administered with an antacid.

[CL: KN]

Rationale: Aspirin's most common side effect is gastrointestinal discomfort, which includes symptoms such as nausea, indigestion, and heartburn.

3. Which statement is true regarding cough suppressants (antitussives)?
a. Self-treatment should be limited to 14 days, so that a serious underlying cause is not overlooked.
*b. Antitussives should be used only if a persistent cough causes pain or lack of sleep or is nonproductive.

c. The only OTC antitussives recognized as safe and effective are Phenaphren and Tempra.
d. Codeine is not commonly used as a suppressant because of its powerful addiction potential.

[CL: KN]

Rationale: Cough is often the means by which bronchial congestion is cleared; therefore, suppression of a cough with antitussives is indicated only if the cough is nonproductive, interferes with sleep, or causes pain.

4. All of the following are expectorants commonly found in OTC cough remedies except:
a. ammonium chloride
b. terpin hydrate
c. guaifenesin
*d. dextromethorphan

[CL: CO]

Rationale: Expectorants commonly found in OTC medications include iodides, ammonium chloride, terpin hydrate, and guaifenesin.

5. Of the following drug characteristics, which one is not appropriate when selecting a liquid form of an antacid?
*a. potassium content
b. palatability
c. volume needed per dose
d. neutralizing capacity

[CL: CO]

Rationale: In choosing an antacid product, sodium content, neutralizing capacity, volume needed per dose, cost, and palatability should be considered.

6. Which of the following OTC medications contains acetaminophen?
a. Alka-Seltzer
b. Anacin
c. Empirin compound
*d. Excedrin

[CL: KN]

Rationale: Excedrin is a combination product which contains both aspirin and acetominophen.

7. Patient guidelines for self-medication include all of the following except:
a. seeking health care provider if no relief obtained
b. using non-drug measures to help treat symptoms
*c. selecting a drug which is nonspecific if currently taking prescription drugs
d. using the OTC medication for only as long as recommended

[CL: CO]

Rationale: Patient guidelines for self-medication include selecting a product which is specific in treating symptoms. Patients should consult a health care provider if taking prescription drugs along with self-care agents.

8. Patients should not self-treat with antacids if the following situation applies:
*a. discomfort associated with sweating and weakness
b. incompatible diet selection
c. excessive stress and tension
d. acute gastritis associated with overeating

[CL: KN]

Rationale: Gastric discomfort associated with weakness or sweating is a situation in which the patient should consult a health care provider.

9. A disadvantage of acetaminophen is the lack of:
   a. anticoagulant activity
   *b. anti-inflammatory activity
   c. analgesic activity
   d. antipyrogenic activity

   [CL: KN]

   Rationale: A disadvantage of acetominophen is the lack of anti-inflammatory activity.

10. The following statement is false regarding self-care measures of a sore throat:
   a. A sore throat due to a streptococcal infection may lead to serious complications if untreated.
   b. A sore throat related to a common cold may be alleviated with self-care measures and local anaesthetics.
   c. A throat culture is needed to definitely establish whether an infection is due to streptococci.
   *d. Topical antibacterial mouthwashes have been proven effective for mouth and throat infections.

   [CL: CO]

   Rationale: Treatment of bacterial infections of the throat and mouth requires systemic medication. None of the OTC topical antibacterials have been proven effective.

Additional Review Questions Not Presented in Text

1. Which of the following statements relative to cough, cold, allergy OTC medication is true?
   a. Expectorants depress the cough reflex in addition to decreasing the viscosity of bronchial secretions.
   *b. Analgesics are used for the treatment of symptoms associated with the common cold.
   c. Oral decongestants facilitate the removal of bronchial secretions from the lower respiratory tract.
   d. Antihistamines are eliminated rapidly from the body due to a short serum half-life.

   [CL: CO]

   Rationale: Analgesics are used to manage the headache, fever, and sore throat associated with a cold.

2. All of the following statements regarding antacids are true except:
   a. Ingestion of large doses of sodium bicarbonate may result in systemic alkalosis.
   b. Antacids are recommended for chronic peptic ulcer and acute gastrointestinal distress.
   *c. Magnesium forms of antacids carry the risk of precipitating hypercalcemia.
   d. Aluminum hydroxide is virtually ineffective unless in liquid form.

   [CL: CO]

   Rationale: Magnesium forms of antacids carry the risk of precipitating hypermagnesemia, especially in patients with renal failure.

3. In developing a nursing care plan for the patient that includes OTC self-medication, the nurse performs the following nursing actions except:
   a. assess if OTC drugs have contributed to the patient's current medical condition
   b. develop nursing diagnoses by synthesizing the patient's information from the assessment.
   *c. formulate a plan of care by matching each OTC medication with a diagnosis
   d. evaluate care by including periodic re-evaluations of outcome criteria

   [CL: CO]

   Rationale: A plan of care is formulated by establishing health goals and interventions designed to achieve the goals.

4. Which statement is false regarding laxatives?

a. Saline cathartics are used when prompt and complete evacuation is required.
*b. Mineral oil enhances the absorption of fat-soluble vitamins from the gut.
c. Osmotic agents increase transit time by increasing intestinal bulk.
d. Laxatives are the most misused and abused of the OTC medications.

[CL: KN]

Rationale: Mineral oil inhibits the absorption of fat-soluble vitamins from the gut.

5. Which of the following is true of dextromethorphan?
a. Related nausea, headache, and drowsiness occur frequently.
b. It is the most commonly found expectorant.
*c. Large doses may cause respiratory depression.
d. As a narcotic derivative, it possesses addictive potential.

[CL: CO]

Rationale: Dextromethorphan, a common cough suppressant, may cause respiratory depression when larger doses are administered. Recommended doses are usually well tolerated, without nausea, headaches, or drowsiness.

CHAPTER 8: TEACHING, LEARNING, AND EVALUATION STRATEGIES FOR COMPLIANCE

Situations from Text

Situation 8-1

Forty-seven-year-old Molly Black, a newly diagnosed diabetic, is prescribed teaching related to insulin administration. The nurse reviews adult teaching-learning principles before working with Ms. Black.

1. The most significant consideration for the nurse to explore prior to teaching the adult patient is:
   *a. readiness to learn
   b. potential medication changes
   c. current health status
   d. age of significant others

   [NP: AS, CL: CO]

   Rationale: An individual will not learn until readiness to learnis displayed.

2. The nurse plans to utilize pamphlets in teaching Ms. Black about insulin. Printed material may have limitations in patient education due to:
   a. publication style
   b. number of illustrations used
   *c. reading level of the patient
   d. number of action words used

   [NP: AN, CL: KN]

   Rationale: If printed material is not readable by the patient, the written information will not be understood.

3. The nurse plans to incorporate the concept of reinforcement during the teaching session with Ms. Black. This concept is inherent in which of the following teaching-learning theories:
   a. cognitive
   *b. conditioning
   c. humanistic
   d. mechanistic

   [NP: PL, CL: KN]

   Rationale: Skinner's conditioning theory focuses on reinforcement as a motivator.

4. The nurse believes that Ms. Black should be totally involved in the teaching-learning of insulin administration. This reflects the following learning style:
   a. extinction
   *b. experiential
   c. programmed
   d. rote

   [NP: AN, CL: CO]

   Rationale: personal involvement in the learning event is a component of experiential learning.

5. Ms. Black's ability to effectively internalize the procedure for self-administration of insulin may be most affected by the:
   a. type of syringe
   b. previous health care experiences
   c. cultural background
   *d. recent diabetic diagnosis

[NP: AS, CL: AN]

Rationale: A recent diagnosis may increase the patient's stress and anxiety level, thus interfering with effective learning.

6. The best way to ensure that responsible learning about insulin administration has occurred would be through:
   *a. self-evaluation
   b. standardized post-test
   c. return demonstration
   d. evaluation by the nurse

   [NP: EV, CL: KN]

   Rationale: One of the major ways by which experiential learning becomes responsible learning is through self-evaluation.

Situation 8-2

Ted Simmons, 56 years old, requires teaching for his cardiac medication therapy following Holter monitor evaluation.

1. In assessing Ted's readiness to learn, the nurse can best utilize this learning theory:
   a. Roger's
   *b. Ausubel's
   c. Skinner's
   d. McLaughlin's

   [NP: AS, CL: CO]

   Rationale: The pre-teaching phase of Ausubel's theory is probably the most useful in assessing the patient's readiness to learn.

2. The nurse assesses that Ted is motivated to learn about his cardiac medication because he:
   a. states that he will take his medication as ordered
   b. avoids having his wife attend the teaching session
   c. misses 50% of the questions on the medication pretest
   *d. asks many questions about his health and medications

   [NP: AS, CL: AN]

   Rationale: By posing questions, an individual displays motivation by desiring greater knowledge about practical health care.

3. Ted is very anxious and overwhelmed at the thought of what he needs to learn to keep healthy. Which of the following nursing diagnoses would be most applicable to Ted's situation?
   a. disturbance in self-concept related to lack of understanding about cardiac medications
   *b. knowledge deficit related to cardiac medications
   c. ineffective family coping related to cardiac medications
   d. alteration in compliance related to cardiac medications

   [NP: AN, CL: AN]

   Rationale: Anxiety may occur when a lack of knowledge regarding a specific event is identified.

4. The nurse understands that the goals of teaching should be achieved:
   *a. several days before the patient is ready for discharge
   b. following instructions on day of discharge
   c. upon arriving home following discharge from the hospital
   d. immediately after presentation of material

   [NP: PL, CL: CO]

Rationale: Teaching goals related to discharge are realized well in advance of discharge to avoid misunderstanding and noncompliance.

5. The nurse would teach Ted about each of the following aspects of his cardiac medications except:
   a. why he is taking the medication
   b. how to measure the correct dosage of the medication
   c. taking the medication in relation to meals
   *d. how much each of the medications costs

   [NP: IM, CL: CO]

   Rationale: Medication teaching responsibilities for the nurse include the purpose of drug therapy as well as method and proper timing of medication administration.

6. In order to promote the desired learning outcomes, the nurse would use the following as a positive reinforcer for Ted:
   a. separation
   b. money
   *c. smiling
   d. punishment

   [NP: IM, CL: AP]

   Rationale: Smiling is an example of a universal non-verbal positive reinforcer.

Additional Situation Not Presented in Text

Melvin Porterfield, a 38-year-old bricklayer with hypertension, requires teaching related to his drug therapy during his hospitalization.

1. Which of the following statements by Mr. Porterfield may indicate noncompliance with his drug therapy prior to this hospitalization?
   a. "I'm responsible for my life and how I'm feeling."
   b. "I always get good treatment from my doctor."
   c. "These pills are costing me a lot of money."
   *d. "My blood pressure isn't as bad as the doctors think."

   [NP: AS, CL: AN]

   Rationale: Subjectively believing the illness is not as severe as perceived by health professionals is a characteristic patient factor that correlates with noncompliance.

2. Mr. Porterfield tells the nurse that he was given a number of pamphlets on hypertension and his medications after his diagnosis. A significant factor which may be related to noncompliance in this case would be:
   a. occupation
   *b. readability level
   c. lifestyle
   d. religious preference

   [NP: AN, CL: AN]

   Rationale: A low readability level may interfere with a patient's ability to understand written materials and may contribute to noncompliance.

3. In teaching Mr. Porterfield about his antihypertensive medication, the nurse utilizes Skinner's teaching and learning principles, which are reflected by the following statement:
   a. The content to be learned must be independently discovered by the patient.
   *b. Behavior is reinforced at each stage in the learning process.
   c. The teacher trusts the student to develop his own potential for learning.

d. Memorization of new ideas occurs without relation to the learner's cognitive structure.

[NP: IM, CL: CO]

Rationale: Skinner's conditioning-behavioristic theory of teaching-learning is based on the principle of reinforcement.

4. A statement by Mr. Porterfield indicating his readiness to learn about his medications is:
   a. "I've lived with this high blood pressure for five years already."
   b. "My father never took pills for his high blood pressure."
   *c. "Could I end up with a stroke if I don't take these pills?"
   d. "I took a pill this morning; is my blood pressure down today?"

[NP: AS, CL: AN]

Rationale: An individual who is motivated to learn asks questions pertinent to his health situation.

5. During the teaching phase, the nurse gives Mr. Porterfield information about self-care and home management of hypertension. Which of the following would <u>not</u> be included in teaching?
   a. avoid bathing in very hot water
   b. observe a low-sodium diet
   c. rise slowly from supine position
   *d. take over-the-counter medications as needed

[NP: IM, CL: AN]

Rationale: It is important for the patient to consult with the pharmacist and/or physician before taking OTC medications.

6. For Mr. Porterfield, each of the following techniques might be effective in reinforcing a medication teaching session <u>except</u>:
   a. a videotape illustrating the drug's purpose
   b. slide presentations on how to take the drug
   *c. specific drug package inserts
   d. a panel presentation on common side effects of the drug

[NP: PL, CL: AN]

Rationale: Oral teachings cannot be reinforced if pamphlets are not written at the learner's reading level.

<u>**Review Questions from Text**</u>

1. In formulating a plan to assess the teaching needs of a patient requiring medication, the nurse knows that the patient's:
   a. cultural traditions have little effect upon the ability to learn
   *b. educational level and reading ability must be determined for successful learning to occur
   c. role in the teaching-learning process is one of subordination
   d. self-esteem should be threatened to ensure rapid learning

[CL: CO]

Rationale: Comprehension of written information depends upon the ability to read.

2. David Ausubel's cognitive/discovery perspective is concerned with all of the following concepts <u>except</u>:
   a. non-observable forms of behavior, thinking, and relationship formation
   b. reception learning where content to be learned is presented in final form
   *c. generalizations that tell the learner that behavior in a given situation continues to be true in future learning experiences
   d. how learners solve problems and form concepts

[CL: KN]

Rationale: The concept of generalizations is inherent in Skinner's learning theory.

3. In developing nursing diagnoses related to the teaching needs of a patient requiring medication, the nurse educator will:
 a. apply the principles of Ausubel's perspective by developing an interpersonal relationship with the patient
 *b. apply Rogers' principles by involving the patient and family in the development of the nursing diagnoses
 c. apply the principles of B. F. Skinner by encouraging questions in an open environment
 d. apply Rogers' principles in dealing with the highly motivated confident learner

[CL: AP]

Rationale: Rogers emphasizes the learner-centered educational approach.

4. In developing teaching techniques specific to the learning needs of the patient requiring medication, the nurse educator knows that all of the following facts are <u>true</u> except:
 *a. The goals of teaching are achieved the day of patient discharge.
 b. Important information is written down by the patient and checked by the nurse for accuracy.
 c. The patient and family see and handle the medications that will be taken at home.
 d. The patient makes the ultimate decision for medication compliance.

[CL: CO]

Rationale: The goals of teaching should be achieved several days before the patient is ready for discharge.

5. Evaluation techniques to assess teaching strategy effectiveness include:
 a. selecting the evaluation criteria as the final step in the evaluation process
 *b. spelling out the evaluation conditions in behavioral objective terms
 c. determining evaluation techniques and methods during the evaluation phase of the nursing process
 d. applying the evaluation process only at the termination of the teaching plan

[CL: CO]

Rationale: Specific behavioral objectives are easily measurable for the attainment of teaching objectives.

6. Which of the following statements is <u>true</u> regarding the SMOG readability formula?
The SMOG formula is:
 a. based on 90 percent comprehension and is the most accurate way of assessing readability
 *b. determined by the square root of the number of polysyllabic words contained within 30 selected sentences
 c. based on dividing the number of complex sentences contained within one paragraph of written material by 3
 d. found to be too complex to be of practical use in the hospital teaching-learing setting

[CL: KN]

Rationale: The SMOG readability formula is based on the square root of the number of polysyllabic words contained within 30 selected sentences. The number 3 is added to the square root, and this score represents the reading grade that a person must have reached in order to understand the material.

7. Compliance can be defined as:
 a. evidence of comprehension of a medical diagnosis and its lifestyle implications
 b. the ability of the patient to repeat information presented in both verbal and written forms
 c. the extent to which a patient's symptoms can be controlled by medication
 *d. the degree to which a patient's behavior regarding the medication plan coincides with medical advice

[CL: CO]

Rationale: Compliance can be defined as the extent to which a patient's behavior with regard to the medication plan coincides with health teaching.

8. According to B. F. Skinner's conditioning behavioristic perspective, EXTINCTION is achieved by:
   a. punishment measures
   *b. withdrawal of reinforcement
   c. rewarding the undesired behavior
   d. refusing to focus on the desired behavior

   [CL: KN]

   Rationale: Extinction is employed to eliminate undesirable behavior and is achieved by withdrawing reinforcement.

9. Patients who would be most suited to Ausubel's learning theory would include the:
   *a. independent, motivated learner
   b. dependent learner with poor reading skills
   c. anxious, shy, or slow learner
   d. unmotivated learner with low readability level

   [CL: KN]

   Rationale: Ausubel's learning theory is best suited to the independent, motivated learner.

10. During the assessment phase of the patient's learning needs, the nurse will focus on all of the following <u>except</u>:
   a. establishing a trusting and nonthreatening relationship
   b. determining educational level and reading ability
   *c. expecting that the patient will demonstrate noncompliance
   d. selecting aspects from all of the learning theories in establishing a data base

   [CL: CO]

   Rationale: The nurse should initially approach the patient with a positive attitude and expect compliance. The nurse must be aware, however, that noncompliance may be demonstrated.

<u>Additional Review Questions Not Presented in Text</u>

1. Which statement describes B. F. Skinner's conditioning perspective?
   *a. Behavior is reinforced at each stage in the learning process.
   b. The patient controls the learning environment.
   c. The patient learns in unified wholes.
   d. The nurse need not be present for learning to occur.

   [CL: KN]

   Rationale: Reinforcement is a central concept of Skinner's learning theory.

2. In Carl Rogers' interpersonal humanistic perspective:
   a. The teacher is the central figure in the teaching-learning process.
   *b. The teacher develops a profound trust in the student to develop his or her own potentiality to learn.
   c. Advance organizers are utilized to facilitate the learning process.
   d. The cognitive and psychomotor domains are the primary focus in the teaching-learning process.

   [CL: KN]

   Rationale: In Rogers' theory, the teacher assumes the role of facilitator of learning; thus, trust in the learner is essential.

3. Of the following statements, which one is <u>not</u> true regarding <u>planning</u> nursing intervention for the patient requiring medication?
   a. Most patients learn best when material is presented visually.
   b. All health team members should work together to educate the patient.

c. Interventions are based upon the patient's pre-assessment needs and nursing diagnoses.
*d. Group discussion or therapy groups are particularly useful for educating acutely ill patients.

[CL: CO]

Rationale: Group therapy is particularly effective for patients with chronic disease.

4. In developing evaluation tools or techniques to measure patient learning, the nurse may use:
   a. formation evaluation to compare the patient's performance to a relatively fixed standard
   b. criterion referenced evaluation to gather information about patient performance and to provide feedback as soon as possible
   *c. informal discussion, formal paper-and-pencil tests, oral quizzes, and return demonstrations
   d. any methodology determined by the nurse during the intervention phase of the nursing process

   [CL: AP]

   Rationale: These methods of evaluation provide input into the attainment of educational goals.

5. In applying teaching-learning theories to the evaluation of patient learning the nurse knows that:
   a. Skinner advocates the exclusive use of self-evaluation
   b. Rogers' theory suggests the use of criterion-referenced evaluation as established by the nurse
   c. Ausubel advocates the use of jointly determined educational goals
   *d. Ausubel's theory suggests pre- and post-tests as the most appropriate evaluation tools

   [CL: CO]

   Rationale: Ausubel emphasizes the importance of pre- and post-testing in the evaluation of educational goals.

CHAPTER 9: DRUGS USED IN DIAGNOSTIC TESTING

Situation from Text

Situation 9-1

Meryl Golden is a 76-year-old female admitted to the medical-surgical unit for diagnostic testing of abdominal pain.

1. In planning the scheduling of barium studies for Mrs. Golden, the nurse is aware that:
   a. the barium swallow should be performed prior to the barium enema
   b. the barium swallow and barium enema cannot be performed during a single patient admission
   c. barium studies should be scheduled before other diagnostic tests
   *d. the barium enema should be performed before the barium swallow

   [NP: PL, CL: CO]

   Rationale: Barium is eliminated unchanged in the feces, requiring several days for evacuation. For this reason, the barium enema should be performed before the barium swallow.

2. Prior to barium studies, if Mrs. Golden should complain of increasing abdominal pain with rigidity or vomiting, the nurse's best response would be to:
   a. administer analgesics and narcotics by intravenous route
   *b. inform the physician and prepare to cancel barium studies
   c. prepare to give barium via intravenous route and keep NPO
   d. prepare to give barium sulfate via a nasogastric tube

   [NP: IM, CL: AN]

   Rationale: Barium administration is contraindicated in patients with perforation of the gastrointestinal tract or intestinal obstruction. If signs of perforation or obstruction are observed, such as increased abdominal pain, rigidity, or nausea, the physician should be informed.

3. All of the following would be included in planning the care for Mrs. Golden after completion of barium studies except:
   *a. limit oral fluid intake
   b. observe for light-colored stools
   c. provide mouth care ad lib
   d. check for bowel sounds

   [NP: PL, CL: CO]

   Rationale: Nursing actions following barium enema include to encourage intake of oral fluids.

4. Due to Mrs. Golden's age, the nurse will be particularly concerned during rectal administration of barium, because of:
   a. hypertension
   b. tachycardia
   c. constipation
   *d. vagal response

   [NP: AS, CL: CO]

   Response: Administration of a barium enema may stimulate a vagal response resulting in bradycardia and hypotension. This occurs more frequently in the older adult.

5. Mrs. Golden has been NPO since midnight and received enemas until clear the morning of the scheduled barium enema. Which of the following nursing diagnoses apply?
   a. knowledge deficit related to events of barium studies

b. ineffective family coping related to stress of diagnostic studies
*c. potential fluid volume deficit related to NPO status and enemas
d. disturbance in self-concept related to enema administration

[NP: AN, CL: AN]

Rationale: Dehydration can occur when elderly patients are kept NPO and receive numerous enemas.

6. Following the barium studies, the nurse is concerned with evaluation. Which of the following is not an aspect of the evaluation phase?
a. Observe for signs of anaphylaxis.
b. Arrange follow-up care as needed.
c. Alter care plan to include post-diagnostic measures.
*d. Record prior experiences with diagnostic testing.

[NP: EV, CL: CO]

Rationale: Determining the effect of the patient's past experiences with diagnostic testing is an aspect of nursing assessment.

Additional Situation Not Presented in Text

As evening charge on a medical-surgical floor in a small community hospital, Estelle Nelson encounters the following patients, who are admitted for diagnostic procedures.

1. Mr. Suarez, a 45-year-old, is being evaluated for possible cholecystitis and will be given the diagnostic agent iopanoic acid (Telepaque). In planning care, Estelle is aware that:
a. the dosage should not exceed 12 gms in 24 hours
*b. 3 gms (6 tablets) are administered p.o. 10 hours before the text
c. the agent is administered intravenously 8 hours before testing

[NP: PL, CL: CO]

Rationale: The adult dosage of Telepaque is 3 gm (6 tablets) administered one at a time in 5 minute intervals 10-14 hours before the test.

2. Estelle prepares Mrs. Henderson for gastric function studies using histamine phosphate. Estelle will withhold all of the following medications except:
*a. beta blockers
b. anticholinergics
c. H_2 antagonists
d. antacids

[NP: IM, CL: CO]

Rationale: In preparation for testing with histamine phosphate, medications should be withheld that inhibit or stimulate gastric secretion, such as anticholinergics, H_2 antagonists, and antacids.

3. Mr. Wheatfield is admitted for congestive heart failure and is scheduled for cardiac function studies with indocyanine green (Cardio-Green). Prior to this testing, Estelle would observe for all of the following except:
a. fluid overload
b. dehydration
*c. histamine sensitivity
d. iodine allergy

[NP: AS, CL: CO]

Rationale: Prior to administration of nonradioactive dye, the patient is assessed for dehydration and fluid overload, which are contraindications. The dye should be used with caution in patients with an iodine allergy.

4. Carol Gillmoore received a PPD by the Mantoux method. When Estelle examines the area for reaction, she will report the following as significant:
   a. induration of 4 mm in diameter without erythema
   b. purplish red erythema (+++) without induration
   c. trace erythema (+) with induration 4 mm in diameter
   *d. induration of 10 mm in diameter without erythema

   [NP: EV, CL: AP]

   Rationale: Induration is the most significant clinical sign of reaction related to PPD. An induration which measures greater than 10 mm is a positive reaction. Erythema as a single finding is not of clinical significance.

5. Mr. Danner is to have cardiac blood pool imaging with Technetium. After this test, Mr. Danner will be taught all of the following <u>except</u>:
   a. to perform proper hygiene after voiding
   b. to urinate frequently
   *c. to limit oral fluid intake
   d. to follow directions regarding body positioning

   [NP: IM, CL: AP]

   Rationale: After studies utilizing Technetium, the patient should be instructed to increase fluid intake and void frequently in order to avoid accumulation of radioactivity in the bladder.

6. Karen Freeman is a 30-year-old undergoing liver function studies with Bromsulphalein (BSP). Estelle will observe for which of the following with regard to BSP?
   a. fluid overload
   *b. extravasation
   c. albumin sensitivity
   d. hypertension

   [NP: IM, CL: CO]

   Rationale: Extravasation with BSP can cause cellular damage and should be avoided.

<u>Review Questions from Text</u>

1. All of the following medications are used in diagnostic testing <u>except</u>:
   a. histamine phosphate
   b. barium sulfate
   c. hypaque sodium
   *d. acetylcholine chloride

   [CL: CO]

   Rationale: Histamine, barium, and hypaque are all used in diagnostic testing. Acetylcholine chloride is a solution used in cataract surgery to obtain complete miosis.

2. Iodine compounds may be:
   a. administered only by the oral route
   b. administered to all patients without adverse reactions
   *c. injected directly into the area to be visualized
   d. limited to use with patients allergic to barium

   [CL: CO]

   Rationale: Iodine diagnostic compounds opacify structures and vessels upon contact. These preparations can be administered orally or intravenously.

3. Of the following statements regarding common diagnostic agents, which one is not correct?

*a. Radioactive isotopes localize only in abnormal tissue.
b. The most common side effect following barium use is constipation.
c. The most serious side effect of iodine testing is anaphylaxis.
d. The diagnostic dosage of radiopharmaceuticals is higher than the therapeutic dosage.

[CL: CO]

Rationale: A radiopharmaceutical is chosen because of its affinity to localize in either normal or abnormal tissue.

4. In developing a nursing care plan for the patient undergoing diagnostic testing, the nurse performs all of the following actions except:
a. schedules barium studies last
*b. administers insulin to the NPO diabetic patient
c. assesses the patient before, during, and after the procedure
d. explains the procedure at a level the patient can understand

[CL: KN]

Rationale: Insulin should be withheld as long as the diabetic patient is NPO. Special scheduling is often necessary for the diabetic patient.

5. Nonradioactive dyes are used to:
a. detect abnormal tissue
*b. measure organ function
c. diagnose adrenal insufficiency
d. delineate soft tissue

[CL: KN]

Rationale: Nonradioactive dyes are used to measure organ function.

6. The following statement is correct with regard to agents which stimulate gland secretion:
a. Agents which stimulate the secretion of enzymes are called tropic hormones.
b. Secretogogues include thyrotropin and adrenocorticotropic hormone.
c. Pentagastrin stimulates duodenal and pancreatic secretion.
*d. Sincalide stimulates gallbladder contraction and bile release.

[CL: KN]

Rationale: Sincalide is a secretogogus agent which stimulates gallbladder contraction and bile release.

7. Diagnostic skin tests are performed for the diagnosis of all of the following except:
*a. rheumatoid arthritis
b. coccidioidomycosis
c. histoplasmosis
d. tuberculosis

[CL: CO]

Rationale: Skin tests are administered for the diagnosis of infections such as tuberculosis, coccidioidonmycosis, and histoplasmosis.

8. Hypaque Sodium is contraindicated in the following patient situation:
a. hyperuricemia
b. intestinal malformations
*c. iodine hypersensitivity
d. peptic ulcer disease

[CL: KN]

Rationale: Hypaque Sodium is contraindicated in patients with iodine hypersensitivity.

9. In diagnostic radiology:
   a. particulate radiation is measured
   b. energy is released by stable electrons
   *c. electromagnetic radiation is measured
   d. alpha and beta rays are emitted

   [CL: KN]

   Rationale: In diagnostic radiology, electromagnetic radiation, the release of gamma or x-rays, is measured.

10. Which of the following agents might be added with the dye preparation in order to reduce the incidence of allergic reactions?
   *a. diphenhydramine
   b. epinephrine
   c. acetominophen
   d. oxygen

   [CL: CO]

   Rationale: Diphenhydramine (Benadryl) may be given prior to testing if a hypersensitivity reaction is anticipated.

Additional Review Questions Not Presented in Text

1. The diagnostic agent barium sulfate is:
   a. administered via the intravenous route
   b. used to diagnose the presence of gastrointestinal fistulas
   c. absorbed through the gastrointestinal tract
   *d. used to aid visualization of the gastrointestinal tract

   [CL: KN]

   Rationale: Barium sulfate is used to visualize the gastrointestinal tract.

2. Which statement is not correct relative to assessing the patient receiving diagnostic drugs?
   a. Many individuals allergic to fish may have an iodine allergy.
   *b. Thyroid function tests can be affected if barium has been administered.
   c. Assessment of all systems should be performed just prior to testing.
   d. Physician and psychological status should be checked prior to testing.

   [CL: CO]

   Rationale: Thyroid function results are affected by iodine-based dye preparations.

3. All of the following are methods of skin testing except:
   a. patch test
   b. scratch test
   *c. subcutaneous test
   d. intradermal test

   [CL: CO]

   Rationale: The methods of skin testing include the patch test, skin test, and intradermal test.

4. A primary nursing intervention for patients receiving provocative agents includes:
   *a. monitoring for physiological responses
   b. administering oral tropic hormones

c. receiving a verbal patient consent
d. interpreting laboratory findings

[CL: KN]

Rationale: Physiological responses to a provocative agent can be serious. Therefore, the primary function of the nurse in caring for the patient is to monitor for physiological responses.

CHAPTER 10: DRUGS USED IN ANESTHESIA

Situations from Text

Situation 10-1

As a unit coordinator in a postanesthesia recovery room, Jill Henderson frequently applies knowledge of anesthetic agents.

1. Bob Wills, a 40-year-old, received halothane (Fluothane) as an induction agent. Jill will observe for all of the following with regard to halothane except:
   a. hepatotoxicity
   *b. skeletal muscle relaxation
   c. respiratory depression
   d. bradycardia and dysrhythmias

   [NP: IM, CL: CO]

   Rationale: Halothane is associated with myocardial and respiratory depressant effects. The drug can also cause hepatotoxicity.

2. Amy Pallet is recovering from abdominal surgery in which Isoflurane (Forane) was used as the anesthetic agent. In planning postanesthesia care, Jill will expect:
   a. nausea and vomiting
   b. postoperative excitation
   c. cardiac dysrhythmias
   *d. depressed mental alertness

   [NP: PL, CL: KN]

   Rationale: Mental alertness is generally depressed for 2 to 3 hours following use of isoflurane. Postanesthesia nausea and excitation are rare. There is less of a tendency to develop dysrhythmias than with other agents.

3. Mrs. Reeves received ketamine hydrochloride (Ketalar) for debridement of a burn. After recovery, Jill teaches Mrs. Reeves about potential effects of the drug, which include:
   a. frequent urination
   b. constipation
   *c. disturbing dreams
   d. decreased muscle control

   [NP: IM, CL: KN]

   Rationale: About 12 percent of patients receiving ketamine experience disturbing dreams.

4. Jill prepares to administer naloxone (Narcan) 0.1 mg IV to Mr. Steiner in order to reverse the effects of narcotics administered preoperatively. It will be important for Jill to assess for the following with regard to Narcan administration:
   a. respiratory difficulty
   b. dry mouth
   *c. intense pain
   d. urine output

   [NP: IM, CL: AP]

   Rationale: Narcan is a narcotic antagonist; when administered, patients can experience intense pain.

5. In order to reintubate Mr. Gardner postoperatively without trauma, pancuronium bromide (Pavulon) is administered. Jill is aware that the antidote for this agent is a mixture of:
   *a. neostigmine and atropine

b. Narcan and neostigmine
c. Benadryl and Robinul
d. epinephrine and Narcan

[NP: PL, CL: CO]

Rationale: When Pavulon, a nondepolarizing block, is no longer needed, it can be reversed by administration of an antidote mixture of neostigmine and atropine.

6. Justine Smith, a 60-year-old, was on Inderal preoperatively. During recovery from general anesthesia, Jill will observe Ms. Smith closely for the following reaction:
   a. anxiety
   *b. hypotension
   c. barbituate potentiation
   d. hypertensive crisis

   [NP: AS, CL: KN]

   Rationale: A possible reaction to general anesthesia related to Inderal taken preoperatively is hypotension.

Situation 10-2

Gerald Moiser is a nurse in an ambulatory surgery unit.

1. When conducting a preoperative nursing history on 18-year-old Steve Adler, Gerald discovers a history of asthma. He is aware that methohexital sodium (Brevital) is to be the anesthetic agent for oral surgery. Due to Steve's history of asthma, Gerald would anticipate:
   a. replacement of Brevital with another agent
   b. no adverse reactions
   *c. administration of Brevital with caution
   d. combining Brevital with an antihistamine

   [NP: AS, CL: AP]

   Rationale: Methohexital sodium (Brevital) is less likely to cause bronchospasm and may, therefore, be administered cautiously to patients with asthma.

2. Gerald assists with an endoscopic procedure using droperidol/fentanyl (Innovar). In the immediate recovery period, Gerald will keep the following drug available:
   *a. Atropine
   b. Demerol
   c. Lidocaine
   d. Compazine

   [NP: PL, CL: CO]

   Rationale: Droperidol/fentanyl can cause bradycardia; therefore, it is essential that atropine be kept readily available.

3. When Mr. Judd experiences respiratory problems postoperatively, Gerald prepares for endotracheal intubation. The anesthesiologist administers succinylcholine in order to facilitate intubation. Gerald is aware that the following will be affected:
   a. sodium
   b. calcium
   c. magnesium
   *d. potassium

   [NP: AN, CL: CO]

   Rationale: After administration of succinylcholine, potassium is forced out of muscle cells and into circulation.

Hyperkalemia is a relative contraindication to its use.

4. Mrs. Hayes is scheduled for removal of a ganglionic cyst, using lidocaine hydrochloride (Xylocaine) with epinephrine for a nerve block. Gerald will review medications which Mrs. Hayes takes, because severe hypertension may result if Xylocaine with epinephrine is given to patients who are taking:
   a. beta blockers
   b. anticholinergics
   *c. MAO inhibitors
   d. H_2 antagonists

   [NP: AN, CL: KN]

   Rationale: Severe hypertension may result if Xylocaine with epinephrine is given to patients taking MAO inhibitors or tricyclic antidepressant drugs.

5. Steve Turner is to receive an epidural using procaine hydrochloride (Novacaine). All of the following statements are correct with regard to Novacaine <u>except</u>:
   a. Use solutions without preservatives for epidural blocks.
   *b. The drug is irritating to soft tissues and nerves.
   c. Procaine should be used with caution in patients with shock.
   d. Use for uncomplicated obstetric delivery only.

   [NP: PL, CL: CO]

   Rationale: Procaine hydrochloride is not irritating to soft tissues or nerves.

6. Mr. Dominick is scheduled for surgery utilizing alfentanil hydrochloride (Alfenta) as an analgesic adjunct. Gerald will assess the following in reference to Alfenta usage:
   *a. creatinine
   b. blood sugar
   c. sodium
   d. potassium

   [NP: AS, CL: AN]

   Rationale: Alfenta should be used with caution in patients with impaired renal function as reflected by creatinine levels.

<u>**Additional Situation Not Presented in Text**</u>

Indu Telek is a nurse on a general surgery floor of a large inner-city hospital.

1. Preanesthetic medication ordered for Mildred Eskew includes Atropine .6 mg IM. Mrs. Eskew questions Indu about the drug. The nurse's best response would be:
   a. "Atropine is given to help relax you."
   b. "Since nausea is a problem after surgery, this will help."
   c. "You will need Atropine to help with breathing."
   *d. "Atropine will reduce the amount of mucous in the lungs."

   [NP: IM, CL: AN]

   Rationale: A major reason for use of Atropine preoperatively is to decrease respiratory tract secretions.

2. For postoperative nausea, promethazine hydrochloride (Phenergan) 50 mg IM has been ordered for Mr. Evans. Indu is aware that this drug possesses all of the following properties <u>except</u>:
   a. antiemetic
   *b. antiarrhythmic
   c. anticholinergic
   d. antipruritic

[NP: AN, CL: CO]

Rationale: Phenergan is a phenothiazine-derivative antihistamine with anticholinergic, antiemetic, antipruritic, and sedative properties.

3. Before giving glycopyrrolate (Robinul) .1 mg IM as a preoperative medication to Mr. Shores, Indu will assess for the following patient condition:
   a. asthma
   b. anxiety
   *c. narrow-angle glaucoma
   d. rheumatoid arthritis

[NP: IM, CL: AP]

Rationale: This synthetic anticholinergic is contraindicated in patients with narrow-angle glaucoma, as well as those patients with unstable cardiovascular status, myasthenia gravis, and obstructive urologic or gastrointestinal diseases.

4. Mrs. Carlson is in the early recovery phase from a cholecystectomy. Which of the following responses indicates successful preoperative and postoperative teaching?
   a. "It hurts too much to move, so I have just stayed in one position."
   *b. "Even though it hurts, I need to turn from side to side."
   c. "The nurse will bring my pain medicine every 4 hours on schedule."
   d. "I'm afraid my incision will open if I turn or sit up."

[NP: EV, CL: AN]

Rationale: Early mobilization is essential to prevent postoperative complications.

5. Maureen Rhodes returns from surgery during which an inhalation anesthetic was used. Indu is aware that Ms. Rhodes may experience the following with regard to inhalation anesthetics:
   *a. rapid onset of pain
   b reduced mobility
   c. confusion and disorientation
   d. respiratory complications

[NP: PL, CL: KN]

Rationale: Inhalation anesthetics leave the system more rapidly; therefore, the patient may experience awareness of pain sensation earlier than with lingering agents.

6. During the postoperative planning phase, Indu takes into consideration all of the following <u>except</u>:
   a. type of anesthetic used
   b. surgical procedure performed
   c. associated anesthetic side effects
   *d. dependence on anesthetic agents

[NP: PL, CL: CO]

Rationale: The postoperative nursing care plan depends on anesthetic agent used, procedure performed, and side effects associated with a particular anesthetic agent.

Review Questions from Text

1. Which of the following medications is commonly used as an anesthetic?
   a. glycopyrrolate (Robinul)
   b. pentobarbital sodium (Nembutal)
   c. promethazine hydrochloride (Phenergan)
   *d. droperidol/fentanyl (Innovar)

[CL: IN]

Rationale: Droperidol/fentanyl (Innovar) is the combination narcotic and anesthetic agent which produces a state of neuroleptic analgesia.

2. Methoxyflurane (Penthrane) is an anesthetic that has which of the following properties:
   *a. long recovery period
   b. few side effects
   c. good induction properties
   d. high vapor pressure

[CL: KN]

Rationale: Methoxyflurane (Penthrane) is a potent inhalation anesthetic with slow induction and recovery times. This drug has numerous side effects and its use is limited.

3. Barbiturates, as intravenously administered anesthetic agents, produce:
   a. good analgesia
   b. respiratory tract irritation
   c. good skeletal muscle relaxation
   *d. rapid recovery period

[CL: KN]

Rationale: Intravenous barbiturates have a rapid recovery period and are, therefore, often utilized for short surgical procedures.

4. Of the following statements, which one is correct regarding local anesthesia?
   a. Field block anesthesia involves injecting the agent directly into the area to be desensitized.
   b. Infiltration anesthesia involves infiltrating the tissue around the area to be desensitized.
   *c. A nerve block is achieved by injecting the anesthetic agent close to a mixed nerve.
   d. Spinal anesthesia is achieved by injecting a drug into a nerve block in the spinal column.

[CL: CO]

Rationale: A nerve block is achieved by injecting the drug close to a mixed nerve in order that the area innervated by the nerve will become insensitive.

5. In planning care for the postoperative patient, the nurse knows:
   a. patients receiving spinal anesthesia are kept supine for 2 to 4 hours postoperatively
   *b. deep muscle relaxation can result in bladder atony or decreased intestinal motility
   c. if voiding has not occurred within 4 hours postoperatively, the patient is catheterized
   d. immobilization of the patient helps to relieve abdominal distention and pain

[CL: KN]

Rationale: The state of deep muscle relaxation of general anesthesia can result in bladder atony or decreased intestinal motility.

6. Depolarizing neuromuscular blocking agents act by depolarization of the:
   *a. motor end plate in order to produce muscle paralysis
   b. nerve axon fiber to create desensitization in muscle fibers
   c. postsynaptic membrane in order to inhibit muscle movement
   d. nerve cell dendrites which then block acetylcholine release

[CL: KN]

Rationale: Depolarizing or noncompetitive neuromuscular blockade is achieved by depolarization of the motor end plate.

7. Which of the following statements is correct regarding anesthesia?
   a. Balanced anesthesia involves utilizing an agent along with its antidote.
   b. Regional anethesia can be achieved by inhalation of certain drugs.
   *c. In order to achieve a painless state, there must be temporary areflexia.
   d. Many drugs are available which meet all of the criteria for an anesthetic.

   [CL: CO]

   Rationale: In order for there to be no pain, there must be an absence of reflexes.

8. Stage III of anesthesia is characterized by:
   a. minimal muscle relaxation
   *b. spinal cord depression
   c. respiratory paralysis
   d. cerebral cortex depression

   [CL: KN]

   Rationale: Spinal cord depression and true muscle relaxation occur during Stage III of anesthesia.

9. Desirable characteristics of a good local anesthetic drug include all of the following except:
   a. action confined to nerve tissue
   b. sufficiently long duration
   c. compatability with vasoconstrictor agents
   *d. solubility in high glucose solutions

   [CL: CO]

   Rationale: Desirable characteristics of a good local anesthetic drug include solubility in saline solution and water, in addition to long duration, compatability with vasoconstrictor drugs, and action confined to nerve tissue.

10. Which of the following local anesthetics is of the ester type?
   *a. piperocaine
   b. dibucaine
   c. lidocaine
   d. etridrocaine

   [CL: KN]

   Rationale: Piperocaine is a local anesthetic of the ester type.

Additional Review Questions Not Presented in Text

1. Fluothane (Halothane) is best known for its:
   a. flammable and explosive properties
   *b. rapid induction and rapid recovery properties
   c. wide safety range of administration
   d. minimal effect upon the heart and liver

   [CL: KN]

   Rationale: A major advantage of Halothane is its rapid induction and rapid recovery.

2. Which characteristic describes isoflurane (Forane)?
   a. antagonizes the effects of neuromuscular blocking agents
   b. produces hepatic and renal toxic effects
   c. causes central nervous system stimulation
   *d. has no adverse effect on intracranial pressure

   [CL: KN]

Rationale: As long as ventilation is maintained, Isoflurane has no adverse effect on intracranial pressure.

3. Which statement is correct regarding drugs used for muscle relaxation?
   a. D-tubocurarine (Tubarine) produces intense muscle contractions post administration.
   *b. Pancuronium bromide (Pavulon) works by competitive inhibition on the postsynaptic membrane.
   c. Succinylcholine (Anectine) stabilizes intraocular pressure and is recommended for glaucoma patients.
   d. Atracurium (Tracrium) achieves its effect by depolarization of the motor end plate.

[CL: KN]

Rationale: Pavulon, a nondepolarizing neuromuscular blocking agent, works by competitive inhibition on the postsynaptic membrane.

4. Preoperative nursing interventions include the following actions except:
   a. teaching about the perioperative period
   b. overseeing patient lab tests
   *c. administering preclinical medication just prior to voiding
   d. allowing the patient to lie quietly after preoperative medication

[CL: CO]

Rationale: The patient should be asked to void just prior to preclinical medication administration.

5. Postoperative evaluation of the success of nursing interventions reveals all of the following responses except:
   *a. absence of flatus
   b. relief of pain
   c. absence of rales
   d. relief of nausea

[CL: CO]

Rationale: The passing of flatus postoperatively indicates proper bowel function. Early mobilization can relieve the discomfort from distension caused by flatus.

CHAPTER 11: INTRAVENOUS THERAPY

Situations from Text

Situation 11-1

Mr. Wells, an 86-year-old, is transferred from a nursing home to an acute care facility. The admitting diagnosis is dehydration.

1. During the admission process, the nurse will be aware of the following clinical sign of dehydration:
   *a. poor skin turgor
   b. moist clammy skin
   c. pink frothy sputum
   d. abdominal cramps

   [NP: AS, CL: AP]

   Rationale: A clinical sign of dehydration is poor skin turgor.

2. Intravenous fluid has been ordered for Mr. Wells. It will be important for the nurse to assess the following prior to initiating therapy:
   a. ability to communicate
   b. patient height
   *c. body weight
   d. cranial nerves

   [NP: AS, CL: CO]

   Rationale: Baseline data, such as patient weights, electrolytes, and laboratory tests, are obtained prior to starting the IV.

3. The report from the nursing home reveals that Mr. Wells has had a fever for the last three days and has not been eating or drinking adequately. The nurse is aware that the following process has probably occurred:
   *a. hyperosmotic contraction
   b. hyperosmotic expansion
   c. iso-osmotic contraction
   d. hypo-osmotic expansion

   [NP: AN, CL: AP]

   Rationale: When intake is less than output, dehydration occurs. This results in greater concentration of particles in the extracellular space. To compensate, fluid moves from the intracellular space to the extracellular space, and the cells become shrunken.

4. Intravenous fluid in the form of 2.5 percent dextrose + 0.45 percent sodium chloride is started for Mr. Wells. This type of solution is:
   a. hydrating and isotonic
   b. replacement and isotonic
   *c. hydrating and hypotonic
   d. replacement and isotonic

   [NP: AN, CL: AN]

   Rationale: 2.5 percent dextrose + 0.45 percent sodium chloride is an example of a hydrating solution which is hypotonic in composition.

5. The rate of infusion of the intravenous fluid 2.5 percent dextrose + 0.45 percent sodium chloride should be given:

a. rapidly in order to rehydrate as quickly as possible
b. slowly due to rapid shift into the extracellular space
c. rapidly in order to increase vascular volume
*d. slowly due to sudden shift of fluid into the cells

[NP: PL, CL: KN]

Rationale: Hypotonic solutions should be given slowly because a sudden shift of fluid into the cells can occur.

6. In evaluating Mr. Wells' intravenous therapy, all of the following outcome criteria are expected except:
a. normal electrolytes and osmolality
*b. urine output less than 30 cc per hour
c. absence of pain at the administration site
d. absence of infiltration, extravasation, or thrombosis

[NP: EV, CL: AN]

Rationale: With adequate hydration and renal function, urine output should exceed 30 cc per hour.

Situation 11-2

As an emergency room nurse, Marianne Holt encounters patients daily who require intravenous therapy and correction of acid-base imbalances.

1. Shelby Andrews presents to the emergency room, complaining of feeling "anxious" and stating that she has tingling in feet and hands. An arterial blood gas reveals respiratory alkalosis. Marianne will be prepared to treat her with:
a. sodium bicarbonate
b. mechanical ventilation
c. oxygen therapy
*d. rebreather bag

[NP: IM, CL: AP]

Rationale: Respiratory alkalosis is caused by excessive loss of carbon dioxide. It is treated by eliminating the cause and helping the patient to breathe more deeply and slowly. A rebreather bag helps to retain carbon dioxide.

2. Mr. Butler, a 72-year-old with chronic renal failure, is short of breath and restless. His wife admits that he has not been adhering to his renal diet. Marianne notes pitting edema at the ankles and crackles in the lung bases. Marianne is aware that edema results from all of the following except:
*a. reduced hydrostatic pressure
b. reduced oncotic pressure
c. increased capillary permeability
d. reduced lymphatic drainage

[NP: AS, CL: KN]

Rationale: Edema results from increased hydrostatic pressure in addition to reduced oncotic pressure, increased capillary permeability, and/or reduced lymphatic drainage.

3. Mrs. Owens, a 62-year-old, is being treated for nausea and vomiting related to the flu syndrome. Marianne draws blood for baseline lab data. An arterial blood gas demonstrates metabolic aklalosis. Related to this, Marianne anticipates the following lab results:
a. high potassium and low chloride levels
*b. low potassium and low chloride levels
c. high potassium and high chloride levels
d. low potassium and high chloride levels

[NP: AN, CL: AN]

Rationale: If metabolic alkalosis is related to gastrointestinal losses, chloride levels will be low. Potassium levels will also be low because potassium will move into the cells in exchange for hydrogen ions.

4. Mr. Klein has been on oral diuretic therapy for one week after discharge from the hospital. He presents with weakness and weight loss. He currently weighs 147 lb, which represents a 7 lb decrease from his normal 154 lb. Marianne calculates this loss as:
   a. mild
   *b. moderate
   c. severe
   d. extreme

   [NP: AS, CL: CO]

   Rationale: A moderate weight loss is 2 to 5 percent of total body weight. In this case 5 percent of 154 lb is 7.7 lb.

5. Melinda Johnson is brought into the emergency room in diabetic ketoacidosis (DKA). An arterial blood gas reveals metabolic acidosis. Marianne is aware that intravenous therapy is ordered to:
   a. provide potassium and other necessary electrolytes
   b. administer calcium chloride to prevent teteny
   *c. restore adequate vascular volume
   d. administer hyperosmotic intravenous fluid

   [NP: PL, CL: AP]

   Rationale: Patients with metabolic acidosis are often severely dehydrated and need to have adequate volume restored.

6. Arterial blood gases on Jim Hartsman, a patient with chronic obstructive lung disease (COPD), reveal a pH of 7.39 despite elevated carbon dioxide levels. In planning nursing care for Mr. Hartsman, Marianne is aware that this represents a:
   a. decompensated state
   b. partially compensated state
   c. mixed acid-base state
   *d. compensated state

   [NP: AN, CL: AN]

   Rationale: In compensated states, the pH approaches normal, while significant changes may exist in the acid-base components.

<u>**Additional Situation Not Presented in Text**</u>

Sister Rose is an RN on a medical intensive care unit. Management of fluid and electrolyte imbalances is of critical importance.

1. Ellen Krane is receiving intravenous therapy for acute pancreatitis. Which of the following responses indicates that patient teaching regarding intravenous fluids has been effective?
   a. "I am not sure why I have this IV; the nurse says I need it."
   b. "It is common to have some pain at the IV site."
   *c. "If I notice any swelling at the IV site, I should tell the nurse."
   d. "Some redness around the IV site is to be expected."

   [NP: EV, CL: AN]

   Rationale: A major complication of intravenous therapy is infiltration. The nurse should observe frequently for this occurrence and, in addition, teach the patient about IV complications.

2. While setting up an IV administration, Sister Rose connects a 5-micron in-line filter to the tubing. Which of the following statements is correct regarding this type of filter?

*a. This device helps to eliminate gross particulate matter.
b. The filter is used to prevent air from entering the system.
c. The device prevents the passage of some bacteria and yeast.
d. The filter removes nearly all bacteria and fungi.

[NP: IM, CL: KN]

Rationale: The 5-micron size in-line filter helps to filter gross particulate material.

3. Mr. Chin returns to the unit after gastrointestinal studies demonstrate a partial bowel obstruction. Mr. Chin has a nasogastric tube to low intermittent suction. Sister Rose will anticipate the following type of intravenous solution:
a. hydrating
b. balanced
*c. replacement
d. carbohydrate

[NP: PL, CL: AP]

Rationale: Replacement solutions are solutions composed of various electrolytes that approximate losses from gastrointestinal suction.

4. Mrs. Headley is admitted for hemodynamic monitoring related to a diagnosis of inappropriate ADH secretion (SIADH). Initial assessment includes observing for clinical signs of hypo-osmotic expansion, which include:
a. abdominal cramps
*b. neuromuscular symptoms
c. dry cracked membranes
d. excessive thirst

[NP: AS, CL: CO]

Rationale: Symptoms of hypo-osmotic expansion are primarily neuromuscular in nature, for example, twitching, hyperirritability and mental disturbances.

5. In planning nursing care for patients with intravenous therapy, Sister Rose will include all of the following except:
a. evaluate lab values daily for abnormal results
b. monitor intake and output and daily weights
c. note caloric intake from dextrose-containing solutions
*d. prepare IV solutions at the patient's bedside

[NP: IM, CL: AP]

Rationale: Intravenous solutions should be prepared in the medication room, where the nurse is free from distraction.

6. Harry Delaune, a 21-year-old, is admitted with diarrhea and weakness associated with AIDS. An isotonic solution is ordered for hydration purposes. Which of the following might be ordered?
*a. 0.9 percent sodium chloride
b. 5 percent dextrose + Lactated ringers
c. 3 percent sodium chloride
d. 5 percent dextrose + 0.2 percent sodium chloride

[NP: AN, CL: KN]

Rationale: Isotonic solutions such as 0.9 percent sodium chloride have concentrations of water and salt equal to those found in the extracellular fluid.

Review Questions from Text

1. Of the following statements, which one is correct regarding water balance in the human body?
   a. The average adult human body is 80 percent water.
   b. Approximately 15 percent of the body water is intracellular.
   c. Approximately 45 percent of the body water is extracellular.
   *d. Lean individuals have a higher percentage of water than fat individuals.

   [CL: CP]

   Rationale: Fat is mostly water free; therefore, the lean individual has more water per kg than the fat individual.

2. All of the following statements are correct regarding the classification of fluid volume imbalances except:
   *a. Hyperosmotic contraction occurs when water and solutes are lost from the extracellular compartment.
   b. Hypo-osmotic contraction occurs when there is a loss of solute in excess of water from the extracellular space.
   c. Iso-osmotic contraction occurs when there is an equal loss of fluid volume along with solutes.
   d. Osmolarity describes the concentration of free particles, molecules, or ions in a solution.

   [CL: CO]

   Rationale: Hyperosmotic contraction results when a greater concentration of particles is present in the extracellular compartment due to water loss. Volume then shifts from the intracellular space to the extracellular space by osmosis, resulting in intracellular contraction.

3. The hydrating solution of 5 percent dextrose plus 0.45 percent sodium chloride contains:
   a. 38.5 mEq/L of chloride and 38.5 mEq/L of sodium
   b. 51 mEq/L of sodium and 38.5 mEq/L of potassium
   *c. 77 mEq/L of sodium and 77 mEq/L of chloride
   d. 77 mEq/L of chloride and 51 mEq/L of potassium

   [CL: KN]

   Rationale: The 5 percent dextrose and 0.45 percent sodium chloride solution contains 77 mEq/L of sodium and 77 mEq/L of chloride.

4. An intravenous replacement solution is:
   *a. a combination of water, carbohydrates, and electrolytes used to replace losses from the gastrointestinal tract
   b. available in both 10 and 20 percent dextrose solutions to correct losses due to hemorrhaging
   c. high in potassium and sodium to approximate electrolyte loss through renal excretion
   d. used to promote renal function, when a fluid deficit exists, by using a balance among cations and anions

   [CL: KN]

   Rationale: Replacement solutions are composed of water, carbohydrates, and electrolytes that are used to replace concurrent losses from the gastrointestinal tract.

5. A patient receiving an intravenous feeding of 3000 ml daily of a 10 percent invert sugar in water solution receives approximately:
   *a. 1100 calories a day
   b. 2000 calories a day
   c. 510 calories a day
   d. 2800 calories a day

   [CL: AN]

   Rationale: A 10 percent invert sugar solution has 380 calories per liter. If 3000 ml of the solution is administered daily, the patient will receive approximately 1100 calories per day (3 x 380).

6. Nursing responsibilities in caring for the patient receiving intravenous therapy include to:

a. examine the intravenous sites at least once every four hours
*b. monitor the patient's intake, output, and body weight daily
c. prepare the solution and admixture using clean technique
d. lower the infusion rate if redness or swelling occurs at the intravenous site

[CL: KN]

Rationale: With intravenous administration, fluid imbalances may occur; therefore, intake, output, and body weight should be monitored.

7. Body buffers operate in all of the following locations except:
 a. body cells through proteins and phosphates
 b. red cells through hemoglobin
 *c. intracellular fluid through glucose exchange
 d. extracellular fluid through bicarbonate

[CL: CO]

Rationale: Buffering occurs in body cells through proteins and phosphates, in red cells through hemoglobin, and in extracellular fluid through bicarbonates.

8. A primary treatment for respiratory acidosis would include:
 a. hemodialysis
 *b. mechanical ventilation
 c. sedation for anxiety
 d. rebreather apparatus

[CL: KN]

Rationale: The primary treatment for respiratory acidosis is to improve ventilation, which may be brought about through mechanical means.

9. Lactated ringers (Hartmann's Solution) is an example of the following type of solution:
 a. hydrating
 b. carbohydrate
 c. balanced
 *d. replacement

[CL: CO]

Rationale: Lactated Ringers Solution is an example of a replacement solution.

10. A nursing goal for the patient with fluid volume deficit would be to restore volume to normal by:
 *a. administering hypotonic solutions
 b. administering high glucose solutions
 c. monitoring hypertonic solutions
 d. restricting fluid intake

[CL: AP]

Rationale: In order to achieve proper hydration in patients with fluid volume deficit, hypotonic solutions should be used to replace extracellular fluid.

Additional Review Questions Not Presented in Text

1. Which statement is correct regarding serum electrolytes?
 *a. The major cation in the extracellular fluid is sodium (NA^+).
 b. The major cation in the intracellular fluid is phosphate (PO_4-).
 c. Bicarbonate (HCO_3-) is the major anion in the intracellular fluid.

d. Potassium (K^+) is the major cation in the extracellular fluid.

[CL: KN]

Rationale: Sodium (NA^+) is the major cation in the extracellular fluid. Potassium (K^+) is the major cation in the intracellular fluid.

2. A hydrating intravenous solution is:
   a. composed of water, protein, and varying amounts of electrolytes
   b. isotonic, thus does not draw water from or pass into the cells
   *c. composed of water, carbohydrate, and varying amounts of sodium chloride
   d. high in potassium, in order to replace electrolyte loss

[CL: KN]

Rationale: A hydrating solution is composed of water, carbohydrate, and varying amounts of sodium chloride. These solutions are used primarily for simple hydration.

3. Carbohydrate solutions may be ordered to assist patients in meeting their energy requirements. The nurse caring for such patients knows that a liter of an intravenous solution containing:
   a. 5 percent dextrose has 190 calories
   *b. 10 percent dextrose has 340 calories
   c. 5 percent invert sugar has 170 calories
   d. 50 percent dextrose has 680 calories

[CL: KN]

Rationale: A 10 percent dextrose solution has 340 calories per liter.

4. An assessable clinical symptom to observe in the patient experiencing a fluid volume deficit is:
   a. pulmonary hypertension
   b. increased urine output
   c. profuse sweating
   *d. concentrated urine

[CL: CO]

Rationale: A concentrated and reduced amount of urine occurs in patients with fluid volume deficit.

5. A balanced intravenous solution:
   a. is isotonic, having balanced concentrations of water and salt equal to the extracellular fluid
   b. contains water, protein, and both cations and anions in a balanced ratio
   *c. contains water, carbohydrate, and both cations and anions in a balanced ratio
   d. is hypertonic, having the ability to balance anions and cations in the fluid compartments

[CL: CO]

Rationale: Balanced solutions are composed of water, carbohydrate as an energy source, and both cations and anions in a balanced ratio.

CHAPTER 12: BLOOD PRODUCTS AND BLOOD SUBSTITUTES

Situations from Text

Situation 12-1

Susan Harrison, a 26-year-old with primary leukemia, is being treated for anemia and leukopenia.

1. Susan's hemoglobin and hematocrit are both decreased, and the physician orders 2 units packed red blood cells to be infused. After carefully checking the blood unit for transfusion, the nurse will:
   a. monitor the flow rate at 100 gtts per minute
   b. infuse the cells with 5 percent dextrose and 0.9 percent sodium chloride
   *c. start the infusion at 20 gtts per minute for the first 10 minutes
   d. observe patient for up to one hour after infusion for signs of reaction

   [NP: IM, CL: AP]

   Rationale: Blood is usually started at 20 gtts per minute for the first 10 minutes. If no reaction is noted, the rate may be increased to 50 to 70 gtt per minute.

2. Due to Susan's low white blood cell count (WBC), orders are given to transfuse one unit of white cells. The nurse plans to:
   a. infuse the white cells slowly over at least one hour
   b. infuse the white cells through a micropore filter
   *c. premedicate with acetaminophen and antihistamines
   d. administer concurrently with an antibiotic

   [NP: PL, CL: CO]

   Rationale: Patients are often premedicated with acetaminophen and antihistamines in order to decrease sensitivity reactions.

3. During administration of packed RBCs, Susan complains of shaking chills. She has a fever of greater than 101 degrees F. The best action by the nurse would be to:
   *a. stop the infusion of RBCs and infuse 0.9 percent sodium chloride
   b. slow the drip rate down to 20 gtts per minute until symptoms subside
   c. continue the infusion and administer acetaminophen and antihistamines
   d. continue infusion, but observe and record vital signs every 15 minutes

   [NP: IM, CL: AP]

   Rationale: If problems develop, the infusion can be stopped and the normal saline solution turned on. When a reaction occurs, hospital policy should be followed.

4. If Susan should receive multiple transfusions, the following may be necessary:
   a. potassium supplementation
   *b. supplemental calcium
   c. ammonia compounds
   d. magnesium replacement

   [NP: AN, CL: CO]

   Rationale: Blood preservatives contain citric acid which binds with free calcium in the blood. Patients who receive multiple blood transfusions may require a calcium supplement.

5. Acquired infections represent potential complications as a result of blood transfusions. All of the following may be transmitted <u>except</u>:
   a. malaria

b. infectious mononucleosis
c. herpes simplex
*d. von Willebrand's disease

[NP: AN, CL: CO]

Rationale: Von Willebrand's disease is a congenital clotting disorder involving a deficiency of factor VIII.

6. The nurse will check laboratory tests performed to determine if Susan's therapy is effective. The nurse would expect:
a. a unit of packed red cells should raise the hematocrit by 6 gms
b. one unit of packed red cells should increase the hemoglobin level by 10 fold
c. one unit of packed red cells should raise the platelet count by 10,000 microliters
*d. one unit of packed red cells should raise the hematocrit by 3 gms

[NP: EV, CL: KN]

Rationale: In evaluating the effectiveness of blood transfusion, a unit of packed red cells should raise the hematocrit by about 3 grams.

Situation 12-2

Stephen Weber is a charge nurse on the evening shift on a medical oncology unit.

1. Mr. Sumner has a platelet count of less than 20,000 per cu mm. Stephen prepares to administer 10 units of platelets at the following rate:
*a. within 10 minutes
b. over an hour
c. within 2 hours
d. over 30 minutes

[NP: IM, CL: AP]

Rationale: Platelets are administered quickly within 10 minutes.

2. When Janet Adams' family discovered that she was receiving a blood transfusion, they became very upset and questioned Stephen as to the reason. Stephen's best response would be:
a. "Janet is very ill right now and needs the blood transfusion. It would be best to let her rest."
b. "I will call the doctor and have her talk to you. Then I am sure that you will understand."
*c. "Janet's red blood cells are low because of the chemotherapy. This will help her feel stronger."
d. "Because of the chemotherapy, she is unable to make new red cells. We hope this works."

[NP: IM, CL: AN]

Rationale: The administration of blood may be traumatic for the family. The nurse will inform the family of the reason for the transfusion and allay their fears.

3. Evan Mitchell is hospitalized with idiopathic thrombocytopenia. He has received multiple blood and platelet transfusions. In preparing for another platelet transfusion, Stephen will anticipate:
a. routine typing and crossmatching for A and B antigens
*b. typing for the human histocompatibility antigen
c. administering Rhogam prior to starting the transfusion
d. gamma globulin administration to prevent Hepatitis B

[NP: PL, CL: AP]

Rationale: After 10 to 15 transfusions with random donor platelets, patients become sensitized and the life span of subsequent transfused platelets is reduced. The platelets will need to be matched for the human histocompatibility antigen.

4. In collecting the equipment necessary to administer 16 units of platelets to Mr. Mitchell, Stephen discovers that Central Supply is out of platelet administration sets. An alternative set would include:
   a. regular 18 gauge needle and syringe
   *b. a filter with a pore size of at least 170 microns
   c. 60 cc leur lock syringe without filter
   d. a filter with a pore size of at least 70 microns

   [NP: IM, CL: KN]

   Rationale: If special platelet administration sets are not available, a filter with a pore size of at least 170 microns may be used. This prevents excess filtration of the platelets.

5. All of the following are considered outcome criteria for the patient needing fluid volume expansion <u>except</u>:
   a. restoration of mental alertness
   b. normal blood pressure
   c. skin warm and dry
   *d. urine output less than 1/2 ml/kg/hour

   [NP: EV, CL: CO]

   Rationale: Urine flow greater than 1/2 ml/kg/hour is an appropriate finding indicating adequate volume expansion.

6. Thomas Winfred has received six units of packed red blood cells during the past 24 hours as the result of a clotting disorder. Stephen is aware of the potential for:
   *a. acid-base disturbances related to the citric acid preservative
   b. increased glucose related to infusion of multiple RBCs
   c. decreased potassium related to diuresis and volume expansion
   d. shortened bleeding times related to increased clotting factors

   [NP: AN, CL: CO]

   Rationale: Patients receiving multiple blood transfusions need to have their acid-base balance checked due to the accumulation of citric acid.

<u>Additional Situation Not Presented in Text</u>

Laura Larson is a staff nurse on a busy surgical intensive care unit. Many patients require volume expansion with blood products and blood substitutes.

1. Mr. Norstram is one day post coronary artery bypass graft surgery. Albumin 25 percent is ordered to help support circulating volume and reduce edema. Laura is aware of the following with regard to albumin infusion:
   a. It is fairly unstable and should be used promptly.
   *b. The suggested rate of infusion is 2 ml/minute.
   c. It should be infused plasma expansion.
   d. Albumin is typed and matched for compatible antibodies.

   [NP: PL, CL: KN]

   Rationale: The suggested rate of infusion for 25 percent albumin is 2 ml/minute.

2. Plasma protein fraction (Plasmanate) has been ordered for Ms. O'Hara, a post craniotomy patient. Laura sets the rate of infusion at:
   *a. 5 to 8 ml/minute
   b. 2 ml/minute
   c. 10 ml/minute
   d. 15 to 20 ml/minute

   [NP: IM, CL: KN]

Rationale: Plasma protein fraction is administered to adults at a rate of 5 to 8 ml/minute.

3. Prior to administering any plasma expander, Laura should be aware of the need for:
   a. an access site with an 18 gauge catheter/needle
   b. assessment of neurological status
   *c. baseline lab data such as hematocrit
   d. typing and crossmatching for all plasma expanders

   [NP: AS, CL: CO]

   Rationale: When administering plasma expanders, it is important for the nurse to be aware of baseline lab data such as the hematocrit. This level will decrease with increasing plasma volume.

4. John Dupree is recovering from a traumatic crush injury of the leg, which he suffered while riding a motorcycle. Dextran 40 has been ordered as an IV infusion. Laura observes crystals in the dextran bottle. Her best course of action would be to:
   a. discard the bottle or return it to pharmacy
   b. infuse with dextran with a 150 micron filter
   c. infuse the solution, as crystallization is expected
   *d. place the solution in warm water to dissolve

   [NP: IM, CL: AP]

   Rationale: If crystallization is noted in the dextran bottle, place the bottle in warm water in order to dissolve the crystals.

5. In managing a patient post emergency surgery for a dissecting aortic aneurysm, Laura monitors an infusion of high molecular weight Dextran (Dextran 70). Laura is aware of the following:
   *a. The expansion of plasma volume lasts 24 hours or longer.
   b. It should not be used if a large volume of blood is lost.
   c. It tends to leak out of the vascular space and into tissues.
   d. The solution has more oxygen-carrying capacity than Dextran 40.

   [NP: AN, CL: KN]

   Rationale: Fifty percent of Dextran 70 is excreted within 24 hours. Volume expansion improves hemodynamic stratus for 24 hours or longer.

6. Laura maintains assessment of laboratory data on patients receiving large amounts of plasma expanders. All of the following findings may be observed with regard to these products <u>except</u>:
   a. altered prothrombin time
   b. decreased hematocrit
   *c. elevated potassium
   d. dilution of plasma protein

   [NP: AS, CL: CO]

   Rationale: Administration of large amounts of plasma expanders may result in transient prolongation of PT and PTT, dcreased hematocrit, and dilution of plasma protein.

Review Questions from Text

1. Of the following statements, which one is correct with regard to whole blood or its derivatives?
   *a. Platelets do not contain the Rh (D) antigen that red cells carry.
   b. White cells must be given within 48 hours after donation.
   c. Whole blood is used to restore a blood loss of greater than 500 ml.
   d. Packed cells contain only red cells in a volume of 250 ml.

   [CL: KN]

Rationale: While platelets share the red blood cell A and B antigens, they do not contain the Rh (D) antigen.

2. Plasma expanders are substances which have the ability to expand a depleted blood volume. These substances:
   a. transmit hepatitis and acquired immune deficiency syndrome
   b. are typed and matched with the patient's blood before administration
   *c. cause anaphylactic reaction in hypersensitive patients
   d. have oxygen-carrying capacity and contain clotting factors

   [CL: KN]

   Rationale: Patients receiving plasma expanders need to be monitored closely, due to the possibility of an anaphylactic reaction.

3. In caring for the patient receiving a blood transfusion, the nurse:
   a. administers the blood concurrently with a dextrose solution to prevent clumping of red blood cells
   b. monitors the patient at least every 2 hours for signs of a reaction to the blood transfusion
   c. administers the blood using a single tubing with a 170-micron filter
   *d. compares the blood group and Rh factor on the label with those of the patient

   [CL: KN]

   Rationale: To ensure accuracy and compatibility, the nurse compares the blood group and Rh factor of the blood for administration with those of the patient.

4. All of the following are usual signs of an anaphylactic reaction <u>except</u>:
   a. chills and fever
   *b. tingling in toes
   c. change in vital signs
   d. chest and back pain

   [CL: CO]

   Rationale: Signs of a reaction to a blood transfusion include backache, change in vital signs, urticaria, chills and fever, headache, flushing, chest pain, and sudden shock.

5. Dextran 40, a low-molecular weight blood substitute:
   *a. is used as a hemodiluent in the heart-lung machine
   b. increases platelet-aggregation and osmotic pressure
   c. causes sludging of blood in the microcirculation
   d. reduces cardiac output and microcirculatory flow

   [CL: KN]

   Rationale: Because Dextran 40 has a low viscosity and an ability to keep red blood cells from sludging in small vessels, it is sometimes used as a hemodiluent in the heart-lung machine.

6. Donated blood is labeled with all of the following information <u>except</u>:
   a. the proper name of the component
   b. method by which component was prepared
   c. temperature range for storage
   *d. type of antibodies present

   [CL: CO]

   Rationale: Donated blood is labeled with information such as proper name of component, method of preparation, and temperature range for storage.

7. Which of the following statements is <u>correct</u> with regard to the Rh factor system?
   a. Persons with Rh antibodies are considered to have Rh-positive blood type.

b. Rh-positive mother will develop antibodies when giving birth to Rh-negative child.
*c. Rh-positive persons may receive blood that is Rh-negative.
d. Type O Rh-negative blood is referred to as the universal recipient.

[CL: AN]

Rationale: An Rh-positive person can receive Rh-negative blood. In the reverse situation, however, the Rh-negative person will produce antibodies when infused with Rh-positive blood.

8. Plasmapheresis is a donor technique with the advantage of:
   a. allowing persons to donate every 48 hours if necessary
   *b. retaining plasma platelets or white blood cells
   c. taking only one hour for the process to be completed
   d. returning the plasma and retaining only the red cells

[CL: CO]

Rationale: In plasmapheresis, only the plasma platelets or white blood cells are retained; the red cells are returned to the donor.

9. Stored whole blood has the following properties:
   a. high pH and calcium levels
   b. low potassium levels
   c. high glucose levels
   *d. low 2,3-DPG levels

[CL: KN]

Rationale: Stored whole blood contains low glucose and 2,3-diphosphoglycerate (2,3-DPG) levels. It is also high in potassium and has a low pH.

10. Plasma protein products are contraindicated in all situations <u>except</u>:
   *a. evidence of repeated infusions
   b. history of allergic reaction to albumin
   c. presence of severe anemia
   d. presence of cardiac failure

[CL: CO]

Rationale: Plasma protein products contain no cellular elements; therefore, there is no risk of sensitization with repeated infusions.

Additional Review Questions Not Presented in Text

1. Albumin is separated from plasma and is administered to:
   a. facilitate oxygen binding capacity
   *b. bind bilirubin in circulation to reduce jaundice
   c. reduce osmotic pressure within the vessel wall
   d. facilitate red blood cell production

[CL: KN]

Rationale: Albumin has the ability to bind bilirubin in circulation and is used to treat infants with erythroblastosis fetalis.

2. All of the following statements are correct regarding cryoprecipitate <u>except</u>:
   a. It is administered to treat hemophilia and von Willebrand's disease.
   b. The component contains factor I (fibrinogen) and factor VIII.
   *c. Cryoprecipitate has all of the clotting factors present.

d. This product does carry the risk of hepatitis.

[CL: CO]

Rationale: Cryoprecipitate contains fibrinogen and factor VIII and is used to treat hemophilia and von Willebrand's disease.

3. The major risk of administering volume expanders is:
*a. pulmonary edema
b. allergic reaction
c. diminished microcirculation
d. hepatic insufficiency

[CL: KN]

Rationale: The major risk of volume expansion with any intravenous fluid is pulmonary edema.

4. Therapeutic goals during acute bleeding include all of the following <u>except</u>:
a. blood volume at 10 percent of normal
b. platelets over 25 percent (50,000) of normal
c. hemoglobin at least 8 gm/dl and hematocrit 24 percent
*d. total serum protein at least 40 percent of normal

[CL: CO]

Rationale: During acute bleeding, therapy is aimed at maintaining total serum protein at least 60 percent of normal.

5. Which of the following statements is <u>correct</u> regarding the use of frozen red cells?
a. To protect red cells from crystallizations at low temperature, they are mixed with normal saline.
*b. The use of frozen red cells can reduce febrile reactions and tissue antigen sensitization.
c. Frozen red cells contain both platelets and plasma in a glycerin substrate.
d. Once the frozen red cells have been prepared, they must be used within 48 hours.

[CL: KN]

Rationale: Approximately 98 percent of the sensitizing lymphocytes are removed through the process of preparation of red cells. The use can reduce febrile reactions and tissue antigen sensitization.

CHAPTER 13: UTILIZING THE NURSING PROCESS WITH PATIENTS WHO ABUSE DRUGS AND ALCOHOL

Situations from Text

Situation 13-1

Mr. Shipley is a 46-year-old cocaine addict admitted by his wife to the acute care unit of a drug rehabilitation center.

1. The nurse admitting Mr. Shipley may observe the following physical effect of acute cocaine intoxication:
   a. pinpoint pupils
   *b. cardiac arrhythmias
   c. slurred speech
   d. drowsiness

   [NP: AS, CL: KN]

   Rationale: Signs of intoxication from cocaine include cardiac arrhythmias.

2. Mr. Shipley admits to drinking a "glass or two" of vodka along with cocaine use daily. The nurse is aware that the combination of alcohol and cocaine use represents:
   a. dual addiction
   b. cross tolerance
   *c. mixed addiction
   d. dual tolerance

   [NP: AN, CL: AP]

   Rationale: Mixed addiction is a condition in which the person is dependent on more than one substance, such as cocaine and alcohol.

3. During the acute phase of intoxication related to stimulant use, the nurse will provide all of the following <u>except</u>:
   a. a safe environment for patient and others
   b. medication (Diazepam) to prevent seizures
   c. referral to the substance abuse team
   *d. in-depth discussion about his drug use

   [NP: IM, CL: CO]

   Rationale: The nurse should obtain information about drug use, but refrain from lengthy interpersonal interactions which might increase agitation.

4. Mr. Shipley experiences sleep disturbances related to withdrawal from cocaine. The best intervention for the nurse to include in planning care would be to:
   a. direct strenuous exercises
   b. administer strong sedatives
   c. allow long periods of privacy
   *d. teach relaxation techniques

   [NP: IM, CL: KN]

   Rationale: Non-pharmacologic nursing interventions such as relaxation techniques promote sleep and rest. Administering strong sedatives may induce dependence.

5. In planning teaching concerning the psychologic and physiologic effects of alcohol and cocaine use, the nurse will:
   *a. focus on education aspects as soon as Mr. Shipley recovers from acute intoxication

b. wait until Mr. Shipley initiates the interaction by asking questions
c. plan initial education as an outpatient in group therapy if he consents
d. initiate teaching concerning drug use only if ordered by the attending physician

[NP: PL, CL: CO]

Rationale: During the acute phase of intoxication, the nurse is primarily concerned with deterring life-threatening effects. Education, however, is an important aspect of care and should be initiated whether or not the patient appears receptive.

6. Which of the following responses indicates an understanding by the wife of the best approach to take with Mr. Shipley?
 a. "He really does not have a bad problem, only when his work is stressful."
 b. "I tell him all the time that taking drugs and drinking will ruin his life."
 *c. "I will no longer make excuses for him; we need to face the problem together."
 d. "He gets mad when I talk about the problem, so it's best to let him quit on his own."

[NP: EV, CL: AN]

Rationale: This response reflects an understanding of the need to confront the problem rather than to deny it.

Situation 13-2

Rebecca Long is a staff nurse working in the chemical dependency unit in a psychiatric hospital.

1. Sherry Trahan, a 17-year-old with a history of substance abuse, is in acute intoxication from Valium (depressant). Rebecca will observe for the following:
 a. increased respiratory rate
 *b. loss of superficial reflexes
 c. hypertension
 d. restlessness and rapid speech

[NP: AS, CL: KN]

Rationale: Signs of intoxication from depressant drugs include loss of superficial reflexes, diminished respiratory volume, and hypotension.

2. Jason Williamson has been admitted with intoxication of unknown substance. He demonstrates severe anxiety and panic, needing to be restrained for violent behavior. Rebecca is aware that these symptoms probably relate to:
 *a. phencyclidines
 b. opioids
 c. sedatives
 d. marijuana

[NP: AN, CL: AP]

Rationale: Signs of phencyclidine intoxication include severe anxiety, feelings of panic, and potential for aggressive/violent behavior.

3. In planning interventions for patients in withdrawal from opioids (heroin, morphine), Rebecca will include the following:
 a. providing a stimulating environment
 b. allowing for periods of isolation
 *c. administering decreasing doses of opioids
 d. producing euphoria with medications

[NP: PL, CL: KN]

Rationale: The nurse will administer decreasing amounts of opioids, usually in the form of methadone, as indicated.

4. Mrs. Bruster is withdrawing from alcohol-benzodiazepine dependence. Rebecca will anticipate the possible occurrence of seizures:
   a. around days 4 to 6
   *b. between days 7 to 14
   c. within 48 hours
   d. after 2 weeks

   [NP: AN, CL: KN]

   Rationale: In patients with mixed alcohol-benzodiazepine (Valium, Librium) dependence, seizures may occur between days 7 and 14.

5. When Samuel Franks, a 16-year-old, is admitted for LSD intoxication, Rebecca prepares to implement all of the following except:
   *a. administer antipsychotic medication
   b. provide reassurance and presence
   c. implement seizure precautions
   d. promote a quiet environment

   [NP: PL, CL: AP]

   Rationale: The use of antipsychotic medications should be avoided in treating patients for hallucinogen intoxication.

6. Rebecca will include all of the following as appropriate nursing goals for patients in acute intoxication induced by depressants except:
   a. prevention of death and the development of further pathology
   b. promotion of health at the level possible for the patient
   c. provision of a safe, non-threatening environment
   *d. evidence of patient's desire to abstain from drug use

   [NP: PL, CL: CO]

   Rationale: The goals associated with acute intoxication induced by depressants include provisions for a safe environment and a stable physiologic status. The patient may or may not verbalize a desire to abstain from further drug use.

Additional Situation Not Presented in Text

Barbara Harrison is the day supervisor of a community mental health clinic. Many of the clients she encounters have substance abuse problems.

1. Roger Irwin is a student nurse who is finding it difficult to discuss substance abuse with clients who display signs of addiction. Barbara is aware that this type of behavior is most likely due to:
   *a. unresolved feelings about substance abusers
   b. desire to deny that any problems exist
   c. inattention to the client's needs
   d. inadequate assessment techniques

   [NP: AN, CL: AN]

   Rationale: This type of behavior is "enabling" and health professionals may engage in enabling behavior due to unresolved personal feelings about substance abusers.

2. In taking a drug history, Barbara will be alert to the potential for alcohol dependence if the following is assessed:
   a. five drinks taken during the period of one week
   b. two or more drinks taken per social occasion
   *c. five or more drinks taken per social occasion

d. one drink daily, taken at night

[NP: AS, CL: KN]

Rationale: The consumption of five or more drinks per social occasion may indicate alcohol dependence.

3. Mr. Call denies alcohol use; however, laboratory studies confirm the presence of alcohol in the blood. The best approach for Barbara to take would be to:
   a. consider the laboratory results to be inaccurate
   *b. discuss lab findings with the family and patient
   c. wait until the patient admits to alcohol use
   d. report the findings to the psychiatrist only

[NP: IM, CL: AP]

Rationale: The appropriate response would be to inform the patient and family of the laboratory findings which contradict his verbal history.

4. Adriana Sanchez brings her 17-year-old son to the clinic in acute PCP intoxication. While Barbara awaits transfer of the patient to the acute unit, she is prepared to administer all of the following except:
   a. antihypertensives
   b. anticonvulsants
   c. major tranquilizers
   *d. amphetamines

[NP: PL, CL: CO]

Rationale: The signs of PCP intoxication can include aggressive, agitated, violent behavior. Amphetamine administration would be contraindicated.

5. In caring for patients withdrawing from amphetamines, Barbara may include the following nursing diagnoses except:
   a. hyperthermia--potential for related to intoxication with amphetamine
   b. alteration in thought processes related to amphetamine intoxication
   *c. diversional activity deficit related to amphetamine intoxication
   d. potential for self-harm related to intoxication with amphetamines

[NP: AN, CL: AN]

Rationale: The patient should be provided with a nonstimulating environment during acute intoxication with stimulants. Diversional activities may increase agitation.

6. In evaluating the effectiveness of interventions for the substance dependent, Barbara is aware that:
   a. drug abuse is a chronic problem that rarely can be resolved
   b. the decision to live a life without the drug remains with the patient's family
   c. individuals who return to drug use are those who cannot be rehabilitated
   *d. recovery from substance abuse is a lifetime process characterized by relapses

[NP: EV, CL: CO]

Rationale: Rehabilitation from substance abuse requires ongoing effort to abstain from psychoactive substances. Periods of relapse may occur and the patient should be encouraged to continue working toward a drug-free lifestyle.

Review Questions from Text

1. Which statement is not correct regarding the definition of terms related to drug abuse?
   a. Dependency refers to a state in which the person needs a specific drug to maintain abilities to function.
   b. Drug abuse is the use of drugs that create legal, emotional, social, and health problems for the individual.
   *c. Tolerance develops when a person requires the drug to experience positive feelings and a sense of self-

esteem.
d. Physical dependence develops when the person experiences physical wihdrawal symptoms when the drug wears off.

[CL: CO]

Rationale: Tolerance is the state in which increased amounts of a substance are necessary to achieve the same effects as previously attained with the use of lesser amounts.

2. Which statement is correct regarding etiologic factors of drug and alcohol dependency?
   a. Physical dependency always has a genetic etiology or causative factor.
   b. Theories exist which adequately explain the causes of drug and alcohol dependency.
   c. Drug and alcohol dependency can be viewed as involving a single factor.
   *d. Scientific understanding of dependency is at an early point in development.

[CL: KN]

Rationale: Many theories are currently proposed which attempt to explain etiologic factors of drug dependency, but none adequately addresses all aspects of the problem. Scientific understanding of addiction is at an early stage of development.

3. In the assessment of the patient who abuses drugs, the nurse will:
   *a. use the street names for drugs during the information-gathering phase
   b. begin the interview with discussion of sensitive information about drug use
   c. note only verbal responses to questions designed to elicit drug and alcohol usage
   d. utilize indirect questioning in order to make the patient feel more comfortable

[CL: KN]

Rationale: The patient may only know drugs by their street names; therefore, the nurse must be aware of such terminology in clarification of which drugs the patient takes.

4. When providing care for the patient who is withdrawing from the effects of alcohol, the nurse will perform all of the following except:
   a. assess mental status
   b. implement seizure precautions
   *c. restrict fluid intake
   d. establish a non-stimulating environment

[CL: CO]

Rationale: In caring for the patient withdrawing from alcohol, the nurse promotes adequate hydration.

5. Nursing intervention for the patient withdrawing from a hallucinogen includes:
   a. leaving the patient alone in order to reduce environmental stimuli
   *b. observing for signs of shock, which include pallor and hypotension
   c. engaging in lengthy conversations in order to decrease patient anxiety
   d. withholding all medications, including those for medical purposes

[CL: CO]

Rationale: The patient experiencing withdrawal from hallucinogens needs to be observed for signs of shock.

6. All of the following statements are correct regarding drug and alcohol abuse except:
   *a. The percentage of deaths related to substance abuse has declined by 10 percent since 1982.
   b. Alcoholism ranks as the third major cause of death in the United States after coronary disease and cancer.
   c. About 20 to 35 percent of persons hospitalized in non-psychiatric settings suffer from alcohol-related illness.
   d. One in four individuals is estimated to have a personal experience with a family member or friend who is substance dependent.

[CL: KN]

Rationale: The prevalence of substance abuse and related health problems is widespread and now ranks as the third major cause of death in the United States.

7. Theories on the individual and family suggest that the following characteristic may place the individual at risk for substance-related problems:
   a. resolved psychological conflict
   *b. family members with substance problems
   c. increased amount of "free" time
   d. economically advantaged status

[CL: KN]

Rationale: Individuals with family members who have substance dependence problems are at risk for the development of a similar dependence.

8. All of the following statements are correct regarding the impaired nurse <u>except</u>:
   *a. Nurses develop addictive illness at a higher rate than people in the general population.
   b. Recognition that addiction is treatable is central to the management of impaired practice.
   c. The trend in employing institutions is to treat the impaired nurse before firing.
   d. Impaired practice is most readily identified by changes in job performance.

[CL: CO]

Rationale: Nurses develop addictive illness at rates comparable to people in the general population.

9. The following is correct regarding dual addiction.
   Dual addiction is:
   a. dependence on more than one substance
   b. tolerance for large amounts of similarly acting drugs
   *c. simultaneous dependence on drugs which have similar effects
   d. the combination of physiological and psychological dependence

[CL: CO]

Rationale: Dual addiction is the simultaneous dependence on psychoactive drugs which have similar effects.

10. The disease model, articulated by E. M. Jellinek, describes behaviors consistent with symptoms of addiction. This model includes all of the following <u>except</u>:
   a. loss of control over intake of drug
   b. compulsive need to continue use
   c. psychologic and behavioral change
   *d. imitation of family members with substance abuse

[CL: KN]

Rationale: The disease model describes addictive behavior as the loss of control over drug use, compulsive need to continue use, and psychological and behavioral change.

<u>Additional Review Questions Not Presented in Text</u>

1. The most addicting and widely used drug in America is:
   a. cocaine
   b. marijuana
   *c. nicotine
   d. alcohol

[CL: KN]

Rationale: Nicotine represents the most addictive and widely used drug in America. Cocaine has the next highest addictive potential.

2. A therapeutic reaction of the nurse to the individual drug abuser includes all of the following except:
   a. developing knowledge related to drug treatment
   *b. shielding the patient from painful realizations
   c. including a drug history in comprehensive assessment
   d. making appropriate referrals for substance abuse

   [CL: CO]

   Rationale: The nurse reacts therapeutically by not engaging in behavior which supports the user's denial that there is a problem.

3. A correctly stated and appropriate nursing diagnosis for the patient recovering from alcohol withdrawal may include:
   a. hallucinations related to long-term drug abuse and withdrawal
   *b. potential for anxiety related to withdrawal from beverage alcohol
   c. continued drug abuse related to anxiety about withdrawal
   d. liver disease and hepatic coma due to substance abuse

   [CL: AN]

   Rationale: The nursing diagnosis should reflect actual and/or potential health problems of the patient. The secondary phase of the diagnosis notes the specific etiology of the problem.

4. Anticipated short-term outcomes related to addiction to alcohol and other drugs include all except:
   a. clear sensorium, absent of marked emotional disturbance
   b. adequate tissue hydration and nutritional intake
   *c. a drug-free lifestyle with rehabilitation adherence
   d. stable physiologic state with vital signs within usual range

   [CL: CO]

   Rationale: Leading a drug-free lifestyle is a long-term outcome. The anticipated outcomes of short-term nursing intervention include stable vital signs, adequate hydration, and stable cognitive and emotional status.

5. The following statement is correct with regard to substance abuse:
   *a. Health professionals demonstrate enabling behavior by failing to discuss the basic problem with substance abusers.
   b. Enabling behavior refers to behavior patterns of such long standing that the person is unaware of them.
   c. Expressions of anger and criticism about drug use serve to encourage substance abusers in attempts to seek treatment.
   d. Family behaviors such as inhibition of emotional expression benefit the substance abuser by preventing confrontation.

   [CL: KN]

   Rationale: By providing medical and nursing care for drug-induced medical illness without discussing the basic problem, health professionals demonstrate enabling behavior.

CHAPTER 14: PHARMACOTHERAPEUTICS FOR THE NEONATE AND THE PEDIATRIC PATIENT

Situations from Text

Situation 14-1

Darla Stevens is a 42-week-gestation newborn transferred from the operating room to the neonatal intensive care unit due to meconium aspiration.

1. Administration of intravenous fluid (5 percent dextrose) has been ordered for Darla at 15 cc per hour. The nurse is aware of the following in preparing to start the IV:
   a. Scalp veins may be used in the neonate, but are difficult to see.
   b. An 18 gauge needle is used for intravenous administration in neonates.
   *c. The needle may be inserted in scalp vein in either direction of blood flow.
   d. Only peripheral veins should be utilized for IV administration in neonates.

   [NP: PL, CL: KN]

   Rationale: While it is preferable to insert the scalp vein needle in the direction of venous flow, the needle may be placed in either direction, since scalp veins have no valves.

2. Darla is receiving ampicillin via intravenous piggyback. It will be best for the nurse to change the IV tubing:
   a. every 24 hours with site care
   b. immediately after medication administration
   *c. per policy before a medication is given
   d. every other morning with site care

   [NP: IM, CL: KN]

   Rationale: After a medication is given via the volume control chamber, a portion of the drug remains in the tubing. For the neonate receiving slow infusion rates, routine IV tubing changes should be performed before the medication is given.

3. When giving Darla medications which are dependent on protein binding for drug distribution, the nurse is aware that it may be necessary to:
   *a. decrease the amount of drug and shorten the dosage interval
   b. increase the amount of drug and give at longer intervals
   c. decrease the amount of drug and give at longer intervals
   d. increase the amount of drug and shorten the dosage interval

   [NP: AN, CL: AP]

   Rationale: The neonate has less albumin available for binding with drugs. Due to the larger proportion of unbound drug, there is greater likelihood of developing a toxic reaction. It may be necessary to decrease the drug and shorten the interval time between dosages.

4. On the fourth day, Darla's laboratory data reveal elevated bilirubin levels. At this time it will be important for the nurse to avoid administering:
   a. ampicillin
   *b. aspirin
   c. acetaminophen
   d. gentamycin

   [NP: AS, CL: CO]

   Rationale: Drugs such as salicylates have a stronger binding power for albumin than bilirubin. This would release free bilirubin to cross the blood-brain barrier, potentially causing brain damage.

5. Knowledge of the biotransformation of drugs is essential for drug administration in the neonate. During the

first week of Darla's life, the nurse will observe for the following response to medication administration:
a. reduced therapeutic effect
b. no observable effect
c. reduced drug half-life
*d. prolonged therapeutic effect

[NP: IM, CL: AP]

Rationale: The neonate's liver is immature at birth and less effective for drug metabolism. A prolonged therapeutic effect may be observed due to an increased half life.

6. After two weeks in the neonatal unit, Darla is placed on digoxin for symptoms related to congestive failure. Repeated serum digoxin tests reveal subtherapeutic levels. The need to increase the dosage in order to reach therapeutic levels may be related to:
*a. increasing glomerular filtration rate
b. incomplete secretory mechanism
c. reduction in liver enzymes
d. elevated bilirubin levels

[NP: EV, CL: CO]

Rationale: Drugs such as digoxin are dependent on glomerular filtration rate (GFR). The GFR increases rapidly during the first weeks of life.

Situation 14-2

Molly Fenderson, a 2-year-old asthmatic, is recovering from pneumonia. She is a patient on a pediatric unit, and her mother stays with her. Present medications include oral penicillin and theophylline.

1. Molly develops gastritis with symptoms of gastric distress. The nurse is aware that administration of oral penicillin at this time may result in:
a. no effect on penicillin absorption
b. increased therapeutic response
c. prolonged therapeutic response
*d. altered timing of the therapeutic effect

[NP: PL, CL: CO]

Rationale: Conditions such as gastritis may cause gastric motility to increase suddenly. When this occurs, the opposite timing of the therapeutic effect may be seen.

2. Oral penicillin has been discontinued, and the drug is to be given by intramuscular injection. In choosing an IM site for Molly, the nurse will avoid the deltoid muscle because of all of the following <u>except</u>:
a. the muscle is small and not well developed
b. it lies close to the radial and ulnar nerves
*c. the muscle has a slow rate of absorption
d. it lies close to the brachial artery

[NP: IM, CL: CO]

Rationale: The deltoid muscle in children less than 3 to 4 years old is not well developed and is usually avoided. The area is small, but has a rapid rate of absorption.

3. Molly receives theophylline twice a day. Concerning the effect of metabolism on theophylline levels, the nurse is aware that it may be necessary to:
*a. decrease the dosage interval
b. increase the dosage interval
c. discontinue a dose every other day
d. decrease the daily dosage

[NP: AN, CL: AP]

Rationale: The rate of metabolism of theophylline can be increased in the child and necessitate a decrease in the dosage interval.

4. Before administering any medication to Molly, the nurse will perform all of the following actions except:
   *a. ask her to identify herself
   b. check the armband for identification
   c. identify safe methods of administration
   d. determine if dosage is appropriate

   [NP: IM, CL: KN]

   Rationale: Young children may not want to identify themselves in order to avoid taking the medication. It is imperative to check the armband for identification prior to administering medications.

5. The best criterion to utilize in evaluating Molly's response to theophylline therapy would be:
   a. evidence of wheezing
   b. elevated urine output
   *c. therapeutic serum levels
   d. presence of shortness of breath

   [NP: EV, CL: KN]

   Rationale: For some medications, such as theophylline, the best method to evaluate effectiveness of the medication is by measuring serum concentration.

6. Which of the responses by Molly's mother indicates an understanding of patient teaching with regard to medication compliance?
   a. "She stays with me during the weekdays, so I make sure she gets the medication then."
   b. "We really don't have the extra money for her medicines, so I space them further apart."
   c. "As long as Molly feels good, I don't worry about missing a pill or two."
   *d. "I can give Molly her medicines before breakfast and at bedtime. That way I won't forget."

   [NP: EV, CL: AN]

   Rationale: This response indicates a desire to fit the medication schedule into the family's routine, thereby increasing compliance.

Additional Situation Not Presented in Text

Jason Hall is a 5-year-old in a pediatric intensive care unit. He has a diagnosis of otitis media, dehydration, and tonsillitis. Currently, he is receiving intravenous fluids and antibiotic therapy.

1. The nurse monitors the infusion of 5 percent dextrose via a line with a volume control chamber. The function of the chamber is to:
   *a. prevent accidental fluid overload
   b. eliminate the need for an infusion pump
   c. contain one 8-hour amount of solution
   d. reduce bacterial and fungal contamination

   [NP: PL, CL: KN]

   Rationale: The volume control chamber functions as a safety device, preventing accidental fluid overload to children receiving IV fluids. No more than a one- to two-hour amount of IV solution is placed in the chamber at a time.

2. To administer ear drops to Jason, the nurse will:
   a. pull the pinna downward and back for instillation

b. place cotton tightly in the ear after instillation
c. keep Jason on the affected side after instillation
*d. pull the pinna upward and back for instillation

[NP: IM, CL: AP]

Rationale: To instill ear drops in children over 3 years old, the pinna is pulled upward and back, as in the adult.

3. Jason is crying and complaining of pain. In assessing the gluteus medius muscle for an intramuscular injection of Demerol, the nurse will consider the following factors except:
a. chronological age
b. body weight
c. tissue perfusion
*d. ability to cooperate

[NP: AS, CL: CO]

Rationale: A 5-year-old may be chronologically old enough for IM injections using the gluteus medius muscle, but if the child is undernourished, the vastus lateralis may need to be used. If tissue breakdown is observed, as in the case of numerous injections, tissue perfusion may be affected.

4. Jason's temperature in the evening elevates to 40 degrees C. With regard to the effect of fever on metabolic rate, the nurse realizes that:
a. for each centigrade rise in temperature, metabolism increases by 5 percent
*b. increased metabolic rate will decrease the duration of the therapeutic effect
c. decreased metabolic rate will decrease the half life of medication
d. because temperature regulation is stable in children, there is no effect on metabolism

[NP: AS, CL: AP]

Rationale: An elevated temperature will increase the metabolic rate and decrease the half life of medications, thereby decreasing the duration of the therapeutic effect.

5. When the nurse enters the room to give him a dose of Tylenol elixir, Jason tries to hide under the blanket. The nurse should perform all of the following actions with regard to this situation except:
a. approach Jason in a calm, pleasant manner
b. take control of the situation if he refuses the medicine
*c. offer Jason the choice of taking the medication
d. offer a drink to be taken after the medication

[NP: IM, CL: CO]

Rationale: Do not offer children the choice of taking medications. Offer choices only when the child can have a choice.

6. Jason is receiving gentamycin via intravenous piggyback every 8 hours. Which of the following statements by Jason's mother should alert the nurse to a potential problem?
a. "He seems to be hungry today, always asking for ice cream."
b. "He still has some pain, but the shots seem to help."
c. "Sometimes he takes a nap and doesn't want to play."
*d. "Jason is ignoring me. He did not look up when I called to him."

[NP: EV, CL: AN]

Rationale: In evaluating, the nurse needs to be in tune to the subtle changes in the child's behavior which the parents may observe. In this case, the child may be demonstrating ototoxicity related to the antibiotic.

Review Quetions from Text

1. Which of the following statements is correct regarding physiological differences in absorption of oral medications in pediatric patients?
   *a. In the newborn, the stomach empties in about three hours.
   b. In the older infant and child, the stomach empties in about two hours.
   c. As an infant matures, the stomach has a less predictable emptying rate.
   d. Conditions such as gastritis cause gastric motility to decrease.

   [CL: KN]

   Rationale: Gastric emptying time varies within the pediatric population. In the newborn, the stomach empties in two-and-one-half to three hours.

2. With regard to intramuscular injections in the pediatric patient, all of the following statements are correct except:
   a. Blood flow and tissue perfusion of the muscle are not fully developed in the neonate.
   b. Drug absorption of intramuscular injections is more unreliable in the neonate than in the child.
   c. Conditions which cause vasoconstriction decrease blood flow to the muscles, inhibiting absorption.
   *d. As the child grows, tissue perfusion decreases, making absorption of injections less reliable.

   [CL: CO]

   Rationale: Tissue perfusion of the muscles is not fully mature in the neonate. As the child grows, however, tissue perfusion to the muscles increases, making absorption of intramuscular injections more reliable.

3. As drugs enter the blood stream, they bind to plasma protein for distribution. One factor influencing protein binding is the:
   a. amount of fat soluble vitamins available
   *b. amount of albumin available for binding
   c. distribution of intracellular fluid and solutes
   d. distribution of enzymes for protein binding

   [CL: KN]

   Rationale: The amount of albumin available for binding is a factor influencing distribution of medications which bind to protein. Other factors include blood pH, binding capacity, and substances which compete for binding sites.

4. Drug absorption via the intestine in the neonate is limited by the following characteristics:
   a. The length of intestinal lumen is short compared to the adult.
   b. There is a relatively small surface area for drug absorption.
   c. Due to neuromuscular immaturity, peristalsis is slowed.
   *d. Intestinal peristalsis is rapid and unpredictable.

   [CL: KN]

   Rationale: Due to neuromuscular immaturity, the intestinal peristalsis in the newborn is rapid and unpredictable. Contact time for absorption of drugs is reduced.

5. In teaching parents about medication safety and prevention of accidental ingestion of medications, the nurse will include the following information:
   a. Use child proof caps, as they are effective in preventing ingestion errors.
   *b. Store medications in a locked container and hide the key.
   c. Store medications in the mother's purse, since it is usually out of reach.
   d. Place all drugs on a high shelf which is beyond the child's reach.

   [CL: KN]

   Rationale: The safest place for medication storage is in a locked container or drawer. The key should then be hidden.

6. The following statement is correct regarding gastric acidity in the period immediately following birth:
   a. Gastric acidity in the first week of life is lower than in the adult.
   b. Drugs which are absorbed at a higher rate in a high pH should be withheld.
   *c. Serum drug levels may be higher for drugs absorbed at a low pH.
   d. Drugs which are deactivated by a high pH should be given by an alternate route.

   [CL: CO]

   Rationale: In the period immediately following birth, the gastric acidity is high. Therefore, drugs which are absorbed at a higher rate in a low pH may produce elevated serum levels.

7. With regard to topical medication administration in the pediatric patient, which statement is correct?
   a. Infants require topical medications for frequent infections due to acidity of the skin.
   b. Children have natural skin barriers which prevent the absorption of topical medications.
   c. Children should not receive topical medication until they are 8 years of age or older.
   *d. Infants absorb greater amounts of topical medications, causing potential side effects.

   [CL: KN]

   Rationale: Because the outer layer of skin (stratum corneum) is thinner in infants than in adults, the infant absorbs greater amounts of topical medications, which may cause undesirable side effects.

8. Which of the following is correct relative to the distribution of fat in the pediatric patient:
   *a. A neonate needs a smaller dosage of a fat soluble drug than an older child.
   b. Because the infant has a high fat content, fat soluble drugs are administered with care.
   c. As children grow, fat content decreases, and they require lesser amounts of fat soluble drugs.
   d. To maintain a therapeutic concentration of fat soluble drugs, infants require increased dosages.

   [CL: CO]

   Rationale: A small portion of the infant's body weight is fat. Therefore, the infant requires smaller dosages of a fat soluble drug.

9. In the neonate, the proportion of body water varies from the adult in the following way:
   a. A higher proportion of body water is intracellular.
   b. Smaller dosages of water soluble drugs per kg are needed.
   c. The proportion of extracellular fluid increases as the infant matures.
   *d. The neonate exchanges extracellular fluid more rapidly than an adult.

   [CL: KN]

   Rationale: A high proportion of body water in the neonate is extracellular fluid, which the neonate exchanges more rapidly each day than the adult. Therefore, higher doses of water soluble drugs per kg of body weight are necessary to reach desired concentrations.

10. For administration of intramuscular drugs, the first muscle of choice for a 4-month-old is:
   a. deltoid
   *b. vastus lateralus
   c. dorsogluteal
   d. ventrogluteal

   [CL: AP]

   Rationale: The choice of muscles for intramuscular (IM) injection is limited in the infant, due to small muscle mass. The muscle of choice for IM injections is the vastus lateralis.

Additional Review Questions Not Presented in Text

1. In assessing the pediatric patient requiring medication, the nurse knows which of the following statements is not correct?

a. Body surface area correlates closely with physiologic function of the child.
*b. Clark's rule is a reliable formula for determining pediatric drug dosages.
c. The dehydrated child is at risk for developing toxic drug accumulation.
d. The blood-brain barrier is incomplete at birth, increasing drug permeability.

[CL: CO]

Rationale: Clark's rule utilizes average adult dosage in combination with the child's weight. This formula is not precise for determining pediatric dosages.

2. Nursing actions in administering pediatric medications include:
*a. checking all drug calculations with another nurse before administering medication
b. using standard measuring teaspoons to determine correct medication amounts
c. administering crushed tablets in water for the child who cannot swallow pills
d. restraining the child, with the aid of the parents, for an intramuscular injection

[CL: CO]

Rationale: In order to maintain safety, all drug calculations should be checked by another nurse, preventing detrimental errors in administration.

3. In assessment of the pediatric patient requiring medication, the nurse will:
a. record the child's age to determine the accuracy of medication dosage
b. question the parents about their ability to care for the child at home
*c. include a developmental assessment of the child for the data base
d. ensure medication compliance and administration by appearing sincere but judgmental

[CL: KN]

Rationale: Developmental data is an important aspect of assessment which is helpful in understanding the child's capabilities.

4. Evaluation of the pediatric patients to gauge nursing interactions includes all of the following factors <u>except</u>:
a. basing evaluations on a predetermined list of outcome criteria
*b. assuming parents will be responsible for administering the medication
c. noting evidence that the parents will keep follow-up appointments
d. observing that the parents understand the causes of the child's condition

[CL: KN]

Rationale: The nurse should not assume that the parent who stays with the child in the hospital will be the one to administer medications at home.

5. The primary reason that a large percentage of drugs on the market is not recommended for children is that:
a. most drugs on the market are not suitable for administration in children
b. inadequate interest exists for research in drug administration in children
*c. ethical factors inhibit research in drug experimentation on children
d. children at various stages are not able to absorb and metabolize drugs

[CL: CO]

Rationale: Many drugs on the market are not recommended for children due to ethical problems related to drug experimentation on children to determine safety.

CHAPTER 15: PHARMACOTHERAPEUTICS FOR THE OBSTETRICAL PATIENT

Situations from Text

Situation 15-1

Paula Larson, a 34-year-old G2P1, is admitted in active labor. She has been pre-eclamptic, with blood pressure controlled well with hydralazine (Apresoline).

1. The nurse will observe for one of the following characteristics of pre-eclampsia:
   *a. proteinuria
   b. oliguria
   c. confusion
   d. dyspnea

   [NP: AS, CL: KN]

   Rationale: Proteinuria is one of the triad of symptoms which characterize pre-eclampsia. Edema and hypertension are the other classic symptoms.

2. During the first stage of labor, Paula's blood pressure increases to 170/100, and she begins to demonstrate confusion and clonic movements. The physician orders a magnesium sulfate drip. The nurse will prepare the infusion in the following manner:
   a. 100 mEq in 100 cc D5W to run at 8 to 10 cc per hour
   b. 40 mEq in 500 cc 0.9 percent sodium chloride to run at 2 ml per minute
   *c. 32 mEq in 250 cc of 5 percent dextrose to run at 1 to 4 ml per minute
   d. 8 mEq in 250 cc 0.9 percent sodium chloride to run at 1.5 ml per minute

   [NP: IM, CL: AP]

   Rationale: For a continuous infusion, 32 mEq of magnesium sulfate is added to 250 cc 5 percent dextrose and given at a rate not to exceed 4 ml per minute.

3. In relation to the magnesium infusion, the nurse will observe for the following:
   a. dry pale skin
   *b. hyporeflexia
   c. agitation
   d. increased respirations

   [NP: AS, CL: CO]

   Rationale: The patient should be observed for diminished neuromuscular functioning, including hyporeflexia, which is associated with hypermagnesemia.

4. In the event that Paula demonstrates symptoms related to hypermagnesemia, the nurse will be prepared to administer:
   a. oxygen
   b. epinephrine
   c. potassium phosphate
   *d. calcium gluconate

   [NP: PL, CL: KN]

   Rationale: Calcium is the antidote for magnesium toxicity.

5. Which of the following outcome criteria would indicate successful management of Paula's condition?
   a. decreased contractions
   b. respiratory rate < 16
   *c. absence of seizures

d. absent reflexes

[NP: EV, CL: AN]

Rationale: The patient with eclampsia should demonstrate an absence of seizure activity.

6. Paula safely delivers a baby boy. The infant should be monitored closely for any indications of:
   a. tachypnea
   b. hypocalcemia
   c. hyperkalemia
   *d. neuromuscular depression

   [NP: IM, CL: KN]

   Rationale: Following delivery, infants of mothers who received magnesium sulfate need to be observed closely for signs of neuromuscular depression during the first 24 to 48 hours.

Situation 15-2

Shirley Green is a 26-year-old G1P0 presenting to the labor and delivery unit with regular contractions. During examination, the nurse confirms that Shirley is dilated 3 cm.

1. As labor progresses, Shirley requests some pain medication. Demerol 12.5 mg to 25 mg IV is ordered for pain. The nurse is aware of the following effect with regard to the administration of meperdine hydrochloride (Demerol) during labor:
   a. reduction in signs of fetal distress
   b. promotion of fetal hyperactivity if given early
   *c. prolongation of the latent stage of labor
   d. increased uterine contractions

   [NP: AS, CL: KN]

   Rationale: Since Demerol prolongs the latent phase of labor, it should be administered after labor is well established.

2. After two hours of strong contractions, examination reveals complete dilation. Fetal heart rate and variability remain stable, and Mrs. Green is prepared for an epidural block. Which position will be best for Mrs. Green after epidural anesthesia?
   *a. sandbag under right hip
   b. semi Fowler's position, right side down
   c. pillow at lower back with head flat
   d. supine with head of bed elevated 30 degrees

   [NP: IM, CL: AP]

   Rationale: Hypotension is a side effect of epidural anesthesia. By placing a noncompressible sandbag under the right hip, the uterus is displaced to the left. This position maintains vena caval blood return.

3. Should Mrs. Green exhibit symptoms of hypotension related to epidural anesthesia, the nurse will be prepared to administer all <u>except</u>:
   a. oxygen
   b. intravenous fluids
   c. epinephrine
   *d. Trendelenburg position

   [NP: PL, CL: CO]

   Rationale: Systemic hypotension related to epidural anesthesia may be treated with the administration of oxygen, epinephrine, intravenous fluids, as well as left lateral positioning. The Trendelenburg position further compounds the problem by reducing uteroplacental blood flow and vena caval blood return.

4. After Mrs. Green delivers a normal infant, the nurse gives her an intramuscular injection of ergonovine maleate (Ergotrate). This drug is given to:
   a. inhibit lactation
   b. facilitate delivery of placenta
   *c. treat uterine atony
   d. relax smooth muscles

   [NP: AN, CL: KN]

   Rationale: The action of Ergotrate is to stimulate smooth muscle, thereby controlling postpartal hemorrhage and uterine atony.

5. The nurse may administer all of the following medications to Mrs. Green's baby <u>except</u>:
   a. Vitamin K
   b. silver nitrate
   c. erythromycin ointment
   *d. RhoGam

   [NP: IM, CL: CO]

   Rationale: Rho(D)immune globulin (RhoGam) is administered intramuscularly to women who are Rh-negative and give birth to Rh-positive infants.

6. Mrs. Green prefers to bottle feed her infant and is to receive bromocriptine (Parlodel). The nurse will include the following information during patient teaching:
   a. The drug will provide protection against pregnancy.
   b. It should be taken only if signs of breast engorgement are noted.
   *c. Hypotension and dizziness are common side effects.
   d. If one dose is missed, then two doses should be taken together.

   [NP: IM, CL: KN]

   Rationale: The patient needs to be aware of the side effects of bromocriptine, which include hypotension, dizziness, headache, and nausea.

Additional Situation Not Presented in Text

Regina Martinez (G3P2) is a 33-year-old who is 24 weeks pregnant. She is an insulin dependent diabetic and is being followed closely by the health clinic nurse.

1. The nurse carefully monitors Regina's blood sugar three days a week. The nurse is aware that an increased insulin dosage may be required during pregnancy due to the presence of:
   *a. HPL
   b. prolactin
   c. oxytocin
   d. progesterone

   [NP: AS, CL: KN]

   Rationale: Human placental lactogen (HPL) exerts an antagonistic effect on insulin action, thereby raising blood glucose levels.

2. At 28 weeks, Regina presents with signs of preterm labor. She is admitted to the hospital for intravenous administration of ritrodrine (Yutopar). The nurse will prepare the initial dose of ritrodrine to infuse at:
   a. 150 to 200 ug per minute
   b. 150 to 350 ug per minute
   *c. 50 to 100 ug per minute
   d. 200 to 400 ug per minute

   [NP: IM, CL: KN]

Rationale: The intravenous dose of ritrodrine is 50 to 100 ug per minute. It should be increased every 10 minutes in 50 μg increments until contractions subside.

3. During ritrodrine administration, the nurse will perform all of the following nursing actions for Regina except:
   a. auscultate breath sounds frequently
   *b. maintain patient on right side
   c. weigh patient daily
   d. provide a calm environment

   [NP: IM, CL: CO]

   Rationale: To maintain uteroplacental blood flow, the patient should be placed on the left side.

4. Uterine suppression is successful and Regina will be discharged on an oral dosage of ritrodrine. Because of the side effects of ritrodrine, Regina may need to:
   a. decrease daily insulin dosage
   b. reduce insulin to every other day
   c. eliminate insulin administration
   *d. increase daily insulin dosage

   [NP: PL, CL: CO]

   Rationale: Patients who are diabetic need to be monitored closely if on ritrodrine, because of the side effect of hyperglycemia. The daily insulin dosage may need to be increased.

5. As discharge planning for the patient going home with oral ritrodrine, the nurse will teach Regina to include the following in her diet:
   a. complex carbohydrates
   b. simple sugars
   *c. potassium-rich foods
   d. low sodium foods

   [NP: IM, CL: AP]

   Rationale: A side effect of ritrodrine is hypokalemia. A diet which includes potassium-rich foods should be stressed.

6. Which of the following statements indicates that Regina understands how to take the uterine suppressant ritrodrine?
   a. "If I forget a dose, I should take the missed dose whenever I remember."
   b. "It is best to keep this drug in the bathroom cabinet, away from the kids."
   c. "Side effects are expected, so I shouldn't worry if I am short of breath."
   *d. "I need to let my nurse or doctor know if I begin any other drugs."

   [NP: EV, CL: AN]

   Rationale: It is important to have the patient inform the nurse or doctor if other drugs are to be taken, due to the potential interaction with ritrodrine.

Review Questions from Text

1. Which of the following statements is correct regarding drug distribution and excretion during pregnancy?
   a. As a result of an increase in plasma albumin, pharmacologic drug effects are increased.
   b. An increase in intracellular fluid volume increases the potential for toxic drug effects.
   *c. Elimination is increased, creating a potential for reduced drug plasma concentrations.
   d. Drug half-life is prolonged due to the increase in blood flow through the liver.

   [CL: CO]

   Rationale: During pregnancy, elimination is increased, reducing drug concentration and therapeutic plasma levels.

2. The variables which determine the transfer of drugs across the placenta include all of the following except:
   a. physicochemical characteristics
   *b. gestational age
   c. placental blood flow
   d. properties of the placenta

   [CL: CO]

   Rationale: Variables which determine whether drugs will pass through the placental barrier include physicochemical characteristics of the drug, physiologic properties of the placenta, and maternal and fetal placental blood flow. Gestational age is a factor in determining the effect that the drug will have on the fetus.

3. According to the Federal Drug Administration (FDA), drugs in Category C represent the following risk if taken during pregnancy:
   a. Studies in women have not indicated a risk to the fetus, and harm is remote.
   b. Human studies have not been completed to support the use in women without fetal risk.
   c. Evidence of fetal risk exists, but the drug may be used only if absolutely necessary.
   *d. Use in women should be limited, unless the benefit outweighs the risk to the fetus.

   [CL: KN]

   Rationale: Category C drugs represent those which may be used in pregnant women only if the benefit of use outweighs the risk to the fetus.

4. All of the following may be used for relief of pain during active labor except:
   *a. barbiturates
   b. analgesics
   c. antiemetics
   d. anesthetics

   [CL: KN]

   Rationale: Active labor with imminent delivery is a contraindication for barbiturate administration.

5. Regarding the use of general anesthesia during delivery, the following statement is correct:
   a. General anesthesia potentiates intense uterine contractions which can cause hemorrhaging.
   b. The interval from induction to delivery can be up to one hour before fetal depression is observed.
   c. The risk of aspiration is reduced with the use of general anesthesia in pregnant women.
   *d. The use of general anesthesia for delivery may result in delayed mother-infant bonding.

   [CL: CO]

   Rationale: After general anesthesia, there is a delay in infant/mother contact in the postpartal period. This separation may result in delayed mother-infant bonding.

6. A risk associated with paracervical block includes:
   a. maternal aspiration
   *b. fetal bradycardia
   c. maternal hypoglycemia
   d. fetal hypertension

   [CL: KN]

   Rationale: Paracervical blocks are not frequently utilized as a labor anesthetic due to the high incidence of fetal bradycardia.

7. Contraindications for the use of beta sympathomimetic drugs include all of the following except:
   *a. mild pre-eclampsia

b. abruptio placenta
c. pulmonary hypertension
d. fetal distress

[CL: CO]

Rationale: Uterine suppression drugs most frequently used are beta sympathomimetics. These drugs should be used with caution in patients with mild to moderate pre-eclampsia, but are contraindicated if prolongation of labor is deleterious to infant or mother.

8. A positive oxytocin challenge test (OCT) indicates:
*a. low placental reserve
b. adequate placental oxygen
c. prolongation of gestation
d. placental hemorrhage

[CL: KN]

Rationale: A positive OCT indicates low placental reserve and the need for termination of the pregnancy.

9. Oxytocin administration is contraindicated in the following condition:
a. cardiovascular disease
b. renal disease
c. hypertension
*d. placenta previa

[CL: CO]

Rationale: Oxytocin is contraindicated in cases of placenta previa. The dosage should be reduced in patients with cardiovascular, renal, or hypertensive disease.

10. The following type of drug is known to be excreted in breast milk:
a. insulin
b. heparin
*c. diazepam
d. oxytocin

[CL: CO]

Rationale: Diazepam should be used with caution in breast-feeding mothers, due to the risk of drug accumulation in the neonate.

Additional Review Questions Not Presented in Text

1. Appropriate nursing actions for the patient receiving oxytocin intravenously include all of the following except:
a. Document vital signs and temperature every 2 hours.
*b. Reduce infusion if uterine hyperactivity occurs.
c. Document correct intake and output.
d. Palpate fundus to evaluate contractions.

[CL: CO]

Rationale: The infusion of oxytocin should be stopped at the first sign of uterine hyperactivity.

2. The following statement is correct about administration of RhoGam:
a. It is given to Rh-positive mothers before antibodies are formed.
b. A positive indirect Coombs test indicates the need for RhoGam.
*c. Patients may experience symptoms of a transfusion reaction.
d. It is not necessary to type crossmatch the RhoGam recipient.

[CL: KN]

Rationale: Rho(D)immune globulin is obtained from human plasma. Rh-negative patients who are to receive the drug are typed and crossmatched. Reactions similar to a blood transfusion may occur.

3. With regard to phenytoin administration during pregnancy, it is usually necessary to:
   a. discontinue the medication
   *b. increase the daily dosage
   c. reduce the daily dosage
   d. maintain the prepregnant dosage

   [CL: KN]

   Rationale: Due to rapid elimination during pregnancy, phenytoin levels may need to be increased in order to prevent seizures.

4. Which of the following agents would be administered in the event of a toxic reaction to ritrodrine (Yutopar)?
   *a. propranolol
   b. calcium gluconate
   c. epinephrine
   d. carboprost

   [CL: KN]

   Rationale: Propranolol, a beta adrenergic blocking agent, would be the drug of choice for a toxic reaction to ritrodrine, a beta sympathomimetic.

5. Acid base balance affects the transfer of drugs across the placenta. In the case of maternal alkalosis, the result will be:
   a. accumulation of drugs with an acid pH in the fetus
   b. rapid utilization of ionized drugs in the fetus
   *c. accumulation of drugs with an alkaline pH in the fetus
   d. rapid utilization of protein-bound drugs in the fetus

   [CL: KN]

   Rationale: In maternal alkalosis, the oxyhemoglobin curve shifts to the left, reducing the amount of oxygen available to the fetus. This creates fetal hypoxia and acidosis, resulting in a build-up of alkaline pH drugs in the fetus.

CHAPTER 16: PHARMACOTHERAPEUTICS FOR THE GERIATRIC PATIENT

Situation from Text

Marian Cantrell, an 84-year-old, is admitted to the medical-surgical floor with a diagnosis of urinary tract infection.

1. An IV is started, and the nurse administers gentamycin via an intravenous piggyback. It will be important for the nurse to assess the following in relation to gentamycin administration:
   a. magnesium level
   *b. creatinine level
   c. sodium level
   d. calcium level

   [NP: IM, CL: AP]

   Rationale: Gentamycin is a nephrotoxic agent; therefore, creatinine levels should be checked as a reflection of renal function.

2. In planning nursing interventions for Mrs. Cantrell, all of the following would be included <u>except</u>:
   a. monitor serum gentamycin levels
   b. measure intake and output
   *c. restrict fluids to 100 cc per day
   d. weigh patient daily

   [NP: PL, CL: AN]

   Rationale: A fluid restriction would potentiate dehydration. Since gentamycin is a water-soluble drug, more would remain in circulation and lead to possible toxicity.

3. The nurse will observe Mrs. Cantrell for the following sensory disturbance indicating a toxic effect of gentamycin:
   a. visual
   b. tactile
   c. olfactory
   *d. auditory

   [NP: IM, CL: CO]

   Rationale: Drugs such as gentamycin can produce ototoxicity.

4. Mrs. Cantrell received a sleeping pill (Nembutal) for the first night in the hospital. The next day she was drowsy and wanted to sleep instead of eating her breakfast. The nurse is aware that this effect is most probably due to:
   *a. reduced hepatic function
   b. reduced cardiac output
   c. gentamycin interaction
   d. delayed toxic effects

   [NP: AS, CL: AP]

   Rationale: The reduced metabolism of barbiturates by the liver is partly responsible for the "hangover" effect seen in the elderly.

5. Mrs. Cantrell has a history of diabetes and is currently taking tolbutamide (Orinase). This drug is an example of one that is affected by:
   a. hypokalemia
   b. hyponatremia
   c. hyperlipidemia
   *d. hypoproteinemia

[NP: AS, CL: CO]

Rationale: Orinase is an example of a medication which is bound to protein for distribution. Hypoproteinemia can cause an increase in the amount of unbound drug, resulting in increased action.

6. On the fourth day of hospitalization, Mrs. Cantrell has an irregular heart rate and is started on oral procainamide (Pronestyl). The nurse will assess the following with regard to this medication:
 a. protein intake
 *b. renal function
 c. folic acid levels
 d. subcutaneous fatty tissue

[NP: IM, CL: KN]

Rationale: Drugs such as procainamide are primarily excreted by the kidneys. Careful monitoring of renal function is important so that possible problems leading to drug toxicity can be identified.

Additional Situation Not Presented in Text

Mr. Summers is a 58-year-old who comes into a health screening unit to get his blood pressure checked. His blood pressure is 150/86 and his heartrate is 96 (regular).

1. The nurse questions Mr. Summers about medications which he takes routinely. Which response indicates the best understanding about self-medication?
 a. "I take a yellow pill once a day and a white pill twice a day."
 b. "My doctor knows what medications I am taking."
 c. "I don't know the name of the pills, but I take them at least twice a day."
 *d. "It is hard for me to remember the names, so I carry a list of what I take."

[NP: AS, CL: AN]

Rationale: This response indicates some understanding of and interest in his health care regimen.

2. The list of medications which Mr. Summers presents to the nurse includes: Aldomet 250 mg twice a day; Lasix 40 mg once a day; potassium supplement 1 tbsp once a day. When asked about the reason for taking each medication, he states that they are all for his blood pressure. An appropriate nursing diagnosis for Mr. Summers would be:
 a. noncompliance related to inability to name medications
 b. impaired home maintenance management related to self-medication
 c. alteration in thought process related to inability to remember medications
 *d. knowledge deficit related to medication regimen for blood pressure control

[NP: AN, CL: AP]

Rationale: The nursing diagnosis of knowledge deficit is most appropriate. Mr. Summers demonstrates a need for education concerning medication regimen.

3. Mr. Summers tells the nurse that he has been having "dizzy spells" after rising from a lying position. He feels that this is due to getting older. The nurse is aware that his symptom is probably due to:
 *a. side effects of blood pressure medication
 b. toxic effects of potassium supplement
 c. natural process of aging
 d. neurological damage related to aging

[NP: AN, CL: AP]

Rationale: Many times, side effects of medications may be mistaken for signs of aging. In this case, dizziness may relate to a side effect of Aldomet, his blood pressure medication.

4. The nurse schedules patient teaching for Mr. Summers. For successful learning, the nurse will plan to do the

following:
a. use medical terminology for greater understanding
b. choose pastel colors for presenting visual aids
*c. refer to the shapes, colors, and sizes of medications
d. use abstract terms along with concrete skills

[NP: PL, CL: KN]

Rationale: Using specific shapes, colors, and sizes of the medications to the nurse's advantage helps in teaching identification of medications.

5. The best criterion for determining effective teaching is to:
a. have the patient repeat instructions
*b. allow for return demonstration
c. have the patient write down the medications
d. allow the patient to recite the material

[NP: EV, CL: CO]

Rationale: Rote memory is generally short-term and items may not be remembered a short time later. A return demonstration will help to incorporate long-term memory and skills.

6. Which of the following statements by Mr. Summers reveals a potential problem with over-the-counter medication?
*a. "I take a laxative every day to keep regular."
b. "I take about 2 aspirins a day for arthritis in my hands."
c. "Whenever I eat spicy foods, I take an antacid."
d. "If I get a headache, I sometimes take Tylenol."

[NP: AS, CL: AN]

Rationale: This statement indicates a potential for laxative abuse.

Review Questions from Text

1. All of the following are correct regarding aging and age-related medication problems <u>except</u>:
a. Some studies suggest that up to 30 percent of older adults suffer adverse drug side effects.
b. The aging process alters the therapeutic and adverse responses to drug therapy.
*c. The major causes of death among elderly patients are cancer and its related drug therapy.
d. Some studies have found that 20 percent of the hospitalization of older adults is due to prescription drug effects.

[CL: KN]

Rationale: The number one cause of death continues to be cardiovascular disease, although other illnesses, such as cancer, are associated with aging.

2. The components of drug disposition include all of the following processes <u>except</u>:
a. absorption
*b. adaptation
c. distribution
d. metabolism

[CL: CO]

Rationale: The principles of drug disposition involve absorption, distribution, metabolism, and excretion.

3. All of the following statements are correct with regard to aging and the drug response <u>except</u>:
*a. Often signs of aging are mistaken for side effects of prescription drugs.

b. In general, medications tend to be overprescribed for the elderly.
c. Drug therapy is often the most risky component of patient care in the elderly.
d. Currently, recommendations are being proposed for medication use in the elderly.

[CL: KN]

Rationale: Many times, side effects of medications are mistaken for symptoms related to the aging process. Most illnesses are treated with drug therapy, but, in the elderly, this can represent a risky component of patient care.

4. The following represents normal physiological changes with aging:
*a. Lean body mass tends to decrease.
b. Subcutaneous tissue tends to increase.
c. Total body water in the elderly usually increases.
d. Muscle mass proportionally increases.

[CL: KN]

Rationale: Lean body mass and total body water tend to decrease in the elderly.

5. In the older adult, fat soluble drugs are:
a. distributed to a smaller portion of tissue than in young adults
b. absorbed at a slow rate due to reduced fat stores
c. released into circulation quickly after being absorbed
*d. associated with increased duration of drug action

[CL: KN]

Rationale: The elderly have increased fat composition and fat soluble drugs are distributed in a greater volume of tissue. After absorption, the drugs are released slowly, resulting in an increased duration of effect.

6. The least desirable site for intravenous infusion of doxorubicin (Adriamycin) in the older adult would be:
*a. hand
b. subclavian
c. forearm
d. antecubital

[CL: AP]

Rationale: Due to the reduction in subcutaneous tissue, intravenous administration of a vesicant drug such as doxorubicin should not be administered via veins in the hand.

7. The following represents the effect of aging on cardiovascular function:
a. increased cardiac output
*b. reduced arterial wall elasticity
c. increased renal plasma flow
d. reduced peripheral vascular resistance

[CL: KN]

Rationale: The elastic fibers in the arteries lose about 30 percent of their stretching ability as a person ages.

8. The effect of aging on hepatic function results in:
a. reduced blood levels of drugs
*b. prolonged drug effect
c. reduced incidence of toxicity
d. decreased intensity of drug effect

[CL: KN]

Rationale: Aging reduces the liver's ability to metabolize certain drugs, resulting in a prolonged drug effect, due to prolonged concentrations of drug in the system.

9. Which statement is correct regarding sensory changes in the older adult?
   a. Eyesight is not affected by visual changes associated with aging.
   b. All hearing loss in the older adult is due to the aging process.
   *c. Sensory changes may affect the elderly person's ability to learn about his medication regime.
   d. Not all senses are affected by aging; for example, olfactory acuity remains stable.

[CL: CO]

Rationale: Sensory and perceptual alterations, such as reduced hearing acuity, may interfere with a person's ability to understand instructions.

Additional Review Questions Not Presented in Text

1. In planning nursing interventions for administering medications to the elderly patient, the nurse knows that:
   *a. adverse drug side effects tend to increase in relation to increasing age
   b. antidepressant drugs are most commonly used to reduce suicide among the elderly
   c. morphine sulfate is the drug of choice for controlling pain in the elderly
   d. fat soluble drugs do not present a problem in metabolism in the elderly

[CL: CO]

Rationale: Due to age-related changes which affect drug disposition, older patients are at greater risk for toxic effects.

2. Which statement is incorrect regarding areas to assess in the elderly patient?
   a. Functional capacity, such as vision or eye-hand coordination, is to be determined.
   b. A medication history should be taken which includes all nonprescription drugs.
   c. A nutritional history, including diet restrictions and food allergies, is assessed.
   *d. Nicotine and alcohol use are assessed only if the patient feels there is a problem.

[CL: CO]

Rationale: All elderly patients need to be assessed for nicotine and alcohol use in a non-threatening manner.

3. Which teaching strategy would be appropriate to gain medication compliance in the elderly?
   a. mixing the older patients with those of younger age groups
   b. teaching at a rapid pace in order to cover all the material
   c. limiting teaching sessions to two-hour time periods
   *d. encouraging the use of adaptive devices when possible

[CL: CO]

Rationale: Encouraging the use of hearing aids or glasses whenever possible enhances the potential for learning and retaining information.

4. Which statement is correct regarding drugs and the older adult?
   a. Elderly patients consume approximately 50 percent of all prescription drugs.
   *b. Little research has been conducted on drug therapy in the over-65 population.
   c. Drug responses are predictable and do not vary from one elderly person to another.
   d. Approximately 85 percent of elderly patients are chronically ill and on major medications.

[CL: CO]

Rationale: Until recently, little has been done to identify the special needs of the elderly in relation to drug therapy.

CHAPTER 17: OVERVIEW OF ANATOMY AND PHYSIOLOGY OF THE CENTRAL NERVOUS SYSTEM

Review Questions from Text

1. The telencephalon consists of both the right and left cerebral hemispheres and the:
   a. substantia nigra
   b. hypothalamus
   *c. basal ganglia
   d. thalamus

   [CL: KN]

   Rationale: The basal ganglia are embedded within the cerebral hemispheres.

2. All of the following statements are correct regarding the anatomy and physiology of the brain except:
   a. The basal ganglia initiate and modulate motor movement.
   *b. The limbic system plays a role in musculoskeletal response.
   c. The hypothalamus coordinates complex reflexes.
   d. The cerebelum coordinates activity of the skeletal muscles.

   [CL: CO]

   Rationale: The limbic system is concerned with the expression of mood, feelings, and emotions. It also is involved in the regulation of rhythms, appetite, and learning.

3. Cerebral spinal fluid is formed across the:
   a. pia mater
   b. sulci
   c. dural sinuses
   *d. choroid plexus

   [CL: KN]

   Rationale: Cerebral spinal fluid is formed across the choroid plexus.

4. Which of the following statements is correct regarding the transmission of nerve impulses?
   a. The action potential crosses directly from nerve to nerve or nerve to muscle.
   *b. The action potential releases a chemical substance which diffuses across the nerve synapse.
   c. When a transmitter binds to its antagonist receptor, nerve conduction is elicited.
   d. By occupying transmitter sites, antagonists prevent the appropriate nerve response.

   [CL: CO]

   Rationale: The action potential does not cross directly from nerve to nerve. As the action potential reaches the nerve ending, it releases a chemical called a transmitter, which diffuses across the nerve synapse and acts on a specific receptor at the post-synaptic membrane.

5. The afferent division of the peripheral nervous system is composed of:
   a. cell bodies which lie within the CNS and convey information about voluntary movement
   b. nerves which lie ouside the CNS and control involuntary movement
   c. cell bodies which lie outside the CNS and direct messages to the periphery about sensation
   *d. nerves which convey sensory information from peripheral receptors to the CNS

   [CL: KN]

   Rationale: The cell bodies of afferent nerves lie outside the CNS. Action potentials are generated at the receptor end and messages about sensory information are transmitted to the CNS.

6. The sympathetic nervous system:
   *a. activates systems which are necessary for rapid energy expenditure
   b. enhances energy conservation and bodily maintenance
   c. activates skeletal or voluntary muscles to contract
   d. facilitates sensory impulses and integrates responses

   [CL: KN]

   Rationale: The sympathetic nervous system enables the body to deal with emergency situations by eliciting the "fight or flight" reaction.

7. The following statement is correct with regard to cholinergic receptors and subtypes:
   a. Muscarinic receptors are located on the ganglia of the sympathetic and parasympathetic systems.
   b. Nicotinic receptors are found only on the effector cell membrane innervated by postganglionic fibers.
   *c. Nicotinic antagonists exert effects which block both muscarinic and adrenergic transmission.
   d. Muscarinic antagonists, such as mecamylamine, affect the entire somatic system.

   [CL: CO]

   Rationale: Nicotinic receptors are found in the somatic system and in the ganglia of the autonomic system. Ganglionic antagonists which block nicotinic receptors cause both muscarinic and adrenergic blockade.

8. $Alpha_1$ adrenergic stimulation causes:
   a. bronchial constriction
   b. vascular vasodilation
   c. constriction of intestinal smooth muscle
   *d. bronchial dilation

   [CL: CO]

   Rationale: In bronchial and intestinal smooth muscle, $alpha_1$ adrenergic stimulation causes relaxation. In vascular smooth muscle, $alpha_1$ adrenergic stimulation causes vasoconstriction.

9. An example of a drug which possesses both $beta_1$ and $beta_2$ activity is:
   a. atenol
   *b. epinephrine
   c. albutanol
   d. phenylephrine

   [CL: KN]

   Rationale: Epinephrine possesses both $beta_1$ and $beta_2$ activity.

10. $Beta_1$ receptors are located in all of the following sites except:
   *a. bronchial smooth muscle
   b. heart
   c. adipose tissue
   d. kidney

   [CL: CO]

   Rationale: $Beta_1$ receptors are located in the heart, kidney, and adipose tissues. $Beta_2$ receptors are located in bronchial smooth muscle.

Additional Review Questions Not Presented in Text

1. All of the following statements are correct regarding cerebral functioning except:
   a. It is the site of awareness and analysis of sensory input.
   b. The cerebral cortex initiates and controls motor movement.

c. It integrates appropriate motor responses to sensory input.
*d. The cerebral cortex influences emotions by associating sensory input.

[CL: CO]

Rationale: The thalamus, not the cerebral cortex, plays a role in influencing emotions by associating sensory input with feelings of pleasantness or unpleasantness.

2. The brain stem performs the following function(s):
*a. contains the vasogenic, cardiac, and respiratory centers
b. serves as the source of all of the cranial nerves
c. participates in water and electrolyte balance
d. coordinates all autonomic activity

[CL: CO]

Rationale: The brain stem is composed of the mesencephalon, pons, and medulla. The medulla contains the vital centers which control cardiac and respiratory functions.

3. The following statement correctly describes a feature of the parasympathetic nervous system:
a. The preganglionic fibers emerge from the thoracic or lumbar sections of the spinal cord.
b. Most of the parasympathetic ganglia are situated close to the spinal cord.
c. In the parasympathetic system, one preganglionic fiber activates many postganglionic fibers.
*d. The parasympathetic system possesses long preganglionic and short postganglionic nerve fibers.

[CL: KN]

Rationale: The parasympathetic ganglia are situated primarily within the effector organ. Therefore, the preganglionic nerve fibers which originate from the craniosacral system are long, while the postsynaptic nerve fibers are short.

4. Nerve receptors which bind with norepinephrine are:
a. cholinergic
*b. adrenergic
c. dopaminergic
d. purinergic

[CL: KN]

Rationale: Adrenergic receptors are those which bind with the neurotransmitter norepinephrine.

5. Which of the following statements is correct concerning peripheral neurotransmitters?
*a. The somatic nervous system utilizes only acetylcholine as the neurotransmitter.
b. All autonomic preganglionic nerve fibers release norepinephrine as the neurotransmitter.
c. The parasympathetic postganglionic nerve fibers release norepinephrine.
d. The sympathetic postganglionic nerve fibers release only acetylcholine.

[CL: KN]

Rationale: The somatic nervous system is completely cholinergic, in that it utilizes only acetylcholine as its neurotransmitter.

CHAPTER 18: DRUGS AFFECTING THE PARASYMPATHETIC NERVOUS SYSTEM

Situations from Text

Situation 18-1

Theresa McNeal is a 60-year-old admitted to the surgical floor and prepared for cataract removal.

1. Acetylcholine chloride (Miochol) will be given to Mrs. McNeal intraocularly during ophthalmic surgery to:
   a. relax the sphincter muscle of the iris
   *b. obtain complete miosis
   c. reduce nasolacrimal secretions
   d. block the flow of aqueous humor

   [NP: AN, CL: KN]

   Rationale: Acetylcholine is given intraocularly during ophthalmic surgery to obtain complete miosis.

2. The nurse will expect the duration of effect of Miochol to be:
   a. one hour
   b. twelve hours
   *c. ten minutes
   d. four hours

   [NP: PL, CL: KN]

   Rationale: The onset of action of Miochol is immediate, with effects lasting 10 minutes.

3. Postoperative recovery for Ms. McNeal is uneventful; however, a recurrent problem of urinary retention is noted. Mrs. McNeal is started on bethanechol (Urecholine). The nurse is aware that this drug should be given:
   *a. orally
   b. intramuscularly
   c. intravenously
   d. topically

   [NP: AN, CL: CO]

   Rationale: Signs of muscarinic excess can occur if Urecholine is given intramuscularly or intravenously. The usual route is oral or subcutaneous.

4. Before giving bethanechol to Mrs. McNeal, the nurse will assess for the following condition, which would indicate a contraindication to its use:
   *a. peptic ulcer disease
   b. abdominal distention
   c. gastric stasis
   d. neurogenic bladder

   [NP: AS, CL: CO]

   Rationale: Due to the cholinergic effect of increased gastric secretions, bethanechol is contraindicated in patients with peptic ulcer disease.

5. In planning for potential toxic effects of bethanechol, the nurse will keep the following drug available:
   a. lidocaine
   b. prostigmin
   c. neostigmine
   *d. atropine

   [NP: PL, CL: KN]

Rationale: Atropine, an anticholinergic drug, is the agent of choice in the event that toxic effects of bethanechol occur.

6. Mrs. McNeal will be discharged home on an oral dose of bethanechol. Which of the following statements indicates successful patient teaching?
   a. "I should keep this drug in a warm, dry place."
   b. "It is best to take this medicine with meals."
   c. "I should not worry if I have any unusual feelings."
   *d. "It is best to keep the drug away from direct light."

   [NP: EV, CL: AN]

   Rationale: Behtanechol should be kept in a light-resistent container. The patient should also be taught to report any adverse side effects immediately.

Situation 18-2

Steven Perry is a 28-year-old accountant admitted to the medical surgical floor due to upper abdominal pain and a history of tarry stools.

1. Endoscopic examination reveals peptic ulcer disease. Which of the following drug therapies would be contraindicated for Mr. Perry?
   a. anticholinergics
   *b. cholinesterase inhibitors
   c. parasympatholytics
   d. muscarinic blockers

   [NP: AN,CL: CO]

   Rationale: Cholinesterase inhibitor drugs block the breakdown of acetylcholine and contribute to the stimulation of cholinergic receptors. This stimulation produces an increase in gastric secretions and is contraindicated in patients with peptic ulcer disease.

2. Mr. Perry is started on a regime of antacids and propantheline bromide. The nurse will observe for all of the following adverse side effects of propantheline bromide <u>except</u>:
   a. photophobia
   b. tachycardia
   c. headache
   *d. urinary urgency

   [NP: IM, CL: CO]

   Rationale: Adverse side effects of propantheline bromide include photophobia, tachycardia, headache, and urinary retention.

3. A nursing diagnosis which would be appropriate for Mr. Perry would be:
   a. alteration in bowel elimination: diarrhea related to propantheline bromide
   b. sexual dysfunction related to the side effects of antacids
   *c. alteration in oral mucous membrane related to side effects of propantheline bromide
   d. hypothermia related to the stress of peptic ulcer disease

   [NP: AN, CL: AP]

   Rationale: A very common side effect of propantheline bromide is dryness of the mouth; therefore, alteration in oral mucous membrane is an appropriate nursing diagnosis.

4. The nurse will plan all of the following interventions for Mr. Perry <u>except</u>:
   a. assess bowel sounds every shift
   *b. restrict oral fluid intake

c. check temperature every four hours
d. monitor intake and output

[NP: PL, CL: CO]

Rationale: Restriction of fluid intake would exacerbate dry mucous membranes. Increasing oral intake is indicated unless ordered otherwise.

5. Medical treatment proves to be unsuccessful, and, after a week of hospitalization, Mr. Perry is prepared for a gastric resection. Glycopyrrolate (Robinul) is given intramuscularly as a preoperative medication. The following is an action of this drug:
 a. decreases risk of regurgitation
 *b. decreases tracheal secretions
 c. increases esophageal sphincter pressure
 d. increases neuromuscular blockade

[NP: AN, CL: KN]

Rationale: Robinul is extremely potent in its ability to decrease pharyngeal, tracheal, and bronchial secretions.

6. When assessing Mr. Perry, the following may be observed in relation to drug therapy:
 *a. dilated pupils
 b. hyperactive bowel sounds
 c. bradycardia
 d. relaxation

[NP: AS, CL: CO]

Rationale: Anticholinergic drugs, such as Robinul and propantheline bromide, produce mydriasis.

<u>Additional Situation Not Presented in Text</u>

Alan Brudowsky, aged 54 years, has been recently diagnosed as having open-angle glaucoma. He is currently being treated with pilocarpine.

1. The nurse is aware, when administering pilocarpine eye drops, that the expected therapeutic action would be to:
 *a. increase outflow of aqueous humor
 b. relax ciliary muscles
 c. relax the sphincter muscle of the iris
 d. achieve complete pupillary dilation

[NP: AN, CL: KN]

Rationale: The mechanism of action is to increase the outflow of aqueous humor via the trabecular meshwork, reducing intraocular pressure.

2. A side effect of pilocarpine for which the nurse will observe is:
 *a. headache
 b. tachycardia
 c. urinary retention
 d. constipation

[NP: IM, CL: CO]

Rationale: Common side effects of pilocarpine include headache, itching of the eyes, and nausea.

3. When assessing Mr. Brudowsky's pupils after instillation of pilocarpine, the nurse will expect to observe:
 a. pupillary dilation
 *b. pupillary constriction

c. unequal accommodation
d. slow response to light

[NP: AS, CL: AP]

Rationale: Constricted pupils will be observed in relation to pilocarpine instillation.

4. When teaching Mr. Brudowsky about the drug, it will be important to include the following information:
   a. A burning sensation indicates an allergic reaction.
   *b. Decreased visual acuity may occur.
   c. Blurred vision should be reported immediately.
   d. Bright lights may worsen vision.

   [NP: IM,CL: KN]

   Rationale: Due to constricted pupils, the patient may experience decreased visual acuity, especially in dim light. Patients should be advised to use caution when driving at night.

5. Expected outcomes for Mr. Brudowsky include:
   a. reduction in ciliary muscle spasm
   b. increased visual acuity
   c. absence of tension headaches
   *d. decreased intraocular pressure

   [NP: EV, CL: KN]

   Rationale: An expected outcome for patients taking pilocarpine for open-angle glaucoma would be decreased intraocular pressure.

6. An appropriate nursing diagnosis for Mr. Brudowsky would be:
   a. noncompliance related to proper use of pilocarpine eye drops
   b. urinary retention related to use of cholinergic drugs
   *c. alteration in sensory perception: visual, related to pilocarpine
   d. alteration in bowel elimination: constipation related to pilocarpine

   [NP: AN, CL: CO]

   Rationale: Visual sensory perceptual problems would be of concern for Mr. Brudowsky, related to common side effects of pilocarpine.

Review Questions from Text

1. All of the following statements regarding the classification of parasympathetic medications are correct except:
   a. Cholinergic agents mimic the effects of the parasympathetic system.
   b. Indirect-acting parasympathetic agents are cholinesterase inhibitors.
   c. Anticholinergic drugs neutralize the effects of the parasympathetic system.
   *d. Depolarizing neuromuscular blockers are reversed by anticholinesterases.

   [CL: CO]

   Rationale: Depolarizing neuromuscular blockers are noncompetitive in that they cannot be reversed by additional acetylcholine.

2. Scopolamine, used in the treatment of motion sickness, is contraindicated in patients with:
   a. bradycardia
   *b. angle-closure glaucoma
   c. hypersensitivity to cholinergics
   d. excessive salivation

   [CL: KN]

Rationale: Scopolamine is contraindicated in patients with angle-closure glaucoma, due to the effect of increased intraocular pressure.

3. A general drug action of a cholinergic agent is:
   a. reduced salivation
   b. increased cardiac conduction
   *c. decreased cardiac contractility
   d. relaxation of bronchial glands

   [CL: CO]

   Rationale: Direct-acting cholinergic drugs produce decreased cardiac contractility, a negative inotropic effect.

4. All of the following conditions contraindicate the use of acetylcholine and its derivatives except:
   *a. neurogenic bladder
   b. myocardial infarction
   c. asthma
   d. peptic ulcers

   [CL: CO]

   Rationale: Acetylcholine-type drugs are indicated for the patient with neurogenic bladder, due to stimulation of micturation.

5. Carbachol (Miostat) may produce the following side effect:
   *a. diarrhea
   b. hypertension
   c. urinary retention
   d. dry skin

   [CL: KN]

   Rationale: Systemic effects of carbachol include increased peristalsis, abdominal cramping, and diarrhea.

6. Neostigmine bromide (Prostigmin) is used to treat all of the following conditions except:
   a. myasthenia gravis
   b. esophageal constriction
   *c. urinary obstruction
   d. abdominal distention

   [CL: CO]

   Rationale: Prostigmin is contraindicated for patients with mechanical obstruction of the urinary tract.

7. Ganglionic blocking drugs act by:
   a. preventing the release of norepinephrine from preganglionic nerve endings
   b. stimulating the production of ganglionic cholinesterases
   c. interfering with the breakdown of the norepinephrine
   *d. preventing the actions of acetylcholine at the receptor sites

   [CL: KN]

   Rationale: One way in which ganglionic blocking agents work is by preventing the action of acetylcholine at the ganglionic receptor sites.

8. An example of a neuromuscular blocking agent is:
   *a. curare
   b. mecamylamine
   c. trimethaphan

d. trihexyphenidyl

[CL: KN]

Rationale: Curare is a nondepolarizing neuromuscular blocking agent used to produce muscle relaxation for intubation and anesthesia.

9. Which of the following statements is correct regarding anticholinesterases?
   a. These drugs block the accumulation of acetylcholine at receptor sites.
   b. Anticholinesterases are only used as agricultural insecticides.
   *c. These agents prolong the action of acetylcholine.
   d. Anticholinesterases mimic the effects of acetylcholinesterase (ACHE).

   [CL: KN]

   Rationale: Anticholinesterases are agents that interfere with the enzymes which normally destroy acetylcholine at the neuromuscular junctions. This creates a build-up of acetylcholine at the cholinergic receptor sites.

10. Atropine, an anticholinergic drug, is contraindicated in all of the following conditions except:
   a. myasthenia gravis
   *b. iritis
   c. prostate hypertrophy
   d. glaucoma

   [CL: AN]

   Rationale: Atropine ophthalmic solution is used to treat iritis (inflammation of the iris) by producing mydriasis.

Additional Review Questions Not Presented in Text

1. A cholinergic crisis will produce all of the following effects except:
   a. intestinal spasm
   b. hypotension
   *c. mydriasis
   d. muscle fasciculations

   [CL: CO]

   Rationale: Excessive acetylcholine results in miosis rather than mydriasis.

2. Important information which should be included when teaching patients who are taking ganglionic blockers (mecamylamine and trimethaphan) would be to:
   *a. change position slowly
   b. suck on hard candy
   c. take an antidepressant
   d. eat foods high in fiber

   [CL: AP]

   Rationale: The effects of ganglionic blockade include hypotension; therefore, patients should be taught to change position slowly.

3. Which of the following statements is correct regarding vecuronium, a nondepolarizing neuromuscular blocker?
   a. It has a long half-life and produces cumulative effects with repeated doses.
   b. Vecuronium is compatible with barbiturates and can be given in the same syringe.
   c. The major central nervous system side effect is clonic movement of the extremities.
   *d. Vecuronium is used with caution in patients with cardiac, hepatic, and renal disease.

   [CL: KN]

Rationale: Vecuronium is used with caution in patients who have cardiac, neuromuscular, respiratory, hepatic, or renal disease. The major CNS side effects are muscle weakness and paralysis. This short-acting drug is incompatible with barbiturates.

4. All of the following are cholinesterase inhibitors <u>except</u>:
   a. demecarium
   b. neostigmine
   c. edrophonium
   *d. propantheline bromide

   [CL: KN]

   Rationale: Propantheline bromide is an anticholinergic agent.

CHAPTER 19: DRUGS AFFECTING THE SYMPATHETIC NERVOUS SYSTEM

Situations from Text

Situation 19-1

Mr. Morris Trehan, a 52-year-old, has been placed on a trial of ergotamine tartrate (Ergomar) for treatment of migraine headaches. He also has a history of diabetes and peptic ulcer disease.

1. The nurse will plan to observe Mr. Trehan for the following adverse side effect of Ergomar:
   a. hypotension
   b. constipation
   *c. vomiting
   d. impaired vision

   [NP: PL, CL: CO]

   Rationale: More common side effects of ergotamine tartrate (Ergomar) are nausea and vomiting.

2. In teaching Mr. Trehan about Ergomar, the nurse will include all of the following information <u>except</u>:
   a. Report any itching, tingling, or numbness in fingers and toes.
   *b. Take the medication with food four times a day.
   c. Lie down in a dark, quiet room after taking the drug.
   d. Have blood pressure checked on a routine basis.

   [NP: IM, CL: CO]

   Rationale: The sublingual tablets should be taken when a headache develops, and the dosage should not exceed three tablets in a 24-hour period.

3. Mr. Trehan will also be managed on a prophylactic dose of propranolol (Inderal) for prevention of migraine headaches. Which of the following conditions represents a contraindication for therapy?
   a. glaucoma
   b. hyperthyroidism
   c. alcohol withdrawal
   *d. congestive heart failure

   [NP: AS, CL: KN]

   Rationale: Beta blockers are contraindicated in patients with congestive heart failure.

4. All of the following behaviors indicate successful patient teaching about Inderal therapy <u>except</u>:
   a. reducing or stopping cigarette smoking
   *b. using antacids to decrease gastric effects
   c. taking propranolol on an empty stomach
   d. avoiding alcohol while taking the drug

   [NP: EV, CL: AP]

   Rationale: Antacids reduce the bioavailability of propranolol.

5. An appropriate nursing diagnosis for Mr.Trehan would be:
   a. Noncompliance related to medication regime for headaches
   b. Anxiety related to the side effects of beta-blocker therapy
   *c. Activity intolerance: fatigue related to propranolol therapy
   d. Potential for violence related to administration of ergot derivatives

   [NP: AN, CL: AN]

Rationale: Fatigue is a common side effect of beta blockers and results from hemodynamic effects or peripheral metabolic effects.

6. In planning Mr. Trehan's medication regime, all of the following drugs would be given cautiously except:
   a. insulin
   b. cimetidine
   c. diabeta
   *d. aspirin

   [NP: PL, CL: CO]

   Rationale: Concurrent administration of cimetidine and furosemide can cause adverse effects. Patients who are diabetic and on insulin or oral hyperglycemic agents need to be assessed for potential for hyperglycemia.

Situation 19-2

Betty Baschner is a 62-year-old with a history of renal insufficiency admitted to the intensive care unit post gastrectomy surgery. She is receiving Lactated Ringers at 100 cc per hour and has a nasogastric tube to low intermittent suction.

1. The physician orders a dopamine (Intropin) drip at 1 μg/kg/min for Mrs. Daschner. At this dosage, the nurse will expect to observe the following effect:
   a. increased blood pressure
   *b. increased urine output
   c. decreased cardiac output
   d. reduced nasogastric drainage

   [NP: EV, CL: AP]

   Rationale: At low doses, 1 μg/kg/min dopamine dilates renal and mesenteric arteries, producing increased urine output and improved creatinine clearance. At the lower infusion rate, blood pressure is not expected to increase.

2. In planning care for Mrs. Daschner, the nurse will include all of the following interventions with regard to dopamine infusion except:
   a. monitor extremities for color and temperature
   b. assess blood pressure and vital signs closely
   c. use micro drip tubing and an infusion pump
   *d. discontinue intravenous infusion of Lactated Ringers

   [NP: PL, CL: CO]

   Rationale: When administering vasopressor agents, such as dopamine, it is important to maintain adequate blood volume in order to ensure tissue perfusion.

3. The nurse notes extravasation at the dopamine infusion site. After discontinuing the infusion, the nurse will:
   *a. infiltrate phentolamine at the IV site
   b. wrap site in warm, moist saline dressings
   c. apply an ice pack to the area
   d. place a tourniquet above the area of infiltration

   [NP: IM, CL: AP]

   Rationale: In the event of extravasation of dopamine, an alpha-adrenergic blocker such as phentolamine hydrochloride is infiltrated into the same location.

4. After four days in the intensive care unit, Mrs. Daschner demonstrates signs of septic shock. The infusion of dopamine is increased to 10 μg/kg/min. At this infusion rate, the expected outcome would be:
   a. reduced body temperature
   *b. increased blood pressure

c. reduced heart rate
d. increased peripheral perfusion

[NP: EV, CL: KN]

Rationale: At infusion rates of 10 to 20 ug/kg/min, dopamine stimulates alpha-adrenergic activity, resulting in increased blood pressure.

5. Due to potential for drug interaction, all of the following agents should be used with caution except:
   a. MAO inhibitors
   b. thyroid hormones
   c. guanethidine
   *d. nitroglycerine

   [NP: PL, CL: CO]

   Rationale: Nitroglycerin ointment may be used with catecholamine infusions to increase peripheral blood flow without affecting blood pressure.

6. When the dopamine infusion is no longer necesary for Mrs. Daschner, the nurse will plan to include the following measures:
   a. turn off infusion and take the blood pressure every hour
   b. restrict total fluid intake before discontinuing
   c. administer a bolus dose of dopamine and then stop infusion
   *d. wean off dopamine at a slow rate, monitoring vital signs

   [NP: IM, CL: AP]

   Rationale: In some cases, discontinuing dopamine may be difficult, due in part to the short half-life of the drug. The dosage should be tapered slowly and vital signs taken frequently.

Additional Situation Not Presented in Text

Mr. Arnold George is a 27-year-old with chronic asthma admitted to the emergency unit in acute respiratory distress.

1. The cause of respiratory distress is status asthmaticus. For this diagnosis, the nurse will be prepared to administer epinephrine (Adrenalin) in the following maner:
   a. 1:1000 solution given via nebulizer
   *b. 1:1000 solution injected subcutaneously
   c. 1:100 solution injected intraveously
   d. 1:10,000 solution administered transbronchially

   [NP: IM, CL: CO]

   Rationale: The parenteral dosage for administration of epinephrine is a 1:1000 solution given subcutaneously or diluted to 1:10,000 for intravenous administration.

2. The nurse will assess Mr. George for the following adverse effect of epinephrine:
   a. hypotension
   b. miosis
   c. sedation
   *d. tachycardia

   [NP: AS, CL: KN]

   Rationale: An adverse effect of epinephrine is tachycardia.

3. All of the following drugs would be contraindicated for Mr. George except:
   *a. Isuprel

b. Inderal
c. Tenormin
d. Opressor

[NP: AN, CL: AP]

Rationale: Isuprel promotes bronchial dilitation. Inderal, Tenormin, and Opressor are beta-adrenergic blockers and are contraindicated in patients with bronchial asthma.

4. The nurse is aware that epinephrine provides the following beneficial action for asthmatic patients:
   a. bronchoconstriction
   b. dilation of nasal passages
   *c. constriction of bronchial vessels
   d. stimulation of cough reflex

[NP: AN, CL: CO]

Rationale: Epinephrine constricts bronchial vessels, thereby decreasing bronchial secretions in asthmatic patients.

5. Mr. George is also started on ephedrine (Ephedra) orally. Before administration of this drug, the nurse will assess for the following condition, which contraindicates its use:
   *a. narrow-angle glaucoma
   b. barbiturate poisoning
   c. narcolepsy
   d. narcotic overdose

[NP: AS, CL: KN]

Rationale: Due to mydriatic effects, ephedrine is contraindicated for patients with narrow-angle glaucoma.

6. Because of the potential for drug interaction with ephedrine, the nurse will teach Mr. George to be cautious of all of the following <u>except</u>:
   a. guanethidine
   b. digoxin
   c. methyldopa
   *d. acetaminophen

[NP: IM, CL: CO]

Rationale: Special precautions or contraindications for use of ephedrine include concurrent administration of digitalis preparations, methyldopa, and guanethidine.

Review Questions from Text

1. Drugs acting positively on the beta-adrenergic receptor sites:
   a. decrease cardiac contractility
   b. constrict bronchial smooth muscle
   *c. increase cardiac rate
   d. constrict arterioles of skeletal muscle

[CL: KN]

Rationale: An effect of beta-adrenergic stimulation is increased heart rate.

2. Which statement is <u>correct</u> regarding drugs acting as adrenergic stimulants?
   a. Levarterenol bitartrate (Levophed) increases blood flow to the kidney and skeletal muscles.
   b. Isoproterenol hydrochloride (Isuprel) produces bronchial constriction and peripheral vasodilation.
   c. Dobutamine hydrochloride (Dobutrex) causes the release of endogenous norepinephrine from adrenergic fibers.
   *d. Epinephrine (Adrenalin) causes vasodilitation in the blood vessels of muscle fibers with mostly $beta_2$

receptors.

[CL: KN]

Rationale: Epinephrine causes vasoconstriction in the peripheral vessels and vasodilitation of blood vessels of muscles with predominantly $beta_2$ receptors.

3. Which statement is correct regarding the interaction of catecholamines and other medications?
*a. Concurrent use of catecholamines with halothane may result in ventricular dysrhythmias.
b. Tricyclic antidepressant agents antagonize the peripheral effect of catecholamines.
c. Catecholamines' pressor effects are reduced when given with MAO inhibitors.
d. Catecholamine effects are blocked with concurrent use with antihistamines.

[CL: KN]

Rationale: Ventricular dysrhythmias may develop during surgery if catecholamines are used with halothane anesthetics.

4. Adverse effects of indirect and mixed adrenergic agents include all of the following except:
*a. drowsiness
b. palpitations
c. headache
d. dysrhythmias

[CL: KN]

Rationale: Adverse effects of indirect and mixed adrenergic stimulants include nervousness, headache, palpitations, and cardiac dysrhythmias.

5. Dihydroergotamine mesylate (DHE45) is an alpha-adrenergic blocking agent which:
a. contains 100 mg of caffeine per dose
*b. constricts cranial blood vessels
c. prevents serotonin activity
d. enhances peripheral vascular circulation

[CL: KN]

Rationale: DHE45 has a direct constricting effect on smooth muscle of peripheral and cranial vessels and is used to prevent or abort vascular headaches.

6. Which of the following statements is correct with regard to the pharmacokinetics of catecholamines?
a. Most of these drugs are metabolized by cholinesterases in the liver and kidney.
b. Catecholamines are concentrated at only selected tissue and organ sites.
c. CNS effects of catecholamines are due to passage across the blood-brain barrier.
*d. Catecholamine drugs are inactivated through uptake at sympathetic nerve endings.

[CL: KN]

Rationale: Catecholamine preparations are inactivated through uptake and metabolism at sympathetic nerve endings. The drugs are metabolized by monamine oxidase in the liver, kidney, and plasma.

7. In the event of beta-blocker overdose, the following drug has been shown to be useful in reversal of life-threatening complications:
a. protamine sulfate
b. phenotolamine
c. atropine
*d. glucagon

[CL: KN]

Rationale: Glucagon has been shown to enhance myocardial contractility in the event of beta-blocker overdose.

8. Adrenergic drugs work at all of the following receptor sites except:
   a. alpha
   *b. muscarinic
   c. dopaminergic
   d. $beta_2$

   [CL: CO]

   Rationale: Adrenergic drugs work at alpha, $beta_1$, $beta_2$, and dopaminergic receptors. Cholinergic drugs work at muscarinic receptor sites.

9. An example of an alpha blocking agent is:
   a. atenolol
   *b. phentolamine
   c. isoproterinol
   d. dobutamine

   [CL: KN]

   Rationale: Phentolamine hydrochloride is an alpha blocking agent used in the management of secondary hypertension due to pheochromocytoma and in the treatment of extravasation of vasopressors.

10. Which of the following statements is correct with regard to dobutamine hydrochloride administration?
   a. This drug is a naturally occurring catecholamine with selective $beta_2$ action.
   b. Even at low doses, dobutamine will increase heart rate significantly.
   c. Dobutamine increases renal and mesenteric blood flow.
   *d. This drug is appropriate for management of cardiogenic shock.

   [CL: KN]

   Rationale: Dobutamine is an appropriate drug for the treatment of cardiogenic shock due to its selective ability to increase myocardial contractile force. In low doses, there is little increase in heart rate. Unlike dopamine, dobutamine does not increase renal or mesenteric blood flow.

Additional Review Questions Not Presented in Text

1. Adrenergic drugs mimic the effects of the sympathetic nervous system and produce:
   a. vasodilation of the blood vessels to the skin
   b. increased intestinal activity
   c. bronchial constriction
   *d. increased cardiac contractility

   [CL: KN]

   Rationale: Adrenergic drugs increase the force of cardiac contraction via $beta_1$ stimulation.

2. The beta-adrenergic blocker propranolol (Inderal) has all of the following effects except:
   a. slows the heart rate
   *b. increases the SA node cycle
   c. controls supraventricular dysrhythmias
   d. lowers the blood pressure

   [CL: CO]

   Rationale: Inderal prolongs the sinus node cycle and reduces heart rate and conduction time. It is used for control of blood pressure and atrial and supraventricular dysrhythmias.

3. Which statement is correct regarding epinephrine (Adrenaline)?

a. A 1:100 solution is administered intracardially in cardiac arrest.
b. Subcutaneous action begins within 30 minutes of injection.
c. Intravenous effect begins within 5 minutes of injection.
*d. Epinephrine can be given transbronchially during cardiac arrest.

[CL: CO]

Rationale: Epinephrine injection of a 1:10,000 solution can be administered transbronchially (through an ET-tube) during cardiac arrest.

4. Alpha-adrenergic blocking agents:
   a. stimulate normal neural or hormonal activity
   *b. interfere with sympathetic stimulation in peripheral vessels
   c. block the vasodilitation of blood vessels supplying the skin
   d. block the receptors in the heart, causing reduced heart rate

   [CL: KN]

   Rationale: Alpha blockers interfere with the sympathetic stimulation of the smooth muscles of peripheral vessels, increasing blood flow to the skin and reducing blood pressure.

5. Which statement is <u>correct</u> regarding isoproterenol hydrochloride (Isuprel)?
   a. This drug acts almost exclusively on alpha-adrenergic receptors.
   b. A therapeutic effect of Isuprel is peripheral vasoconstriction
   *c. Isuprel lowers peripheral vascular resistance.
   d. This drug reduces cardiac contractility and conduction.

   [CL: CO]

   Rationale: Isuprel lowers peripheral vascular resistance by vasodilating skeletal muscle and mesenteric circulation.

CHAPTER 20: DRUGS THAT PROVIDE PAIN RELIEF

Situations from Text

Situation 20-1

Celia Harrington has been admitted to the surgical unitwith acute cholecystitis. She is being prepared for a cholecystectomy.

1. In planning for preoperative pain relief, the nurse is aware that the following medication may cause adverse effects in Ms. Harrington's case:
   a. oxycodone
   b. codeine
   c. nalbuphine
   *d. meperidine

   [NP: PL, CL: AP]

   Rationale: Meperidine (Demerol) may cause biliary tract spasm.

2. Butorphanol (Stadol) 2 mg IM is ordered for pain. The nurse will observe for all of the following adverse reactions with regard to this drug <u>except</u>:
   a. nausea
   *b. diarrhea
   c. euphoria
   d. agitation

   [NP: AS, CL: CO]

   Rationale: The most common adverse reactions include nausea, euphoria, agitation, and constipation.

3. Postoperatively, Ms. Harrington will receive morphine via an epidural catheter. For management of pain control using this method, the nurse is aware that epidural morphine:
   *a. demonstrates a slow onset of action
   b. provides a short duration of relief
   c. has decreased receptor affinity
   d. is quickly cleared through the CSF

   [NP: PL, CL: KN]

   Rationale: Epidural morphine is more water soluble than lipid soluble, and the onset of action is related to the slow diffusion through the lipid neural membrane.

4. When observing Ms. Harrington for side effects related to epidural morphine, the nurse will be aware of the following:
   a. urinary urgency
   b. polyuria
   *c. pruritis
   d. tachypnea

   [NP: IM, CL: KN]

   Rationale: Pruritis or rash is commonly associated with the administration of epidural opiates, which may be due in part to histamine release.

5. Epidural catheter malposition is a complication of this type of pain therapy. The nurse will notify the physician of all of the following signs <u>except</u>:
   a. paresthesia

b. occipital headache
c. poor pain relief
*d. drowsiness

[NP: PL, CL: CO]

Rationale: Signs and symptoms of paresthesia may be related to nerve tissue compression caused by catheter migration. Throbbing occipital headache may indicate dural puncture. Poor pain relief may be a sign that the catheter is malfunctioning. Drowsiness is more likely related to a side effect of morphine rather than catheter malposition.

6. Ms. Harrington recovers from surgery without complications. For discharge, Tylenol with codeine 30 mg PO has been ordered for pain. The nurse will teach the patient to:
   a. take the drug every three to four hours with meals
   *b. initiate measures to prevent constipation, such as drinking fluids
   c. observe for signs of analgesic neuropathy, which occur early
   d. continue the medication, if needed, for symptoms of arthritis

   [NP: IM, CL: AP]

   Rationale: Constipation is a commonly reported adverse effect of codeine.

Situation 20-2

Mr. Van Chin is a 26-year-old who injured his back in an accident five years ago. He is admitted to the orthopedic floor for evaluation of recurrent back pain.

1. During the assessment phase, the nurse questions Mr. Chin about current medications. He states that he is taking Percodan, which used to help, but now the effect lasts for only an hour. The nurse is aware that this probably indicates:
   a. psychological addiction
   b. hepatic insufficiency
   c. opiate inactivation
   *d. drug tolerance

   [NP: AS, CL: AP]

   Rationale: A sign of tolerance is the report that a drug is not as effective as it once was.

2. During the assessment, Mr. Chin describes his pain as nagging and burning. He states that it has become the "focus of [his] life." These symptoms are characteristic of which type of pain?
   *a. chronic
   b. psychological
   c. phantom
   d. acute

   [NP: AN, CL: AP]

   Rationale: Chronic pain is usually burning or nagging and may become the pathology, altering the patient's lifestyles.

3. Spinal evaluation reveals two herniated discs, and Mr. Chin undergoes a lumbar laminectomy. Postoperative orders include Dilaudid 2 mg IM every 4 hours as needed for pain. The nurse is aware of the following with regard to this drug:
   a. Dilaudid is less potent than morphine when given intramuscularly.
   b. As a partial opiate antagonist, it has less potential for abuse and addiction.
   c. Dilaudid has fewer central nervous system effects than morphine.
   *d. It may have an addictive effect if given with general anesthetics.

   [NP: PL, CL: KN]

Rationale: Dilaudid may exert an addictive effect if used with general anesthetics. In addition, this drug is a semi-synthetic derivative of morphine which is ten times more potent.

4. Mr. Chin requests medication for back pain. When administering Dilaudid to Mr. Chin, all of the following actions are appropriate except:
   a. maintain a positive outlook in anticipation of pain relief
   b. encourage the patient to relax and allow the drug to work
   *c. wait until Mr. Chin shows signs of pain before administering
   d. take advantage of the placebo effect of the drug

   [NP: IM, CL: AP]

   Rationale: Pain medication should be given promptly when needed. Nurses should not rely on their own perception of the pain experience. Pain medication will not be as effective if given after the patient is in severe pain.

5. In evaluating Mr. Chin to determine effectiveness of the pain medication regime, the nurse is aware of the following factor:
   a. Sedation is always linked with signs of an overdose.
   b. Ambulation is encouraged for patients with nausea.
   *c. Symptoms such as vomiting may indicate poorly controlled pain.
   d. Addiction is rarely a problem in patients with "real" pain.

   [NP: EV, CL: KN]

   Rationale: Nausea and vomiting usually are related to adverse effects of the medication, but may indicate poor pain control.

6. If Mr. Chin has problems with urinary retention postoperatively, the following drug may be given:
   a. droperidol
   *b. neostigmine
   c. levallorphan
   d. naloxone

   [NP: IM, CL: KN]

   Rationale: Neostigmine reduces urinary spasms which may cause urinary retention.

Additional Situation Not Presented in Text

Mr. Chester Monroe is a 57-year-old who is admitted to the oncology unit for pain management related to metastatic cancer of the bowel.

1. Mr. Monroe is scheduled to a trial of the patient-controlled analgesic (PCA) therapy using morphine sulfate. When assessing him with regard to pain, the nurse will:
   a. consider that valid pain has an identifiable physical cause
   *b. rely on the patient as the authority on his pain experience
   c. base the assessment on stereotypical pain related to culture
   d. depend on his family for assessment of pain experience

   [NP: AS, CL: KN]

   Rationale: The patient is the authority on his pain experience. The nurse should focus on pain experienced by the patient. Family assessment and cultural aspects are important, but the key component in assessment is the patient's individual experience.

2. In planning interventions for Mr. Monroe and PCA utilizing morphine, the nurse will include all of the following except:
   *a. initiating patient teaching the day before hospital discharge

b. observing the pump device for malfunction or dosage error
c. checking for side effects related to morphine administration
d. assessing dose-effect relationship at one to three hour intervals

[NP: PL, CL: CO]

Rationale: Patient teaching should begin early, particularly since the patient is to be "in charge" of his pain control. The patient needs to be taught all aspects of PCA administration.

3. The nurse will observe for all of the following side effects of morphine except:
 a. constipation
 b. urinary retention
 c. nausea
 *d. mydriasis

[NP: IM, CL: CO]

Rationale: Morphine sulfate causes pupillary constriction due to stimulation of the oculomotor center.

4. The nurse is aware of the potential for drug interaction with morphine and will be cautious when administering:
 a. anti-inflammatory agents
 b. aluminum-containing antacids
 *c. skeletal muscle relaxants
 d. stool softeners

[NP: IM, CL: KN]

Rationale: Concurrent use of skeletal muscle relaxants with morphine can enhance the neuromuscular blocking action.

5. Mr. Monroe says to the nurse, "I'm afraid I will give myself too much medication." The best nursing diagnosis for Mr. Monroe would be:
 a. Impaired Adjustment related to need to control chronic pain
 b. Alteration in Thought Process related to misunderstanding of PCA
 *c. Knowledge Deficit related to pain management using PCA
 d. Powerlessness related to need to rely on the nurse for pain control

[NP: AN, CL: AN]

Rationale: Many of the patient's fears about PCA can be minimized through appropriate patient teaching about PCA.

6. Which of the following statements represents successful patient teaching with regard to morphine administration via PCA?
 *a. "It is better to give more medication at night than in the daytime."
 b. "The nurse said I would be dizzy while walking around and not to worry."
 c. "I don't think this method of pain relief is working; I still have some pain."
 d. "I don't pay much attention to the settings; I let the nurse take care of it."

[NP: EV, CL: AP]

Rationale: Giving less medication during waking hours reduces sedation. Maximizing the dosage during sleeping hours allows for enhanced restful periods.

Review Questions from Text

1. All of the following are opiate partial antagonists except:
 a. palbuphine hydrochloride (Nubain)
 b. butorphanol tatrate (Stadol)
 *c. naloxone hydrochloride (Narcan)

d. pentazocine (Talwin)

[CL: CO]

Rationale: Narcan is an opiate antagonist without an agonist effect.

2. Propoxyphene hydrochloride (Darvon) 65 mg is:
   a. a Schedule II narcotic used for chronic pain
   b. best suited for the suicidal addiction-prone patient
   *c. equivalent to 30 to 45 mg of codeine
   d. recommended for lactating mothers and children

[CL: KN]

Rationale: Propoxyphene hydrochloride 65 mg is equivalent to 30 to 45 mg of codeine.

3. All of the following statements regarding methyl morphine (codeine) are correct except:
   *a. Codeine is contraindicated in patients with high intracranial pressure.
   b. The average adult dosage is 15 to 60 mg four times daily prn.
   c. The drug is classified as a Schedule II controlled substance.
   d. Common side effects include constipation, drowsiness, and nausea.

[CL: CO]

Rationale: Codeine is the analgesic drug of choice for patients with high intracranial pressure.

4. A physiological effect of the opiate kappa receptor is:
   a. dysphoria
   b. respiratory stimulation
   *c. miosis
   d. vasomotor stimulation

[CL: KN]

Rationale: Miosis is an effect of kappa receptor stimulation, while dysphoria and respiratory and vasomotor stimulation are associated with sigma receptors.

5. The endorphin peptides are found in the:
   a. adrenal medulla
   *b. pituitary
   c. stomach
   d. spinal cord

[CL: KN]

Rationale: The endorphin peptides are found in the pituitary gland.

6. All of the following are correct regarding non-opiate narcotics except:
   *a. These drugs stimulate the formation of prostaglandins in inflamed tissue.
   b. Non-opiate agents affect the hypothalamus to lower body temperature.
   c. This type of drug is generally well absorbed from the gastrointestinal tract.
   d. The non-opiate analgesics are metabolized in the liver and excreted in the urine.

[CL: CO]

Rationale: Non-opiate analgesics act peripherally by preventing the formation of prostaglandins in inflamed tissues. This prevents stimulation of pain receptors.

7. The antidote for an overdose of acetaminophen (Tylenol) is:

a. syrup of ipecac
b. sodium bicarbonate
c. haloxone hydrochloride
*d. acetylcysteine

[CL: KN]

Rationale: Acetylcystein (Mucomyst) forms an inactive compound with the reactive metabolite of acetaminophen.

8. Aspirin interacts adversely with all of the following except:
a. corticosteroids
b. pyrazolines
*c. synthetic narcotics
d. sulfonylurea agents

[CL: CO]

Rationale: Aspirin is often combined with synthetic narcotics such as propoxyphene hydrochloride (Darvon).

9. Which of the following statements is correct regarding methadone hydrochloride (Dolophine)?
a. This naturally occurring opiate is used to relieve pain in the terminally ill.
b. Methadone is administered subcutaneously for detoxification and maintenance.
*c. This synthetic opiate is very effective after oral administration.
d. Methadone may be administered five days after MAO inhibitor therapy.

[CL: KN]

Rationale: Methadone is a synthetic opiate which is very effective after oral administration. The oral form is preferred for detoxification, but methadone can be given intramuscularly.

10. All of the following are correct with regard to butorphanol (Stadol) except:
*a. This drug is less potent than morphine when given IM.
b. It is a synthetic opiate agonist-antagonist analgesic.
c. There is less potential for addiction than with morphine.
d. The recommended IM dose is 2 mg every 3 to 4 hours prn.

[CL: CO]

Rationale: Stadol is more potent than morphine sulfate. The opiate antagonistic properties of Stadol reduce the potential for physical addiction.

Additional Review Questions Not Presented in Text

1. Which statement is correct regarding acetylsalicylic acid (aspirin)?
a. Aspirin is one of the most effective narcotic analgesics.
b. This drug has many adverse side effects and can be addictive.
*c. Aspirin can potentiate increased uric acid levels and bleeding times.
d. ASA suppositories are suitable for long-term pain control.

[CL: KN]

Rationale: Aspirin has a potent antiplatelet effect resulting in prolonged bleeding times. This drug also increases uric acid levels.

2. Which statement is correct regarding narcotic agents?
a. Common signs of narcotic toxicity include dilated pupils and agitation.
b. Dosages of oral and parenteral forms of the same drug are interchangeable.
c. Intramuscular injection of narcotics is recommended for cancer patients.
*d. Narcotics interfere with the perception of pain at higher brain centers.

[CL: CO]

Rationale: Narcotics alter the perception of pain and reaction to the pain response.

3. All of the following are advantages of patient-controlled analgesia except:
   a. allows the patient to overcome variations in pharmacodynamic and pharmacokinetic factors
   b. minimizes the time interval between perception of pain and administration of the drug
   c. provides an opportunity for patients to become actively involved in their pain control
   *d. produces continual and complete pain relief during the postoperative recovery period

[CL: CO]

Rationale: Patient-controlled analgesia does not provide complete pain relief, but is successful in minimizing distressing pain.

4. Which of the following statements is correct regarding meperidine HCL (Demerol)?
   a. It is contraindicated in patients less than 14 years of age.
   b. The usual adult dosage is 200 mg every four hours.
   c. The drug may be administered along with MAO inhibitor therapy.
   *d. Meperidine is contraindicated for patients with a head injury.

[CL: KN]

Rationale: Demerol is contraindicated for patients with head injury or increased intracranial pressure.

5. All of the following statements are correct regarding the pain pathways except:
   *a. Nociceptors are efferent fibers which respond to pain stimuli.
   b. Stimulation of myelinated fibers evokes a pricking pain.
   c. Stimulation of unmyelinated fibers evokes a burning pain.
   d. The reticular formation and thalamus are components of pain pathways.

[CL: CO]

Rationale: Nociceptors are afferent fibers which respond to mechanical, thermal, and chemical sensations.

CHAPTER 21: CENTRAL NERVOUS SYSTEM STIMULANTS

Situations from Text

Situation 21-1

Rodney Alterman is a 7-year-old who is exhibiting signs of attention deficit disorder (ADD). The clinic nurse is preparing teaching sessions for Rodney's parents about the disorder and its treatment.

1. Rodney will be started on methylphenidate (Ritalin) 5 mg po. The nurse will instruct the parents to administer the drug:
   a. after each meal
   *b. before breakfast and lunch
   c. after lunch and dinner
   d. before breakfast and retiring

   [NP: IM, CL: AP]

   Rationale: The usual initial dosage for Ritalin, as the treatment for ADD, is 5 mg po before breakfast and lunch.

2. The nurse will plan to include the following when teaching about psychomotor drugs:
   a. Stimulants will always demonstrate therapeutic effects.
   *b. Drug hoidays will be used to evaluate behavioral response.
   c. Habituation will occur in children under the age of 12.
   d. Self-image and learning ability may diminish with drug use.

   [NP: PL, CL: KN]

   Rationale: Usually the drug is given only on school days. Drug holidays are planned to evaluate behavioral response to the agents.

3. In gathering information about Rodney's status in relationship to ADD, the nurse will include the following:
   a. the parents' sexual history
   b. usual eating patterns
   c. parents' future plans for pregnancy
   *d. prenatal and perinatal information

   [NP: AS, CL: KN]

   Rationale: Prenatal, perinatal, and postnatal information should be obtained in order to determine factors contributing to ADD.

4. Due to the adverse effects of Ritalin, the following nursing diagnostic category applies to Rodney:
   *a. Altered Growth and Development
   b. Potential for Infection
   c. Impaired Swallowing
   d. Alteration in Urinary Elimination

   [NP: AN, CL: AP]

   Rationale: Adverse effects of Ritalin use in children include retarded growth and development.

5. In planning patient outcomes, the following goals would be included for Rodney <u>except</u>:
   a. increase attention span
   b. improve physical coordination
   *c. eliminate behavioral problems
   d. enhance peer relationships

[NP: PL, CL: CO]

Rationale: Therapy for children with attention deficit disorders is not a panacea, but usually does improve attention span and coordination and may enhance peer relationships.

6. The nurse will instruct the parents to select the following snack for Rodney:
   a. soft drink
   *b. carob milkshake
   c. chocolate milk
   d. iced tea

   [NP: IM, CL: KN]

   Rationale: Reducing caffeine-containing products may help in controlling hyperactvity and behavioral problems.

Situation 21-2

David Webb is a 46-year-old successful businessman complaining of a tendency to sleep at odd times during the day. A diagnosis of narcolepsy is made, and Mr. Webb is to be started on a trial of amphetamines.

1. The nurse will elicit patient information which will determine contraindications to amphetamine therapy. The following condition applies:
   *a. glaucoma
   b. cataplexy
   c. hypothyroidism
   d. chronic bronchitis

   [NP: AS, CL: CO]

   Rationale: Amphetamine therapy is contraindicated for patients with glaucoma, due to mydriatic effects.

2. Mr. Webb will be started on amphetamine sulfate (Benzedrine) for treatment of narcolepsy. The nurse is aware that the usual dosage of this drug is:
   a. 200 to 250 mg 1/day
   b. 2.5 to 10 mg once a week
   *c. 20 to 60 mg 1/day
   d. 100 to 200 mg every other day

   [NP: AN, CL: KN]

   Rationale: The dosage for Benzedrine as treatment for narcolepsy is 20 to 60 mg 1 pay do. The dosage is age-specific and dependent on severity of the condition.

3. The following data are included in the assessment phase for Mr. Webb:
   *a. neurological baseline
   b. growth and development
   c. diet history
   d. reading and writing ability

   [NP: AS, CL: AP]

   Rationale: For the patient with narcolepsy, the nurse should perform a baseline neurological assessment.

4. The nurse will instruct Mr. Webb to be alert to the following adverse effects of amphetamines <u>except</u>:
   a. depression
   b. headaches
   c. increased motor activity
   *d. rebound bradycardia

[NP: IM, CL: CO]

Rationale: Patients who are taking amphetamines report tachycardia and palpitations. Other effects include depression, headache, and increased motor activity.

5. For Mr. Webb, the following nursing diagnostic category best applies in reaction to the side effects of amphetamine therapy:
   a. Potential Altered Body Temperature
   b. Alteration in Cardiac Output: decreased
   *c. Potential for Alteration in Nutrition
   d. Alteration in Patterns of Urinary Elimination

   [NP: AN, CL: AP]

   Rationale: Anorexia is a frequently reported side effect of amphetamine therapy and represents a potential nutritional problem.

6. Which of the following statements indicates successful teaching with regard to therapy for narcolepsy?
   a. "It does not matter how I take my medicine, as long as I do not skip a dose."
   b. "Since I should not to any office work, I will stay at home and do simple chores."
   *c. "I will plan to go for walks twice a day and vary my daily routine."
   d. "I have decided to do business travel for the company; the air travel will make me feel better."

   [NP: EV, CL: AN]

   Rationale: Patients should be taught to plan a varied and interesting daily schedule and to incorporate recreational activity. They should avoid monotony and routines at home which may be boring. Air travel can precipitate narcolepsy attacks.

Additional Situation Not Presented in Text

Janice Simpson is a 23-year-old who is approximately 150 pounds overweight. She presents with the desire to try medical intervention to lose weight.

1. In assessing Janice, the nurse will include the following important information:
   a. childbearing history
   b. sleep irregularities
   c. previous head trauma
   *d. psychological profile

   [NP: AS, CL: AP]

   Rationale: Assessment of social and psychological profile may reveal insight into the need to overeat.

2. Janice is placed on metamphetamine hydrochloride (Desoxyn) for treatment of obesity. The nurse is aware of the following with regard to Desoxyn:
   *a. The use of this drug for obesity is recommended for only two weeks.
   b. The dosage for administration is 10 to 15 mg po three times a day.
   c. Metamphetamine is best taken at least two hours prior to a meal.
   d. The drug dosage for the oral extended-release tablet is 20 to 30 mg.

   [NP: PL, CL: KN]

   Rationale: The use of metamphetamine for the treatment of obesity is recommended for only two weeks. This type of agent has high abuse potential.

3. In planning patient teaching for Janice, the nurse will include the following information:
   a. eat only two meals a day
   b. take medication after meals

c. record weight monthly
*d. exercise regularly

[NP: PL, CL: KN]

Rationale: Obese patients should be encouraged to exercise daily in addition to decreasing oral intake.

4. The nurse is aware that an important aspect of control of obesity involves a structured routine. The following intervention is vital:
   a. Establish an ideal weight loss goal.
   *b. Offer verbal encouragement.
   c. Plan monthly diet and drug checks.
   d. Set up a standardized drug schedule.

[NP: IM, CL: KN]

Rationale: An important aspect of successful treatment of obesity involves close nurse-patient contact and the provision of verbal support and encouragement.

5. During the evaluation phase, the nurse will include all of the following except:
   a. evaluates for signs such as paranoia and psychosis
   b. reviews teaching and patient treatment goals
   *c. expects long-term results with drug therapy
   d. observes for indications of noncompliance

[NP: EV, CL: CO]

Rationale: The patient and the nurse should not expect long-lasting results with drug therapy alone.

6. With regard to the side effects of Desoxyn, the following would be the most appropriate nursing diagnosis category for Janice:
   a. Altered Growth and Development
   b. Self-Care Deficit
   *c. Sleep Pattern Disturbance
   d. Ineffective Thermoregulation

[NP: AN, CL: AP]

Rationale: For patients taking CNS stimulants, insomnia is a common adverse effect. For this reason, patients should not take the drug up to six hours before the hour of sleep.

Review Questions from Text

1. Central nervous system stimulants produce their pharmacological action by:
   a. decreasing the effect of excitatory neurotransmission
   b. increasing or stimulating inhibitory neurotransmission
   c. enhancing the uptake of catecholamines at adrenergic synapses
   *d. modifying neurotransmitter response by altering cAMP

[CL: KN]

Rationale: One way in which CNS stimulants produce their action is to modify the neurotransmitter response by altering cAMP.

2. The reason for decreased therapeutic use of CNS stimulants is that:
   a. the extremely long duration of action potentiates adverse side effects
   b. more powerful drugs are now used for reversal of CNS depression
   c. the use of these stimulating drugs remains highly controversial
   *d. they are ineffective in reducing pharmacologically induced CNS depression

[CL: KN]

Rationale: Because CNS stimulants are nonspecific antagonists of depressant drugs, they are not effective in reducing pharmacologically induced CNS depression.

3. Analeptic stimulants produce the following adverse effect:
   a. hypercapnea
   *b. clonic-tonic seizures
   c. reduced respirations
   d. severe hypotension

[CL: KN]

Rationale: An adverse effect of analeptic stimulants is the production of clonic-toxic seizures.

4. Doxapram is contraindicated in the following patient condition:
   a. postanesthesia respiratory depression
   b. chronic pulmonary disease
   *c. cerebral vascular accident
   d. drug-induced CNS depression

[CL: KN]

Rationale: Doxapram is contraindicated in patients who are experiencing stimulation of the CNS, such as those with cerebral vascular accidents.

5. The following statement is correct with regard to drug interactions with amphetamines:
   *a. Acetazolamide increases the amphetamine effect by altering renal excretion.
   b. Amphetamines used with quanethidine results in severe hypertension.
   c. The use of phenothiazines causes an exaggerated amphetamine response.
   d. Tricyclic antidepressants decrease the effects of amphetamines.

[CL: CO]

Rationale: The concurrent use of amphetamines and acetazolamine results in an increased amphetamine effect. This is due to the production of an alkaline urine by acetazolamine which inhibits renal excretion of amphetamines.

6. The combined effect of cocaine used with anticholinergic agents results in:
   *a. hypertension and tachycardia
   b. drowsiness and apnea
   c. sweating and nausea
   d. confusion and memory loss

[CL: KN]

Rationale: Using anticholinergic agents with cocaine results in hypertension and tachycardia.

7. Caffeine produces all of the following actions except:
   a. exerts a positive chronotropic effect
   b. stimulates pepsin secretion
   *c. depresses the cerebral cortex
   d. decreases reabsorption of sodium

[CL: CO]

Rationale: Caffeine stimulates the cerebral cortex, reducing fatigue.

8. Important nursing measures when caring for the patient taking cloxapram include:

a. checking for bradycardia
*b. assessing deep tendon reflexes
c. noting skin turgor and hydration
d. palpating peripheral pulses

[CL: AP]

Rationale: The adverse effects of doxapram include increased deep tendon reflexes. Altered deep tendon reflexes may indicate overdose and should be reported immediately.

9. Which of the following statements is correct regarding the use of amphetamines?
a. The overall effect of these drugs on the bladder is sphincter dilation.
b. These drugs stimulate bronchoconstriction and reduced secretions.
c. Amphetamines enhance the sense of smell and taste.
*d. Amphetamines cause respiratory stimulation and mydriasis.

[CL: KN]

Rationale: The overall effect of CNS stimulants is respiratory stimulation and mydriasis, in addition to bronchodilation, loss of taste and smell, and contraction of the urinary bladder sphincter.

Additional Review Questions Not Presented in Text

1. The mechanism of action of caffeine is to:
a. stimulate the release of phosphodiesterase
b. depress the reticular activing system
c. block the action of adenosine
*d. produce increased levels of cAMP

[CL: KN]

Rationale: Caffeine interferes with the enzyme phosphodiesterase, which degrades cAMP, resulting in increased cAMP levels.

2. When administering analeptic drugs to patients with respiratory depression, all of the following actions are included except:
a. check airway and make initial respiratory assessment
b. check arterial blood gases to monitor effectiveness
*c. increase the dosage if hypotension or dyspnea develops
d. institute seizure precautions to maintain patient safety

[CL: CO]

Rationale: If hypotension or dyspnea develops while administering analeptic drugs for respiratory depression, discontinue the infusion.

3. When educating the patient about the implications of caffeine use, the nurse will stress the following:
a. The use of caffeine is not considered to be in the abused drug category.
b. Evidence supports the development of tolerance to the CNS effects of caffeine.
c. Caffeine can be discontinued abruptly without any adverse effects.
*d. Caffeine should not be abruptly stopped in patients who exhibit side effects.

[CL: CO]

Rationale: In order to reduce the effects of withdrawal from caffeine, the patient should be taught to gradually reduce consumption before discontinuation.

4. When following patients who are taking pemoline (Cylert), the following should be checked routinely:
*a. liver function

b. hematocrit
c. sodium and potassium
d. stools for occult blood

[CL: AP]

Rationale: Liver enzymes have been shown to be elevated in patients on pemoline. If evidence of impaired hepatic function occurs, the drug should be discontinued.

CHAPTER 22: UTILIZATION OF ANTICONVULSANTS

Situations from Text

Situation 22-1

Randall Johnson, a 16-year-old, is admitted to the intensive care unit with clonic/tonic seizures. He has a history of a head injury due to a childhood accident. Because he had no evidence of seizures, Randall stopped taking phenytoin (Dilantin) over a year ago.

1. Randall is to receive a loading dose of phenytoin intravenously. The nurse will administer the drug at the following rate:
   a. 100 mg/minute
   b. 20 mg/minute
   *c. 50 mg/minute
   d. 5 mg/minute

   [NP: IM, CL: KN]

   Rationale: Phenytoin should be given slowly at a rate of 50 mg/minute via the intravenous route.

2. When giving the loading dose intravenously, the nurse will observe Randall closely for:
   a. allergic reaction
   b. apnea
   *c. hypotension
   d. anuria

   [NP: IM, CL: KN]

   Rationale: Phenytoin can cause hypotension when given intravenously.

3. Two days later, the serum Dilantin level for Randall is 12 μg/ml. He is on dosage schedule of 100 mg IV every 8 hours. The nurse will expect to:
   *a. continue the dosage as ordered
   b. decrease the daily dosage
   c. hold the drug until further orders
   d. increase the daily dosage

   [NP: EV, CL: AP]

   Rationale: The therapeutic range for serum phenytoin (Dilantin) is 10 to 20 μg/ml; therefore, the nurse will anticipate continuing the dosage as ordered.

4. In the event that Randall has continuous seizures (status epilepticus), the nurse will be prepared to administer:
   a. clonazepam (Klonopin)
   b. carbamazepine (Tegretol)
   c. phenacemide (Phenurone)
   *d. diazepam (Valium)

   [NP: PL, CL: CO]

   Rationale: The standard drug of choice for status epilepticus is diazepam (Valium).

5. Randall is to be discharged home on a maintenance dosage of Dilantin 100 mg PO tid. When performing patient teaching, the nurse will include the following information:
   a. Take the medication on an empty stomach.
   b. Discontinue the drug immediately if side effects occur.
   *c. Maintain a good oral hygiene program.

d. Use any over-the-counter medications as needed.

[NP: IM, CL: KN]

Rationale: Due to the side effect of gingival hyperplasia related to Dilantin therapy, patients should be taught to perform good oral hygiene.

6. Related to the endocrine effects of phenytoin, the nurse will plan to observe for the following:
   a. hypoglycemia
   *b. glycosuria
   c. hypercalcemia
   d. hyperkalemia

[NP: AS, CL: KN]

Rationale: Glycosuria is a secondary endocrine effect of phenytoin, due to the inhibition of insulin secretion.

Situation 22-2

Marvel Carson is a 38-year-old who has a history of simple partial seizures. She is admitted to the medical floor for evaluation because of increased symptoms.

1. Ms. Carson has been on phenobarbital for control of partial seizures. The expected therapeutic serum concentration of phenobarbital is:
   *a. 10 to 25 μg/ml
   b. 15 to 30 μg/ml
   c. 25 to 50 μgml
   d. 30 to 60 μg/ml

[NP: EV, CL: KN]

Rationale: For therapeutic results, a serum concentration of 10 to 25 μg/ml is recommended.

2. When giving phenobarbital, the nurse will be aware of the following major adverse effect:
   a. tachycardia
   b. diarrhea
   c. photophobia
   *d. drowsiness

[NP: IM, CL: CO]

Rationale: The major side effects of phenobarbital relate to neurotoxicity.

3. A realistic outcome for Ms. Carson would include:
   *a. control of partial seizures
   b. absence of drug side effects
   c. elimination of seizure medications
   d. cure of the cause of seizures

[NP: PL, CL: KN]

Rationale: Control of partial seizures is an example of an outcome or goal for patients on anticonvulsants.

4. In planning interventions for Ms. Carson related to phenobarbital administration, the nurse may include all of the following <u>except</u>:
   a. opening capsules and mixing with food
   b. shaking suspensions well before giving orally
   *c. drawing trough levels after drug distribution
   d. implementing seizure and safety precautions

[NP: IM, CL: CO]

Rationale: Trough levels are obtained prior to administration to determine if the minimum effective serum concentration is present.

5. Ms. Carson continues to have simple partial seizures despite phenobarbital therapy, and carbamazepine (Tegretol) is to be started. The nurse will anticipate:
   *a. reducing the phenobarbital in order to prevent interactions.
   b. discontinuing the phenobarbital in order to prevent interactions
   c. administering diazepam prior to discontinuing phenobarbital
   d. discontinuing the phenobarbital, but observing for withdrawal

   [NP: PL, CL: AP]

   Rationale: To reduce the risk of status epilepticus, the phenobarbital should be reduced gradually before discontinuing.

6. Concerning Tegretol administration, the nurse will monitor the following lab result:
   a. calcium
   *b. sodium
   c. magnesium
   d. potassium

   [NP: IM, CL: CO]

   Rationale: Tegretol affects the secretion of ADH, causing a decrease in serum osmolality and sodium levels.

<u>**Additional Situation Not Presented in Text**</u>

Carol Simmons is a 4-year-old recently diagnosed with absence seizures. She has cerebral palsy and has been cared for at home by her mother.

1. Carol is admitted to the medical unit for seizure control. During the assessment phase, the following applies:
   *a. Documentation of behaviors after a seizure is helpful in diagnosis.
   b. Nurse's approval of the treatment plan is critical.
   c. Information must be obtained only from the patient.
   d. The nurse-patient relationship has no effect upon seizure management.

   [NP: AS, CL: CO]

   Rationale: Behaviors which occur around the time of a seizure may aid the physician in diagnosing the type of seizure.

2. Carol is started on a trial of valproic acid (Depakene). Before administering this drug, the nurse will note a baseline for:
   a. thyroid studies
   *b. liver function
   c. cardiac status
   d. renal sufficiency

   [NP: AS CL: AP]

   Rationale: Hepatotoxicity is a common reaction to valproic acid therapy and baseline liver function should be obtained.

3. A nursing action which should be included in managing Carol's seizures with valproic acid would be to monitor:
   a. ionized calcium
   b. T_4 levels
   c. serum osmolarity
   *d. bleeding time

[NP: IM, CL: CO]

Rationale: Reactions related to valproic acid include inhibition of the secondary phase of platelet aggregation, resulting in altered bleeding times.

4. The nurse will expect to give valproic acid by the following route:
   *a. oral
   b. subcutaneous
   c. intramuscular
   d. intravenous

   [NP: PL, CL: KN]

   Rationale: Valproic acid is only administered via the oral route.

5. Carol's mother will be taught to observe and report the following side effect related to valproic acid:
   a. hiccups
   b. increased salivation
   c. agitation
   *d. vomiting

   [NP: IM, CL: KN]

   Rationale: Gastrointestinal disturbances are the most commonly occurring side effects related to valproic acid.

6. To help ensure compliance to the anticonvulsant therapy, the nurse will stress:
   a. stopping the medication if seizures are no longer observed
   b. encouraging Carol to manage her own medication schedule
   *c. reporting the occurrence of a sore throat, fever, or bruising
   d. contacting the physician once a year for a routine check-up

   [NP: IM, CL: AP]

   Rationale: It will be important for Carol and her mother to report symptoms such as a sore throat, fever, or bruising, indicating hematologic dysfunction. At 4 years of age, Carol is too young to be completely responsible for taking the medications as prescribed.

Review Questions from Text

1. An agent which blocks enkephalinergic-induced seizures is:
   a. clonazepam
   b. phenobarbital
   c. diazepam
   *d. valproic acid

   [CL: KN]

   Rationale: Valproic acid is an anticonvulsant drug which blocks enkephalinergic-induced seizures. The enkephalinergic system is thought to be involved in absence epilepsy.

2. Close monitoring during the labor of women on phenobarbital therapy is important because of the potential for:
   a. toxicity
   *b. hemorrhage
   c. withdrawal symptoms
   d. febrile seizures

   [CL: KN]

   Rationale: Depression of clotting factors occurs with pregnant women on primidone, phenobarbital, or phenytoin, resulting in a potential for hemorrhage.

3. Primidone (Mysoline) is similar in chemical composition to the following drug:
   a. phenytoin
   *b. phenobarbital
   c. methadone
   d. diazepam

   [CL: KN]

   Rationale: Primidone is similar in chemical composition to phenobarbital.

4. Which of the following statements is correct with regard to the interaction of phenytoin (Dilantin) and other agents?
   a. Corticosteroid metabolism is decreased when administered with phenytoin.
   b. Isoniazid action inhibits phenytoin, resulting in low serum levels.
   *c. Phenytoin serum levels increase when administered with nifedipine.
   d. Alcohol use with phenytoin results in an enhanced anticonvulsant effect.

   [CL: KN]

   Rationale: Drugs, such as nifedipine, which work by enzyme inhibition increase serum phenytoin levels.

5. Which of the following is a characteristic of phenobarbital?
   a. Phenobarbital is useful in the control of absence seizures.
   *b. Phenobarbital should not be given to comatose patients.
   c. A decrease in drug level occurs with propoxyphene.
   d. The dosage should be increased in the elderly patient.

   [CL: KN]

   Rationale: Due to CNS depression, phenobarbital should not be given to comatose patients.

6. Phenytoin is indicated in the following cardiac-related disorder:
   a. sinus bradycardia
   b second degree A-V block
   c. Stokes-Adams syndrome
   *d. digitalis-induced arrhythmias

   [CL: KN]

   Rationale: Phenytoin has been shown to be useful in controlling arrhythmias related to digoxin toxicity.

7. Carbamazepine (Tegretol) acts by:
   a. increasing the threshhold for neuronal firing
   b. decreasing the discharge of nonadrenergic neurons
   *c. reducing polysynaptic responses
   d. decreasing the influx of calcium during depolarization

   [CL: KN]

   Rationale: Tegretol acts by blocking the post-tetanic potentiation and by reducing polysynaptic responses.

8. An agent which may be used to control myoclonic seizures is:
   a. acetazolamide (Diamox)
   b. ethosuximide (Zarontin)
   *c. clonazepam (Klonopin)
   d. mephenytoin (Mesantoin)

   [CL: CO]

   Rationale: Clonozepam (Klonopin) has been shown to be useful in controlling myclonic seizures.

9. Which of the following plays a major role in the pharmacokinetics of the benzodiazepines?
   a. availability of glutamate
   b. percentage of extracellular water
   c. degree of plasma acidity
   *d. extent of lipid solubility

   [CL: CO]

   Rationale: Lipid solubility plays a major role in the rate at which benzodiazepines enter the central nervous system. Drugs with greater lipid solubility have a faster onset of action.

Additional Review Questions Not Presented in Text

1. The benzodiazepines should be used with caution in patients with:
   a. cardiac dysrhythmias
   *b. narrow-angle glaucoma
   c. myoclonic seizures
   d. leukopenia

   [CL: KN]

   Rationale: Effects of the benzodiazepines include pupillary dilation and increased intraocular pressure; therefore, these drugs are used with caution in patients with narrow-angle glaucoma.

2. For an intravenous drip, diazepam is prepared in the following way:
   a. 100 mg diluted in 250 ml of 5 percent dextrose
   b. 25 mg diluted in 250 ml of normal saline
   *c. 100 mg diluted in 500 ml of 5 percent dextrose
   d. 50 mg diluted in 100 cc of normal saline

   [CL: KN]

   Rationale: For an intravenous drip, diazepam is prepared by diluting 100 mg in 500 ml of 5 percent dextrose and given at a rate of 40 ml/hour.

3. The usual adult therapeutic levels for carbamazepine (Tegretol) are:
   a. 10 to 20 μg/ml
   b. 15 to 30 μg/ml
   c. 20 to 45 μg/ml
   *d. 4 to 12 μg/ml

   [CL: KN]

   Rationale: Therapeutic levels for carbamazepine (Tegretol) range from 4 to 12 μg/ml.

4. A reported side effect of clonazepam (Klonopin) is:
   *a. increase in salivation
   b. hiccups
   c. photophobia
   d. tachypnea

   [CL: KN]

   Rationale: Effects such as increase in salivation and respiratory depression have been reported with clonazepam use.

CHAPTER 23: SKELETAL MUSCLE RELAXANTS AND DRUG THERAPY FOR SPECIFIC DISORDERS OF THE NERVOUS SYSTEM

Situations from Text

Situation 23-1

Edmond Meyer is a 63-year-old recently diagnosed with Parkinson's disease. His condition is being managed on an outpatient basis.

1. The clinic nurse obtains a patient history and reviews Mr. Meyer's symptoms. He describes shakiness and an inability to hold items "steady." He complains that his neck and shoulders are stiff. The nurse is aware that these symptoms relate to:
*a. excitatory effect of the cholinergic system
b. stimulation of excess dopamine at nerve junctions
c. build-up of toxic substances in the substantia nigra
d. lack of acetylcholine for neurotransmission

[NP: AS, CL: AP]

Rationale: The tremors and rigidity of Parkinson's disease relate to the excitatory effect of the cholinergic system.

2. Mr. Meyer is to begin trihexyphenidyl (Artane) 1 mg daily PO. Prior to administration, the nurse will assess for the following condition, which contraindicates its use:
a. diarrhea
b. excessive salivation
c. peptic ulcer
*d. tachycardia

[NP: AS, CL: CO]

Rationale: The use of anticholinergics is contraindicated in patients with tachycardia.

3. In teaching Mr. Meyer about the drug trihexyphenidyl (Artane), the nurse will stress avoiding the concurrent use of:
a. aspirin compounds
*b. antihistamines
c. antacids
d. acetaminophen

[NP: IM, CL: KN]

Rationale: Antihistamines give additive anticholinergic effects.

4. In addition to trihexyphenidyl, Mr. Meyer will begin taking Sinemet 25/100 po tid. The nurse will include the following when teaching about the drug:
a. The drug will eliminate symptoms related to Parkinson's disease.
*b. Long-term therapy with this agent may cause movement disturbances.
c. The patient should take this drug along with a high-protein meal.
d. A multivitamin supplement will help in providing necessary B-vitamins.

[NP: IM, CL: CO]

Rationale: Long-term therapy with levodopa agents may produce adverse effects such as abnormal involuntary movements, akinetic spells, and behavioral disturbances.

5. The concurrent use of trihexyphenidyl and Sinemet can help to alleviate Mr. Meyer's parkinsonian symptoms. However, the nurse is aware of a potential for altered absorption of Sinemet, due to the following effect of

trihexyphenidyl (Artane):
a. reduced lipid solubility
b. enhanced first-pass effect
c. rapid intestinal motility
*d. delayed gastric emptying

[NP: AN, CL: CO]

Rationale: Trihexyphenidyl delays gastric emptying, thereby delaying absorption of Sinemet.

6. When formulating the care plan for Mr. Meyer, the nurse will observe for the following adverse reaction related to therapy with Sinemet:
*a. cardiac dysrhythmias
b. hypertensive crisis
c. constipation
d. photophobia

[NP: PL, CL: KN]

Rationale: Cardiac dysrhythmias are common cardiovascular effects of Sinemet therapy.

Situation 23-2

Debra Paddington, a 45-year-old, is admitted to the medical intensive care unit for evaluation and treatment of myasthenia gravis.

1. During the assessment, the nurse finds which of the following to be an indication of myasthenia gravis?
a. tremor and dyskinesia with intentional movement
*b. weakness which improves with rest
c. complete paralysis of the lower extremities
d. spasticity of large skeletal muscle groups

[NP: AS, CL: KN]

Rationale: Myasthenia gravis is characterized by muscle weakness which becomes severe with activity and improves with rest.

2. Ms. Paddington is scheduled for a Tensilon test. Edrophonium (Tensilon) is administered intravenously by the physician. The nurse will expect the onset of action to be:
a. 10 minutes
*b. 30 to 60 seconds
c. 2 to 4 minutes
d. 5 seconds

[NP: Pl, CL: KN]

Rationale: The onset of action of edrophonium is 30 to 60 seconds.

3. Close monitoring of Ms. Paddington is important during the Tensilon test. The nurse will observe for the following:
*a. bradycardia
b. dry cough
c. sore throat
d. sedation

[NP: IM, CL: AP]

Rationale: When giving an anticholinesterase, the build-up of acetylcholine may cause bradycardia and decreased cardiac output.

4. The diagnosis of myasthenia is confirmed, and Ms. Paddington is started on pyridostigmine (Mestinon) orally. The nurse will be alert to the following adverse effect of Mestinon:
   a. constipation
   b. urinary retention
   *c. diarrhea
   d. dry mouth

   [NP: IM, CL: KN]

   Rationale: Adverse effects of Mestinon include those due to stimulation of cholinergic receptors, such as diarrhea, nausea, and vomiting.

5. In preparing Ms. Paddington for discharge, all of the following as clinically significant will be stressed effects <u>except</u>:
   *a. worsening of symptoms
   b. delayed therapeutic response
   c. chemically-induced hypoglycemia
   d. poor skin turgor

   [NP: PL, CL: AP]

   Rationale: With higher doses of corticosteroids, a period of "early worsening" of the signs and symptoms of myasthenia will occur. And, although the patient may notice this, it is not usually cause for concern.

Additional Situations Not Presented in Text

Jonathan McBride is a 40-year-old with multiple sclerosis. Due to increasing muscle spasticity, he is being placed on a trial of dantrolene sodium (Dantrium).

1. The nurse will note the following baseline information before administering dantrolene sodium:
   a. thyroid studies
   *b. liver function
   c. creatinine clearance
   d. lipid profile

   [NP: AS, CL: AP]

   Rationale: Due to the potential of dantrolene to cause drug-induced hepatitis, patients should have baseline liver function studies.

2. Additional information which may need to be evaluated prior to administration of dantrolene is:
   *a. muscle strength
   b. mental status
   c. cardiac status
   d. bowel and bladder function

   [NP: AS, CL: CO]

   Rationale: Dantrolene sodium does produce muscle weakness and should be used with caution in patients with muscular weakness.

3. Assessment reveals that Mr. McBride is to be started on dantrolene as planned. The nurse is aware that the usual initial dosage is:
   a. 100 mg daily
   b. 75 mg tid
   c. 10 mg bID
   *d. 25 mg daily

   [NP: PL, CL: KN]

Rationale: Dantrolene is started at 25 mg daily and increased to around 400 mg per day.

4. When teaching Mr. McBride about the effects of dantrolene, the following is stressed:
   a. Refrain from activities which involve alertness.
   *b. Report symptoms such as nausea and vomiting to physician.
   c. Take the medication as needed for pain related to spasms.
   d. Avoid milk products within an hour of the oral dosage.

   [NP: IM, CL: KN]

   Rationale: The patient should report signs such as nausea and vomiting, which may indicate drug-induced hepatitis.

5. To evaluate effectiveness of treatment with dantrolene sodium, the nurse is aware of the following:
   a. Symptoms such as drowsiness and dizziness are very common.
   *b. Therapy is discontinued if no response in 45 days.
   c. The drug acts by depressing the central nervous system response.
   d. Studies have shown the drug to be ineffective for painful spasms.

   [NP: EV, CL: KN]

   Rationale: If no observable positive effect is noted within 45 days of treatment, the drug should be discontinued.

6. The nurse overhears Mr. McBride tell his wife that the medication will prevent worsening of his multiple sclerosis. An appropriate nursing diagnosis for Mr. McBride would be:
   a. Impaired Adjustment related to chronic disease status
   b. Alteration in Thought Process related to side effects of dantrolene
   *c. Knowledge Deficit related to the action and use of dantrolene
   d. Impaired Verbal Communication related to implications of medical management

   [NP: AN, CL: AN]

   Rationale: Mr. McBride demonstrates a lack of understanding about the use and action of dantrolene. Further patient teaching is indicated.

Review Questions from Text

1. The management of Parkinson's disease is primarily accomplished by:
   a. reducing the dyskinesias through central skeletal muscle relaxants
   b. inhibiting the excitatory action of dopamine at neuron junctions
   *c. restoring dopamine levels in the central nervous system
   d. stimulating cholinergic activity through the use of dopaminergic drugs

   [CL: CO]

   Rationale: Control of symptoms related to Parkinson's disease is dependent primarily on restoring dopamine levels in the brain.

2. Cortical-adrenal autologous transplantation has been performed as a treatment for patients with:
   a. multiple sclerosis
   *b. Parkinson's disease
   c. myasthenia gravis
   d. Huntington's chorea

   [CL: KN]

   Rationale: The surgical procedure involving transplantation of autologous adrenal cortex tissue to the basal ganglia is performed to treat Parkinson's disease. The adrenal tissue contains dopamine cells which restore dopaminergic function.

3. The rationale for administering carbidopa with levodopa is that:
*a. carbidopa inhibits the breakdown of levodopa in the peripheral tissue
b. levodopa reduces the CNS side effects of carbidopa
c. the drug combination enhances the uptake of pyroxidine for muscular control
d. carbidopa counteracts the muscarinic effects of levodopa

[CL: CO]

Rationale: Carbidopa inhibits the peripheral breakdown of levodopa, thereby increasing the amount which crosses the blood-brain barrier for conversion to dopamine.

4. Central skeletal muscle relaxants are <u>most</u> effective in relieving muscle spasm caused by:
a. multiple sclerosis
b. cerebral palsy
c. pain receptor stimulation
*d. inflammation or trauma

[CL: KN]

Rationale: Muscle spasms of local origin caused by inflammation or trauma are best treated by central skeletal muscle relaxants.

5. Which of the following is an example of a direct-acting skeletal muscle relaxant?
a. diazepam (Valium)
b. methocarbamol (Robaxin)
*c. dantrolene sodium (Dantrium)
d. carisoprodol (Soma)

[CL: KN]

Rationale: Dantrolene sodium (Dantrium) acts directly on skeletal muscle to produce relaxation.

6. Which of the following drugs should not be used for patients with myasthenia gravis?
*a. antihistamines
b. corticosteroids
c. cytotoxic agents
d. carbamates

[CL: KN]

Rationale: Antihistamines have anticholinergic properties which worsen myasthenia symptoms.

7. In patients with the neuromuscular disorder myasthenia gravis:
a. nerve impulses are not present at the neuromuscular junction
b. destruction of dopaminergic receptors occurs, altering voluntary motor control
*c. reduced availability of receptor sites for acetylcholine results in motor weakness
d. excess acetylcholine stimulates extrapyramidal tracts, creating dyskinesias

[CL: CO]

Rationale: In myasthenia gravis, receptor sites for acetylcholine are blocked by antibody complexes, reducing the nerve impulses generating muscle contraction.

8. Patients on levodopa who demonstrate the "on/off" phenomenon may benefit from:
a. increased levodopa dosages
b. corticosteroid therapy
*c. amantadine therapy
d. antihistamine therapy

[CL: KN]

Rationale: Amantadine therapy may prove useful in controlling the "on/off" phenomenon associated with long-term levodopa therapy.

9. An initial adverse effect of bromocriptine is:
   *a. cardiovascular collapse
   b. erythromelalgra
   c. end-of-dose failure
   d. mottled skin

   [CL: CO]

   Rationale: Patients taking bromocriptine may demonstrate a "first-dose phenomenon" manifested by sudden cardiovascular collapse.

<u>**Additional Review Questions Not Presented in Text**</u>

1. Anticholinesterase drugs used to treat myasthenia gravis:
   a. are well absorbed from the gastrointestinal tract
   *b. lead to cholinergic crisis if given in excess
   c. stimulate the breakdown of acetylcholine
   d. produce tolerance and an end-of-dose failure

   [CL: CO]

   Rationale: If given in excess, anticholinesterase drugs can lead to a build-up of acetylcholine, potentiating a cholinergic crisis.

2. Diuretics are not recommended for patients with myasthenia due to:
   *a. the potential for hypokalemia
   b. inhibition of acetylcholine
   c. weakness caused by frequent urination
   d. additive cholinergic effects

   [CL: KN]

   Rationale: Diuretics potentiate hypokalemia, which causes muscle weakness and complicates the clinical picture in patients with myasthenia.

3. Amantadine hydrochloride (Symmetrel) has all of the following characteristics <u>except</u>:
   a. It is an antiviral agent.
   b. The drug crosses the blood-brain barrier.
   *c. Excretion is increased in an alkaline urine.
   d. Onset of action after an oral dose is 15 minutes.

   [CL: CO]

   Rationale: Symmetrel excretion is increased in an acidic urine.

4. Dopaminergic agents, such as levodopa, are contraindicated in the following condition:
   *a. melanoma
   b. cerebral vascular accident
   c. paralysis agitans
   d. pyrexia

   [CL: KN]

   Rationale: Levodopa stimulates the growth of skin melanomas; therefore, patients with a history of melanoma should not be given levodopa.

CHAPTER 24: SEDATIVES AND HYPNOTICS

Situations from Text

Situation 24-1

Julia Abad has been seen in the clinic frequently for difficulty sleeping after a traumatic event. She is 26 years old and is currently in counseling. In addition to insomnia, she complains of feeling "panicked" when in crowded situations.

1. Ms. Abad is to begin treatment with alprazolam (Xanax) 0.5 mg po three times a day. The clinic nurse will focus on the following during the assessment stage:
   *a. response to phobic situations
   b. physiological symptoms only
   c. response to counseling
   d. psychological symptoms only

   [NP: AS, CL: AP]

   Rationale: During the assessment, it is important for the nurse to determine the physical as well as psychological symptoms that the patient is experiencing. The nurse should focus on the response to the anxiety as the core of the illness.

2. The nurse will include the following when teaching Ms. Abad about the use of anxiolytic therapy:
   a. Discontinue if symptoms of drowsiness appear.
   *b. Refrain from alcohol consumption.
   c. Increase dosage at night if unable to sleep.
   d. Take the medication as needed for anxiety.

   [NP: IM, CL: KN]

   Rationale: Alcohol enhances the effect of the anxiolytic agent and should not be used in combination.

3. Ms. Abad is concerned about the types of side effects that she may experience while taking alprazolam. The following effect applies to this agent:
   a. epilepsy
   *b. slurred speech
   c. exfoliative dermatitis
   d. photophobia

   [NP: IM, CL: CO]

   Rationale: A common adverse reaction associated with this agent is slurred speech. Other neurological effects include dizziness and confusion.

4. On a follow-up visit one week later, Ms. Abad states that she is sleeping at night now, but does not feel "rested." The nurse is aware that this probably relates to reduction in:
   a. Stage I sleep
   b. Stage II sleep
   c. Stage III sleep
   *d. REM sleep

   [NP: AN, CL: AP]

   Rationale: Patients taking anxiolytic agents may spend less time in REM sleep, resulting in continued altered sleep patterns and a sense of not sleeping well.

5. A response by Ms. Abad that reflects adequate learning about alprazolam therapy would be:

a. "This drug will keep me from having panic attacks in public."
b. "I should limit my fluid intake to prevent swelling."
*c. "It would be best for me to quit smoking to receive optimal benefits."
d. "This drug will not cause addiction, so I can take it indefinitely."

[NP: EV, CL: AP]

Rationale: Cigarette smoking may decrease the effectiveness of the benzodiazepine by enhancing its metabolism.

6. In planning follow-up care, the nurse will stress that Ms. Abad should not abruptly stop taking alprazolam because of the potential for:
*a. seizures
b. headaches
c. dermatitis
d. rebound tachycardia

[NP: IM, CL: KN]

Rationale: Because alprazolam clears the system rapidly, abruptly stopping the drug may result in seizures.

Situation 24-2

Karen Smith is a 70-year-old who is admitted to the surgical floor for left breast biopsy.

1. During the assessment, Ms. Smith reveals that her mother died of breast cancer. Ms. Smith is withdrawn and tense. The nurse notes that respiration, pulse, and blood pressure are elevated in comparison to admission vital signs. The nurse suspects that Ms. Smith is experiencing which of the following levels of anxiety:
a. mild
b. panic
c. moderate
*d. severe

[NP: AS, CL: AP]

Rationale: Patients with severe levels of anxiety will demonstrate physiologic responses such as increased respirations, pulse, and blood pressure.

2. The nurse informs the physician regarding signs of anxiety. After an examination of Ms. Smith, the physician orders diazepam (Valium) 5 mg q 4 hours prn anxiety. As the initial dose, the nurse is to give 5 mg intramuscularly. The nurse will plan to give the drug in the following IM site:
a. dorsofluteal
*b. deltoid
c. ventrogluteal
d. vastus lateralis

[NP: PL, CL: KN]

Rationale: When diazepam is to be given intramuscularly, the deltoid muscle provides rapid and complete absorption.

3. Of the following outcomes, which indicates successful therapy in Ms. Smith's situation?
a. decreased interaction with family and friends
b. enhanced focusing on mother's death
*c. decreased respirations, pulse, and blood pressure
d. denial of feelings of relaxation and well-being

[NP: EV, CL: AP]

Rationale: In this situation, a measurable outcome of anxiolytic therapy is reduction of blood pressure, respirations, and pulse to preanxiety levels.

4. In planning nursing care for Ms. Smith, the nurse will include the following intervention:
   a. withholding the diazepam if patient appears calm
   b. providing a stimulating environment for distraction
   c. questioning the patient at length concerning feelings
   *d. monitoring for unusual signs of excitement

   [NP: PL, CL: CO]

   Rationale: Unusual excitement may indicate a paradoxic reaction, which may occur with benzodiazepines, especially in elderly patients.

5. A nursing responsibility associated with the care of Ms. Smith includes:
   *a. encourage oral fluids
   b. limit all visitors
   c. restrict music
   d. encourage solitude and reflection

   [NP: IM, CL: AN]

   Rationale: Due to the potential for dry mouth and constipation associated with diazepam therapy, patients should be encouraged to maintain adequate hydration.

6. When evaluating Ms. Smith after several days of diazepam therapy, the nurse is aware of the possibility for the following laboratory result:
   a. reduced albumin
   b. elevated creatinine
   *c. elevated bilirubin
   d. reduced platelets

   [NP: EV, CL: KN]

   Rationale: Benzodiazepines may elevate bilirubin levels. Patient evaluation should include monitoring this laboratory result.

<u>**Additional Situation Not Presented in Text**</u>

Jacob Warner is a 55-year-old postoperative bowel resection on the medical-surgical unit. He has a gastrostomy tube to low intermittment suction, is receiving intravenous fluids, and is NPO.

1. Postoperative orders include secobarbital (Sconal) 100 mg IM HS prn sleep, which Mr. Warner requests. The nurse will anticipate the desired effect within:
   *a. 15 minutes
   b. 90 minutes
   c. 45 minutes
   d. one hour

   [NP: PL, CL: KN]

   Rationale: As a short-acting barbiturate, secobarbital promotes sleepiness within 10 to 15 minutes.

2. The nurse will be alert to the potential for a paradoxical reaction with patients on barbiturates, as manifested by:
   a. sore throat
   b. drowsiness
   *c. hostility
   d. angioneurotic edema

   [NP: IM, CL: KN]

   Rationale: Paradoxical reactions may be seen; symptoms include hostility, confusion, and excitement.

3. When planning appropriate nursing interventions for Mr. Warner, the nurse will include:
   *a. observing for evidence of dreaming
   b. withholding sleeping medication if he is calm
   c. placing him on standard suicide precautions
   d. restraining wrists to prevent pulling of tubes

   [NP: PL, CL: CO]

   Rationale: Patients taking barbiturates should be monitored during and after sleep for evidence of dreaming, indicating REM sleep.

4. On the fourth postoperative day, Mr. Warner is able to take liquids and is switched to secobarbital orally. Important assessment data pertaining to this medication would be:
   a. type of diet
   b. discharge plans
   c. number of visitors
   *d. suicide potential

   [NP: AS, CL: AP]

   Rationale: The nurse should assess the patient's potential for suicide if the patient is taking barbiturate drugs.

5. For discharge, Mr. Warner requests a mild sleeping pill "just in case" he needs it. The physician prescribes chloral hydrate (Noctec) HS prn. The expected dosage range would be:
   a. 250 mg to 2 gms
   *b. 500 mg to 1 gm
   c. 50 mg/kg
   d. 8.3 mg/kg

   [NP: AN, CL: KN]

   Rationale: The usual adult dosage as a hypnotic agent is 500 mg to 1 gm daily HS.

6. When teaching Mr. Warner about proper administration, the nurse will stress:
   a. taking pulse rate daily before each dose
   *b. drinking a full glass of water with each dose
   c. withholding the medication if patient feels drowsy
   d. breaking the capsules before taking each dose

   [NP: IM, CL: KN]

   Rationale: An adverse effect of chloral hydrate is gastritis. This can be reduced by ensuring that each dose is taken with at least a full glass of water.

<u>Review Questions from Text</u>

1. An example of a drug that produces relaxation of skeletal muscles is:
   a. alprazolam (Xanax)
   *b. diazepam (Valium)
   c. meprobamate (Equanil)
   d. talbutal (Lotusate)

   [CL: CO]

   Rationale: In addition to promoting sleep and reducing anxiety and tension, diazepam produces skeletal muscle relaxation.

2. Anxiolytic drugs, such as benzodiazepines, have the following effect:
   *a. potentiate effects of other CNS depressants

b. produce little dependence when given as recommended
c. are associated with gastritis when given with meals
d. are absorbed slowly when given orally

[CL: CO]

Rationale: When benzodiazepines are combined with other CNS depressants, the result is increased CNS depression.

3. With regard to the absorption and fate of barbiturates, the drugs are:
a. used safely for two months without dependence
*b. absorbed through the colon and may be given rectally
c. used safely during pregnancy and lactation
d. excreted as active metabolites via the kidney

[CL: KN]

Rationale: In addition to oral absorption, barbiturates are absorbed through the colon and may be given rectally.

4. Barbiturates would be the drug of choice for:
a. pain
*b. anxiety reaction
c. hepatic encephalopathy
d. paradoxical reaction

[CL: CO]

Rationale: Barbiturates are useful for daytime management of anxiety. These agents should not be used for the patient in pain because they increase the reaction to painful stimuli.

5. When comparing the use of barbiturates with that of benzodiazepines, the following is correct:
a. Benzodiazepines cause more dermatitis than barbiturates.
b. Barbiturates are more economical than benzodiazepines.
c. Barbiturates cause less drowsiness than benzodiazepines.
*d. Benzodiazepines are less addicting than barbiturates.

[CL: CO]

Rationale: The barbiturates have an even greater potential for dependency than the benzodiazepines.

6. Chlordiazepoxide (Librium) is:
a. absorbed rapidly by the intramuscular route
b. known to have no accumulative effects
*c. used as a treatment for alcohol withdrawal
d. known to be useful for situational anxiety

[CL: KN]

Rationale: Because of the prolonged half-life, chloridazepoxide (Librium) is useful in patients with alcohol withdrawal.

7. A sedative/hypnotic associated with a high degree of memory impairment is:
a. chlorazepate dipotassium (Tranxene)
b. chloral hydrate (Noctec)
c. oxazepam (Serax)
*d. triazolam (Halcion)

[CL: KN]

Rationale: Memory impairment has been very frequently reported by patients taking triazolam (Halcion).

8. All benzodiazepines are contraindicated if the following condition exists:
   *a. coma
   b. senile agitation
   c. alcohol withdrawal
   d. psychosomatic disorders

   [CL: KN]

   Rationale: Because of central nervous system depression, benzodiazepines are contraindicated in comatose patients.

9. Colorful dreams and nightmares may take place during which sleep stage?
   a. Stage III
   b. Stage II
   *c. REM
   d. Stage IV

   [CL: KN]

   Rationale: During REM sleep, colorful dreams and nightmares take place.

Additional Review Questions Not Presented in Text

1. A possible result of benzodiazepine drug interaction would be:
   *a. blocked therapeutic response of levodopa
   b. inhibited phenytoin response
   c. facilitated biotransformation of cimetidine
   d. reduced CNS effect with tricyclic antidepressants

   [CL: KN]

   Rationale: Benzodiazepines may block the therapeutic response of levodopa and should be avoided in patients with Parkinson's disease.

2. The greatest percentage of rapid eye movement (REM) sleep occurs in the:
   a. adolescent
   b. older adult
   c. toddler
   *d. newborn

   [CL: KN]

   Rationale: The newborn experiences a high percentage (50 percent) of REM sleep during the sleep cycle.

3. An example of an intermediate-acting barbiturate is:
   a. pentobarbital (Nembutal)
   *b. amobarbital (Amytal)
   c. phenobarbital (Luminal)
   d. secobarbital (Sconal)

   [CL: KN]

   Rationale: Intermediate-acting barbiturates such as amobarbital (Amytal) have a duration of six to eight hours and act within 45 to 60 minutes.

4. Essential to understanding the therapeutic use of sedatives or hypnotics is that these drugs:
   a. alter factors causing the need for such agents
   b. eliminate feelings of distress
   *c. aid in symptomatic relief

d. produce a cure for anxiety reactions

[CL: KN]

Rationale: Hypnotics and sedatives alleviate symptoms of anxiety or sleep problems, but do not provide a cure.

CHAPTER 25: ANTIPSYCHOTIC MEDICATIONS

Situations from Text

Situation 25-1

Patty Lawson, a 22-year-old with a history of nonspecific psychiatric disorders, is admitted to the acute psychiatric unit after disrupting the peace and demonstrating delusional ideations.

1. Patty is disoriented, fearing that she is being followed and persecuted. She requires restraints and attempts to bite an orderly. It will be important for the nurse to perform the following:
   a. Question the patient about her feelings concerning drug therapy.
   b. Wait until the patient has calmed down before doing any type of assessment.
   *c. Formulate a list of symptoms which the patient is exhibiting.
   d. Demonstrate aggressive, forceful behavior in order to control the patient.

   [NP: AS, CL: AP]

   Rationale: It may be difficult to question the patient about her history or her feelings at this time. It will be important for the nurse to list the symptoms which the patient is exhibiting to be used as a baseline for evaluation of drug therapy.

2. Patty is to receive chlorpromazine (Thorazine) IM as a loading dose for acute agitation. The nurse is aware that the usual range for the loading dose is:
   a. 60 to 400 mg/day
   *b. 400 to 1500 mg/day
   c. 50 to 100 mg/day
   d. 20 to 80 mg/day

   [NP: PL, CL: KN]

   Rationale: The intramuscular loading dose for Thorazine is 400 to 1500 mg/day.

3. When the nurse administers Thorazine to Patty, the following approach is appropriate:
   a. Talk with the patient in order to distract her.
   *b. Demonstrate a kind but firm approach.
   c. Ask the patient at what site she would like the injection.
   d. Demonstrate an ability to read her mind.

   [NP: IM, CL: KN]

   Rationale: The best approach with psychotically ill patients is to be kind, firm, and positive. It is best not to have the patient make any decisions at this time or carry on lengthy conversations.

4. The nurse will expect the onset of action of intramuscular Thorazine to be:
   a. 2 to 3 hours
   b. 5 to 10 minutes
   *c. 30 minutes
   d. 1 hour

   [NP: PL, CL: KN]

   Rationale: The predicted onset of action for intramuscular Thorazine is 30 minutes.

5. An expected early side effect of the antipsychotic in this case would be:
   a. secondary anxiety reaction
   b. diaphoresis
   *c. sedation

d. hypothermia

[NP: EV, CL: CO]

Rationale: In the early period of drug therapy, sedation is the predominant side effect.

6. Which of the following behaviors would indicate an expected positive response to the antipsychotic medication after two days of therapy?
   a. return to premorbid level of functioning
   b. absence of delusions
   c. decreased attention span
   *d. increased socialization

[NP: EV, CL: CO]

Rationale: After two days from the initial dose, the nurse can anticipate increased socialization.

Situation 25-2

Ryan David, a 45-year-old, has a long-term history of schizophrenia and frequent readmissions to the acute psychiatric unit. He is currently admitted for a trial with new drug therapy.

1. Mr. David is scheduled to receive thiothixene (Navane). The nurse is aware that the usual route of administration of this drug is:
   a. intravenous
   b. oral
   c. subcutaneous
   *d. intramuscular

[NP: PL, CL: KN]

Rationale: Thiothixene is available only in intramuscular forms.

2. When administering this antipsychotic medication to Mr. David, the nurse includes all of the following <u>except</u>:
   a. changing the needle after filling the syringe with medication
   b. injecting the medication deeply into the muscle tissue
   *c. mixing the drug with an antiemetic to reduce side effects
   d. massaging the site following injection to promote absorption

[NP: PL, CL: KN]

Rationale: Antipsychotic agents are often incompatible with other injectable drugs and should be administered separately.

3. The nurse will include the following when teaching Mr. David about his medication regimen:
   a. The drugs are highly addictive and require withdrawal sedation.
   *b. Most psychotic reactions will recur unless he follows the treatment plan.
   c. Side effects such as sedation are rationale for stopping the drug.
   d. As he begins to feel better with the drug, he may be able to stop counseling.

[NP: IM, CL: CO]

Rationale: Patients need to understand that they must adhere to long-term therapeutic measures despite feelings of well-being. Most psychotic reactions will recur unless patients follow the treatment schedule.

4. The nurse will plan to promptly report the following symptom related to neuroleptic therapy:
   a. mild rash
   b. dry mouth
   *c. sore throat

d. photosensitivity

[NP: PL, CL: CO]

Rationale: Symptoms such as a sore throat may be related to problems of agranulocytosis and should be reported immediately.

5. After three weeks of therapy, Mr. David complains of difficulty chewing and swallowing food. The nurse informs the physicians and is aware that these symptoms relate to:
   a. excessive anticholinergic effects of neuroleptics
   *b. extrapyramidal reactions of neuroleptic agents
   c. manifestations of oculogyric crisis
   d. psychotic effects of schizophrenia

   [NP: EV, CL: AP]

   Rationale: Difficulty swallowing and chewing food may indicate extrapyramidal side effects related to neuroleptic therapy.

6. Should Mr. David experience right upper quadrant pain, jaundice, and clay-colored stools, the nurse will plan to:
   a. provide fresh air and exercise
   b. continue the neuroleptic at a reduced dosage
   *c. encourage a high protein/carbohydrate diet
   d. place an n/g tube for enteral feedings

   [NP: PL, CL: CO]

   Rationale: Symptoms described are related to cholestatic jaundice. The treatment for this condition includes discontinuing the neuroleptic drug, providing bedrest, and encouraging a high protein, carbohydrate diet.

Additional Situation Not Presented in Text

Jordan Oshner is a 68-year-old with symptoms related to increasing depression since the loss of his wife six months ago. He is withdrawn and despondent. Currently Mr. Oshner lives with his son and daughter-in-law.

1. Plans are made to provide counseling twice a week and to begin thioridazine (Mellaril). The nurse is aware that the loading dose is:
   a. 50 to 100 mg/day
   *b. 400 to 800 mg/day
   c. 20 to 600 mg/day
   d. 20 to 100 mg/day

   [NP: PL, CL: KN]

   Rationale: The loading dose of Mellaril is 400 to 800 mg per day.

2. The nurse will provide patient and family teaching about thioridazine. The following information will be stressed:
   a. Discontinue the drug if symptoms of dizziness and drowsiness occur.
   b. Take the medication with an antacid to reduce gastric distress.
   *c. Use a sunscreen and wear protective clothing when out in the sun.
   d. Take an extra pill at night if agitation or restlessness occurs after a dosage.

   [NP: IM, CL: KN]

   Rationale: Due to the side effect of photosensitivity, patients should wear a sunscreen and protective clothing when out in the sun.

3. Mr. Oshner and his family will be instructed to promptly report the following:
   ***a. heart rate over 120 bpm**

b. drowsiness
c. cold sensitivity
d. increased appetite

[NP: IM, CL: AP]

Rationale: An increased heart rate may relate to serious conditions which may occur as a result of neuroleptic agents, for example, neuroleptic malignant syndrome.

4. Mr. Oshner is to be on a maintenance dose of Mellaril 50 mg twice a day. The nurse will instruct the family and patient that the span of time after which a dosage is missed and should not be taken is:
   a. 2 hours
   b. 24 hours
   c. 18 hours
   *d. 8 hours

   [NP: IM, CL: CO]

   Rationale: If a dosage is missed on a twice-a-day schedule of neuroleptics and then remembered after eight hours, the missed dose should not be taken.

5. Related to the strong anticholinergic effects of thioridazine, the following nursing diagnostic category would be applicable in Mr. Oshner's case:
   *a. Potential for Infection: urinary tract
   b. Altered Growth and Development
   c. Alteration in Bowel Elimination: diarrhea
   d. Noncompliance

   [NP: AN, CL: AN]

   Rationale: Anticholinergic effects such as urinary retention place the elderly patient at greater risk for urinary tract infection.

6. A complication for which the nurse will observe related to high doses of Mellaril is manifested in the following symptom:
   a. strong extrapyramidal effects
   b. inability to sit down
   *c. brownish coloration of the vision
   d. clay-colored stools

   [NP: IM, CL: KN]

   Rationale: Pigmentary retinopathy occurs with the use of thioridazine in daily dosages of 800 mg or more. An early symptom related to this condition is a brownish coloration to the vision.

Review Questions from Text

1. Which of the following statements is correct regarding absorption and fate of oral neuroleptics?
   a. Oral concentrates are mixed with 4 ounces of pineapple juice before administration.
   b. Rate of absorption is increased if given concurrently with antacids.
   *c. Most oral concentrates are well absorbed from the gastrointestinal tract.
   d. Criteria for oral dosage is dependent on therapeutic serum levels.

   [CL: KN]

   Rationale: Most oral concentrates are well absorbed from the gastrointestinal tract. Metabolism and biodegradation of antipsychotic drugs are highly variable; therefore, therapeutic serum concentrations have not been established.

2. The antipsychotic drugs have proven to be effective in:

*a. controlling symptoms
b. reducing side effects
c. producing a sense of euphoria
d. preventing psychosis

[CL: KN]

Rationale: While antipsychotic agents are not curative, they have been shown to be effective in controlling symptoms.

3. Which of the following statements is correct regarding elimination of antipsychotic agents?
   a. The drugs are highly distributed in the extracellular fluid compartments.
   b. Most of the agents have a short half-life which is less than 24 hours.
   c. Hemo-dialysis or peritoneal dialysis is the suggested method for treating overdose.
   *d. When discontinued, the drugs may continue to be released from the tissues.

[CL: CO]

Rationale: Antipsychotic drugs are highly lipophilic and are stored in fatty tissues. After the drugs are discontinued, they are slowly released by the tissues and excreted.

4. Cholinergic sites, which are blocked by neuroleptic drugs, produce the following effect:
   a. akathesia
   *b. impaired memory
   c. rigidity
   d. tongue thrusts

[CL: KN]

Rationale: Impaired memory is likely to be produced by blockage of cholinergic sites within the brain.

5. Tardive dyskinesia, a syndrome associated with antipsychotic drugs, is most likely caused by:
   a. cholinergic receptor blockade
   *b. dopamine receptor blockade
   c. short-term drug use
   d. subtherapeutic drug levels

[CL: CO]

Rationale: Tardive dyskinesia is thought to be linked to dopamine receptor blockade, which is the same mechanism responsible for the positive effects of neuroleptic agents.

6. Which of the following descriptions is correct concerning the extrapyramidal side effects of antipsychotic medications?
   a. Akathisia is characterized by a shuffling gait.
   b. Acute dystonic reactions are characterized by puffing the cheeks.
   *c. Pseudoparkinsonism is characterized by motor retardation.
   d. Tardive dyskinesia is characterized by difficulty sitting still.

[CL: KN]

Rationale: A characteristic of pseudoparkinsonism is motor retardation.

7. Haloperidol is contraindicated in patients with:
   *a. Parkinson's disease
   b. severe anxiety reaction
   c. senile dementia
   d. Alzheimer's disease

[CL: KN]

Rationale: Patients with Parkinson's disease may demonstrate worsened symptoms when they take haloperidol.

8. Which of the following drugs is classified as an aliphatic phenothiazine?
   a. trifluoperazine (Stelazine)
   b. thioridazine (Mellaril)
   c. fluphenazine (Prolixin)
   *d. chloropromazine (Thorazine)

   [CL: KN]

   Rationale: Chloropromazine (Thorazine) is classified as an aliphatic, a subgroup of the phenothiazines.

9. Which of the following statements is correct with regard to drug interactions with antipsychotics?
   a. Amphetamines decrease the effects of neuroleptics.
   *b. Alcohol prolongs the effect of neuroleptics.
   c. Neuroleptics prolong the effects of epinephrine.
   d. Antimuscarinics prolong plasma levels of neuroleptics.

   [CL: CO]

   Rationale: Alcohol potentiates and prolongs the effects of antipsychotic medications. For this reason, patients taking neuroleptic agents should avoid alcohol.

Additional Review Questions Not Presented in Text

1. An unwanted autonomic nervous system side effect manifested by orthostatic hypotension is due to:
   a. nicotinic receptor blockage
   *b. alpha-adrenoreceptor blockade
   c. dopamine receptor blockage
   d. tuberoinfundibular tract blockade

   [CL: KN]

   Rationale: Orthostatic hypotension related to antipsychotic drugs is a result of alpha-adrenergic blockade.

2. Patients who are taking an anticonvulsant medication and an antipsychotic medication concurrently may need to:
   a. reduce the dosage of the anticonvulsant
   b. gradually discontinue the anticonvulsant
   *c. increase the dosage of the anticonvulsant
   d. increase the dosage of the antipsychotic

   [CL: KN]

   Rationale: Since neuroleptic drugs lower seizure threshholds, patients on anticonvulsant therapy tend to require higher doses to prevent seizures.

3. The neuroleptic drug of choice for cardiac patients is:
   *a. haloperidol (Haldol)
   b. chlorpromazine (Thorazine)
   c. thioridazine (Mellaril)
   d. promazine (Sparine)

   [CL: KN]

   Rationale: Haldol is the neuroleptic drug of choice for cardiac patients, due to the low incidence of anticholinergic effects.

4. When high doses of phenothiazines are discontinued suddenly, nausea and vomiting frequently occur. A possible cause of these symptoms is:

a. dopaminergic stimulation
b. extrapyramidal stimulation
*c. cholinergic rebound
d. dopaminergic rebound

[CL: KN]

Rationale: Gastrointestinal symptoms associated with discontinuation of high doses of phenothiazines are thought to be caused by cholinergic rebound.

CHAPTER 26: MEDICATIONS FOR MOOD DISORDERS

Situations from Text

Situation 26-1

Emma Ravy, a 33-year-old with recurrent depression, is an outpatient in the county mental health clinic. She is a single mother of three small children and has been unable to maintain a job for the past year.

1. Ms. Ravy is to begin psychotherapy and medication therapy with imipramine (Tofranil). During the assessment, the nurse will pay particular attention to:
   *a. suicidal ideation
   b. ages of her children
   c. verbal expression
   d. occupational factors

   [NP: AS, CL: AP]

   Rationale: Depressed patients are particularly prone to suicide. The nurse needs to be aware of cues, both verbal and nonverbal, which indicate suicidal tendencies.

2. The nurse is aware that the following manifestation is indicative of a major depressive episode:
   a. pressured speech
   b. feelings of omnipotence
   *c. decreased energy
   d. impulsive behavior

   [NP: AS, CL: KN]

   Rationale: Behavior which indicates major depression includes decreased energy and loss of interest in activities.

3. Ms. Ravy is to begin taking imipramine 100 mg orally at night. Prior to administering this agent, the nurse will check for which of the following, which represents a contraindication to use?
   a. history of dysmenorrhea
   *b. evidence of breastfeeding
   c. history of diabetes mellitus
   d. presence of pulmonary disease

   [NP: AS, CL: CO]

   Rationale: Nursing mothers should not take imipramine because it is excreted in the breast milk in low concentrations.

4. The nurse will teach Ms. Ravy to avoid taking her daily dosage with:
   *a. orange juice
   b. milk
   c. coffee
   d. water

   [NP: IM, CL: AP]

   Rationale: Tricyclic antidepressives should not be taken with substances containing ascorbic acid, which causes decreased effectiveness.

5. Which of the following would be included in patient teaching regarding imipramine therapy?
   a. Take the drug as needed for depression.
   b. Expect beneficial results within 2 days.
   c. Use a strong antiseptic mouthwash.
   *d. Avoid driving motor vehicles.

[NP: IM, CL: CO]

Rationale: Side effects such as sedation and drowsiness are common; therefore, the patient should avoid driving or operating machinery.

6. When evaluating Ms. Ravy at a return check-up, which of the following behaviors represents successful treatment?
   a. flight of ideas
   b. decreased response to pain
   c. sensitivity to criticism
   *d. attention to personal hygiene

   [NP: EV, CL: KN]

   Rationale: Evidence of successful treatment of depression includes demonstration of interest in personal appearance.

Situation 26-2

Herbert Voss is a 46-year-old with a long history of severe depression and anxiety. He is currently a patient in the chronic unit of a mental hospital. After various tricyclic antidepressant agents have proven to be ineffective alone, Mr. Voss is to begin treatment with isocarboxazid (Marplan). He is currently taking amoxapine (Asendin) 200 mg daily.

1. Before beginning therapy with isocarboxazid, the nurse will expect to:
   a. withhold all medications for at least 24 hours
   *b. maintain a low monoamine diet for 1 to 2 weeks
   c. keep patient NPO for 12 hours
   d. restrict fluid intake to 1000 cc per day for 1 week

   [NP: PL, CL: CO]

   Rationale: Due to the potential for drug interactions, the patient should be maintained on a low monoamine diet for 1 to 2 weeks prior to isocarboxazid therapy.

2. Mr. Voss is to begin isocarboxazid 30 mg po HS daily. The nurse will observe for the following during initial therapy:
   a. weight loss
   *b. orthostatic hypotention
   c. difficulty urinating
   d. increased salivation

   [NP: IM, CL: KN]

   Rationale: A common adverse reaction to isocarboxazid therapy is orthostatic hypotension. This side effect is less pronounced as therapy continues.

3. Evidence of toxic effects which would indicate altering the dosage of isocarboxazid therapy includes:
   *a. headache
   b. impotence
   c. bradycardia
   d. diarrhea

   [NP: EV, CL: CO]

   Rationale: Toxic symptoms related to overdose include neurological symptoms such as headache or confusion.

4. The addition of isocarboxazid to Mr. Voss' present medication regime may result in:
   a. reduced effect of isocarboxazid
   *b. increased effect of amoxapine

c. increased effect of isocarboxazid
d. reduced effect of amoxapine

[NP: AN, CL: AP]

Rationale: An increased effect of amoxapine may be seen with the addition of an MAO inhiabitor drug.

5. With regard to food and drug interactions involving isocarboxazid, Mr. Voss is at risk for:
   a. septic shock
   b. bradycardia
   *c. hypertensive crisis
   d. urticaria bullosa

   [NP: AN, CL: KN]

   Rationale: A hypertensive crisis can arise after contraindicated food or medication is taken. Hypertension is the result of supranormal release or catecholamine stores.

6. When teaching Mr. Voss about dietary restrictions related to isocarboxazid therapy, the nurse will stress eliminating:
   a. oranges
   b. chicken
   c. eggs
   *d. cheese

   [NP: IM,CL: KN]

   Rationale: The patient taking an MAO inhibitor needs to avoid foods high in tyramine, such as cheeses, red wines, and smoked meats.

Additional Situation Not Presented in Text

Shelby Minor, a 29-year-old medical student, is admitted by his parents to the acute unit a of psychiatric center. An initial diagnosis of an acute manic episode is made.

1. Which of the following symptoms correlates with an acute manic episode?
   *a. lack of judgment
   b. somnolence
   c. withdrawn reaction
   d. self-deprecation

   [NP: AS, CL: KN]

   Rationale: Symptoms related to an acute manic episode include demonstration of a lack of judgment in personal and financial matters.

2. A loading dose of lithium carbonate 1800 mg is ordered to be given orally. Prior to initiating therapy, the nurse will include the following in baseline data:
   a. total serum protein
   b. protein electrophoresis
   c. chest x-ray
   *d. T_3, T_4

   [NP: AS, CL: CO]

   Rationale: Thyroid function studies, including T_3, T_4, need to be obtained prior to initiating therapy with lithium, due to the potential for hypothyroidism.

3. A nursing responsibility associated with caring for Mr. Minor is to:

a. evaluate patient response according to laboratory data
*b. monitor fluid and electrolyte balance
c. schedule blood lithium levels in the evening
d. provide a stimulating atmosphere

[NP: IM, CL: KN]

Rationale: The patient should be monitored for electrolyte and fluid imbalances which might alter lithium effectiveness or potentiate toxicity.

4. When teaching Mr. Minor and his family about the necessary diet restrictions, the nurse will stress that he must avoid:
a. protein
*b. coffee
c. salt
d. cheese

[NP: IM, CL: KN]

Rationale: Caffeine reduces lithium levels by increasing renal excretion. The patient should avoid coffee and caffeine products.

5. Included in evaluating effective lithium treatment is obtaining serum lithium concentrations. Laboratory data for Mr. Minor reveal a serum concentration of 1.2 mEq/L. The nurse is aware that this represents a:
a. severe toxicity
b. subtherapeutic level
*c. therapeutic level
d. moderate toxicity

[NP: EV, CL: AP]

Rationale: For acute manic episodes, a lithium serum concentration of 0.8 to 1.2 mEq/L represents a therapeutic level.

6. Mr. Minor complains of a fine hand tremor occurring a day after lithium is started. The nurse's best action would be to:
*a. assure him that this usually subsides
b. administer a sedative agent as ordered
c. hold the lithium until the tremor subsides
d. administer an anticholinergic drug as ordered

[NP: IM, CL: AP]

Rationale: Initial side effects such as a fine hand tremor usually subside after the first few weeks.

Review Questions from Text

1. The action of tricyclic antidepressants is thought to be achieved by:
a. increasing storage sites of acetylcholine for presynaptic nerves
b. reducing the levels of dopamine available for receptor transmission
*c. prolonging the presence of norepinephrine within the nerve synapses
d. inactivating serotonin production at the neurotransmitter site

[CL: CO]

Rationale: Although the action of antidepressants is not completely understood, they are thought to act by regulating the processes which inactivate norepinephrine and serotonin. This results in prolonging the presence of norepinephrine (and serotonin) within the nerve synapses.

2. Antidepressant drugs are widely distributed because they are predominantly:

a. inactive metabolites
*b. lipid-soluble
c. ionized
d. unbound

[CL: KN]

Rationale: Antidepressants are highly lipid-soluble and are extensively distributed throughout body tissue.

3. Which of the following is a common anticholinergic symptom associated with antidepressants?
a. dysrhythmias
b. photophobia
*c. blurred vision
d. diarrhea

[CL: KN]

Rationale: Anticholinergic symptoms associated with antidepressants include blurred vision, dry mouth, constipation, and urinary hesitancy.

4. An example of a monoamine oxidase (MAO) inhibitor is:
a. trimipramine maleate
b. doxepin hydrochloride
*c. phenelzine sulfate
d. zimelidine

[CL: KN]

Rationale: Phenelzine sulfate is an example of a monoamine oxidase (MAO) inhibitor).

5. MAO inhibitors should be given cautiously to patients with the following condition:
*a. pheochromocytoma
b. asthma
c. reverse vegetative symptoms
d. severe anxiety

[CL: KN]

Rationale: MAO inhibitors are contraindicated in conditions for which increasing circulating sympathomimetic amines would be deleterious, such as pheochromocytoma.

6. Which of the following statements is <u>correct</u> with regard to drug interactions with tricyclic antidepressants?
a. A decreased effectiveness of antidepressants is seen when given with phenothiazines.
b. Ammonium chloride increases the effect of tricyclic antidepressants.
*c. Sodium bicarbonate increases the effect of tricyclic antidepressants.
d. A decreased effectiveness of antidepressants is seen when given with acetazolamide.

[CL: CO]

Rationale: The effectiveness of tricyclic antidepressants is enhanced when given with sodium bicarbonate.

7. A symptom of severe lithium toxicity is:
*a. hyperreflexia
b. vertigo
c. polydipsia
d. muscle weakness

[CL: KN]

Rationale: Signs/symptoms of severe lithium toxicity include hyperreflexia, stupor, or seizures.

8. Which of the following narcotic agents would be contraindicated for patients on MAO inhibitors?
   a. hydromorphone
   *b. meperidine
   c. morphine
   d. codeine

   [CL: KN]

   Rationale: A potentially life-threatening interaction exists between meperidine (Demerol) and MAO inhibitors; therefore, the drugs should not be administered together.

9. Some diagnostic tests are altered by tricyclic antidepressants. Which of the following represents a correct example?
   a. reduced serum bilirubin
   b. increased VMA excretion
   c. reduced excretion of catecholamines
   *d. increased blood glucose

   [CL: CO]

   Rationale: Tricyclic antidepressants may increase blood glucose levels.

10. Lithium exerts its therapeutic action by:
   a. stimulating the production of dopamine in the substantia nigra
   *b. reducing the release of norepinephrine from synaptic vesicles
   c. inhibiting the breakdown of serotonin at the postsynaptic junction
   d. decreasing the reuptake of norepinephrine by synaptosomes

   [CL: KN]

   Rationale: Lithium is thought to act by reducing the release of norepinephrine and increasing its reuptake. This results in a dampened effect at the synaptic junction.

Additional Review Questions Not Presented in Text

1. Patients taking MAO inhibitors should be taught to recognize and report symptoms of hypertensive crisis, which include:
   a. pinpoint pupils
   *b. neck stiffness
   c. drowsiness
   d. dizziness

   [CL: CO]

   Rationale: Symptoms related to hypertensive crisis include neck stiffness, occipital headache, nausea, vomiting, palpitations, and sweating.

2. Which of the following statements is correct regarding cyclic antidepressant overdose?
   a. Hemodialysis is effective in the treatment of cyclic antidepressant overdose.
   b. Symptoms of cyclic antidepressant overdose are limited to cardiovascular effects.
   c. Drugs such as atropine are indicated in cyclic antidepressant overdose.
   *d. Exchange transfusions are ineffective in the treatment of cyclic antidepressant overdose.

   [CL: KN]

   Rationale: Exchange transfusions and hemodialysis are ineffective in treating cyclic antidepressant overdose, due to the extensive tissue distribution of the drug. Atropine is contraindicated for cyclic antidepressant overdose because of synergistic effects.

3. Psychomotor stimulants such as methamphetamine are:

a. classified as Schedule I drugs
b. used to prevent rebound depression
c. found to be effective for major depression
*d. used as secondary agents to treat depression

[CL: CO]

Rationale: Psychomotor stimulants have been used as adjunctive therapy for depression. However, since they tend to potentiate addiction and rebound depression, their therapeutic use is controversial in most depressive states.

4. Doxepin (Sinequan) liquid is incompatible with:
a. fruit juice
*b. cola
c. milk
d. tea

[CL: CO]

Rationale: Doxepin liquid should not be diluted with carbonated beverages because of incompatibility.

CHAPTER 27: OVERVIEW OF ANATOMY AND PHYSIOLOGY OF THE CARDIOVASCULAR SYSTEM

Review Questions from Text

1. The layer of the heart in which the major blood vessels are located is the:
   a. pericardial sac
   b. epicardium
   *c. myocardium
   d. endocardium

   {CL: KN]

   Rationale: The myocardium is the tissue layer in which the major blood vessels are located.

2. The tricuspid valve lies between the:
   *a. right atrium and right ventricle
   b. right ventricle and pulmonary artery
   c. left atrium and left ventricle
   d. left ventricle and aorta

   [CL: CO]

   Rationale: The tricuspid valve separates the right atrium from the right ventricle.

3. Which of the following statements is correct regarding the action potential curve of the cardiac cell?
   a. During Phase I, a fast influx of potassium ion moves into the cell.
   b. During Phase 4, only a strong stimulus will precipitate an action potential.
   *c. During Phase 2, a slow influx of calcium ions moves into the cell.
   d. During Phase 3, a fast influx of sodium ions moves into the cells.

   [CL: CO]

   Rationale: Phase 2 of the action potential curve is the point at which calcium enters the cell via slow channels.

4. The following description applies to the conduction system of the heart and the EKG pattern:
   a. The P waves reflects atrial repolarization.
   b. The PR interval represents atrial contraction.
   *c. The QRS complex represents ventricular depolarization.
   d. The T wave represents ventricular depolarization.

   [CL: CO]

   Rationale: Ventricular depolarization is represented by the QRS complex on the electrocardiogram.

5. Which of the following pacemaker areas initiates a heart rate of 60 to 40 per minute?
   a. AV node
   b. SA node
   *c. bundle of His
   d. Purkinje fibers

   [CL: CO]

   Rationale: The bundle of His or AV junction initiates a heart rate of 60 to 40 beats per minute. The AV node has no pacemaking cells.

6. Cardiac output is measured by stroke volume and:
   a. preload
   *b. heart rate

c. conductivity
d. elasticity

[CL: KN]

Rationale: Contractility refers to the ability of the heart to generate enough force to eject blood volume at a particular fiber length.

7. The right coronary artery supplies oxygenated blood to the:
   a. SA node in 60 percent of the population
   b. AV node in 10 percent of the population
   c. lateral portion of the left ventrical
   *d. posterior leaflet of the mitral valve

[CL: KN]

Rationale: The right coronary artery supplies the posterior leaflet of the mitral valve.

8. Which of the following statements is correct regarding capillary pressures?
   a. Capillary hydrostatic pressure ranges from 10 mmHg at the arterial end to 30 mmHg at the venous end.
   *b. When capillary hydrostatic pressure is normal and colloid osmotic pressure is low, edema results.
   c. When capillary hydrostatic pressure is normal and colloid osmotic pressure is low, dehydration results.
   d. The higher the colloid osmotic pressure, the higher the gradient of fluid moving into interstitial tissues.

[CL: KN]

Rationale: Capillary filtration increases when capillary hydrostatic pressure is normal and colloid pressure is low, resulting in fluid shifts into the interstitial spaces (edema).

9. Coronary artery perfusion occurs during:
   *a. ventricular diastole
   b. atrial repolarization
   c. ventricular systole
   d. ventricular depolarization

[CL: KN]

Rationale: Approximately 90 percent of coronary artery perfusion occurs during diastole.

Additional Review Questions Not Presented in Text

1. The following represents a normal pressure within the heart:
   a. right atrial pressure of 20/0 mmHg
   *b. right ventricle pressure of 25/5 mmHg
   c. pulmonary artery pressure of 50/20 mmHg
   d. left ventricle pressure of 80/5 mmHg

[CL: CO]

Rationale: The right ventricle generates a pressure of around 25/5 mmHg.

2. The sequence of normal electrical conduction through the heart is:
   a. SA node, bundle branches, AV node, bundle of His, Purkinje fibers
   *b. SA node, AV node, bundle of His, bundle branches, Purkinje fibers
   c. SA node, AV node, bundle branches, Purkinje fibers, bundle of His
   d. SA node, bundle of His, AV node, bundle branches, Purkinje fibers

[CL: CO]

Rationale: Normal electrical conduction through the heart follows the pathway of: SA node, AV node, bundle of His, bundle branches, Purkinje fibers.

3. Atrial tachycardia is characterized by the following:
   a. irregular atrial rate of 100 (+/-50) beats per minute
   b. F waves with a variable atrial rate of 200 (+/-50)
   c. atrial beats which arise from the AV node at a variable rate
   *d. regular atrial rhythm with a rate of 200 (+/-50)

   [CL: KN]

   Rationale: Atrial tachycardia is a fast regular rhythm arising from atrial tissue at a rate of 20 (+/-50) beats per minute.

4. An example of a conduction defect is:
   *a. first degree AV block
   b. atrial tachycardia
   c. ventricular premature beats
   d. sinus bradycardia

   [CL: CO]

   Rationale: Conduction defects occur when the transmission of impulses is somehow altered, as in the case of first degree AV blocks.

5. Which of the following is <u>correct</u> with regard to second degree AV block?
   a. The AV node is unable to conduct an impulse from the SA node.
   b. There are two pacemakers in the heart, each controlling its own rate.
   c. Cardiac output increases in response to greater cardiac demand.
   *d. There are more P waves than QRS complexes on the EKG.

   [CL: KN]

   Rationale: In second degree AV block, not all of the impulses are transmitted through the AV node; therefore, there are more P waves than QRS complexes.

CHAPTER 28: CARDIAC GLYCOSIDES

Situations from Text

Situation 28-1

Juliana Fortham, a 66-year-old, is admitted to the coronary care unit with symptoms of nausea, vomiting, and a heart rate of 43 beats per minute. Medications which Ms. Fortham currently takes include digoxin, Lasix, and a potassium supplement.

1. A diagnosis of digoxin toxicity is made according to serum digoxin concentrations. The nurse is aware of the following:
   a. Digoxin will be decreased slowly to prevent rebound dysrhythmias.
   *b. Acid-base and electrolyte values should be checked.
   c. High doses of potassium will be necessary to restore automaticity.
   d. Cardioversion is the treatment of choice for digoxin toxicity.

   [NP: PL, CL: KN]

   Rationale: Electrolytes and acid-base imbalances are corrected in the case of digoxin toxicity. Potassium may or may not need to be supplemented.

2. Within a few hours, Ms. Fortham begins to have atrial dysrhythmias. Which of the following drugs would be the most appropriate in this situation?
   a. cholestyramine
   b. phenobarbital
   c. Fab fragments
   *d. phenytoin

   [NP: PL, CL: CO]

   Rationale: Atrial dysrhythmias related to digoxin toxicity can be treated with phenytoin (Dilantin).

3. The nurse will check Ms. Fortham's laboratory results for the following condition which would potentiate digoxin toxicity:
   a. hyperkalemia
   b. hyperthyroidism
   c. hypocalcemia
   *d. hypomagnesemia

   [NP: AS, CL: KN]

   Rationale: Hypomagnesemia tends to increase the sensitivity to digitalis preparations.

4. After a few days of close observation, serum digoxin levels are reassessed. The nurse will check for the following therapeutic range of digoxin:
   *a. 0.5 to 2.0 ng/ml
   b. 6 to 10 ng/ml
   c. 2.5 to 4.5 ng/ml
   d. 14 to 26 ng/ml

   [NP: EV, CL: KN]

   Rationale: Therapeutic range of digoxin is 0.5 to 2.0 ng/ml of serum.

5. Ms. Fortham's serum digoxin reflects a therapeutic level, and she is to be discharged on 0.125 mg po daily. Which of the following would be included in patient teaching?
   a. taking the medication in the morning before rising
   *b. monitoring pulse rate daily

c. discontinuing the medication if pulse rate is stable
d. eating a diet high in bran fiber

[NP: IM, CL: AP]

Rationale: It will be very important for the patient to monitor her pulse rate daily and to report a pulse rate <60 or >110 before taking the medication.

6. Ms. Fortham asks the nurse why the digoxin level was high. She states, "I thought my heart was supposed to slow down with the medicine." Which of the following represents the most appropriate nursing diagnosis for Ms. Fortham?
   a. Noncompliance related to failure to report signs and symptoms of digoxin toxicity
   *b. Knowledge Deficit related to understanding of the potential toxic effects of digoxin
   c. Impaired Home Maintenance Management related to inability to take digoxin correctly
   d. Alteration in Thought Processes related to understanding the signs and symptoms of toxicity

   [NP: AN, CL: AN]

   Rationale: Patient education about digoxin administration is critical to preventing toxic manifestations of the drug and expensive hospital costs. The patient in this case demonstrates a lack of understanding concerning the potential for toxic effects.

Situation 28-2

Bob Norman, 49 years old, is recovering from an inferior myocardial infarction. The nurse on duty in the coronary care unit notes a change in rhythm from sinus rhythm to atrial fibrillation, heart rate of 130 bpm.

1. The physician orders a loading dose of digoxin (digitalization). The nurse is aware that the loading dosage is approximately:
   a. .0012 to .0050 mg/kg
   *b. .010 to .020 mg/kg
   c. .5 to 1.0 mg/kg
   d. .25 to 1.0 mg/kg

   [NP: AN, CL: KN]

   Rationale: The loading dose in adults is approximately .010 to .020 mg/kg, administered as three to four equally divided doses over 24 hours.

2. Mr. Norman is complaining of difficulty breathing and weakness. The nurse will expect to administer the digoxin by the following route:
   a. subcutaneous
   b. oral
   c. intramuscular
   *d. intravenous

   [NP: PL, CL: AP]

   Rationale: The usual route of digoxin administration is by intravenous injection if the patient is symptomatic.

3. When giving the digoxin, the nurse will observe for the following potential effect:
   a. hypoglycemia
   b. confusion
   *c. hypertension
   d. seizures

   [NP: IM, CL: CO]

   Rationale: Blood pressure may be increased in patients with limited cardiac reserve who are receiving digoxin by the intravenous route.

4. After successful digitalization, serum levels of digoxin are within a therapeutic range. The maintenance dose will be determined by:
*a. creatinine clearance
b. liver function
c. body weight
d. potassium levels

[NP: AN, CL: CO]

Rationale: Because the primary elimination of digoxin is by renal mechanisms, the maintenance dose is based on creatinine clearance.

5. A nursing responsibility related to the care of Mr. Norman includes:
a. administering digoxin in the deltoid muscle
*b. notifying the physician of a heart rate of 120 bpm
c. relying only on patient assessment for therapeutic response
d. drawing serum levels 10 hours after an oral dose of digoxin

[NP: IM, CL: CO]

Rationale: A rapid pulse may indicate that the patient needs to have the digoxin dosage increased or to have serum levels evaluated.

6. Which of the following statements indicates successful patient teaching concerning digoxin use?
a. "I will only have to take this drug for a month or two, until my heart heals."
*b. "If I miss a dose, I should eliminate it and not take two in one day."
c. "If I have any nausea or vomiting, I should stop taking the medicine."
d. "A little swelling in my feet or ankles is not uncommon with this medicine."

[NP: EV, CL: AN]

Rationale: Patients should be taught not to try to "catch up" on missed dosages by taking two pills in one day. If a dosage is missed, then it should be eliminated.

Additional Situation Not Presented in Text

Gerald Langston is admitted to the intensive care unit in severe congestive heart failure. He is a 76-year-old with a long history of recurrent heart failure. The medications which he takes at home include digoxin, Lasix, Capoten, and Micro-K.

1. During the nursing assessment, the nurse notes that Mr. Langston has no peripheral edema and complains of fatigue, weakness, and shortness of breath during the night. Currently he must sit completely upright in order to breathe. The nurse is aware that these symptoms correspond with which of the following types of heart failure?
a. acute left heart failure
b. acute right heart failure
*c. chronic left heart failure
d. chronic right heart failure

[NP: AS, CL: AP]

Rationale: Symptoms such as fatigue, weakness, and nocturnal dyspnea relate to chronic left side heart failure. Peripheral edema is associated with right side heart failure.

2. Invasive cardiac monitoring lines are placed, and Mr. Langston is to be started on amrinone lactate (Inocor). Prior to administering this agent, the nurse will assess the following:
a. white blood cell count
*b. fluid volume status
c. sodium level

d. neurological function

[NP: AS, CL: CO]

Rationale: Prior to administering amrinone, the patient's fluid volume status should be assessed, particularly those on diuretic therapy.

3. Mr. Langston is to receive a bolus dose of amrinone intravenously. The nurse will prepare to give:
*a. .75 mg/kg
b. .05 mg/kg
c. .025 mg/kg
d. .45 mg/kg

[NP: IM, CL: KN]

Rationale: The initial or bolus dose of amrinone is .75 mg/kg IV given over 2 to 3 minutes.

4. The nurse will mix the intravenous drip of amrinone in the following solution:
a. sterile water
b. Ringer's lactate
c. 5 percent dextrose
*d. normal saline

[NP: PL, CL: KN]

Rationale: Amrinone should be diluted in normal saline for intravenous infusion because the drug reacts with glucose solutions over a 24-hour period.

5. To achieve therapeutic effects, the nurse will plan to maintain the following range of dosages:
a. 2 to 5 mcg/kg/minute
b. .25 to 1 mcg/kg/minute
c. 20 to 25 mcg/kg/minute
*d. 5 to 10 mcg/kg/minute

[NP: PL, CL: KN]

Rationale: The maintenance dosage of amrinone is 5 to 10 mcg/kg/minute.

6. While administering this drug, the nurse will observe for the following side effect, which is related to its use:
a. agitation
b. seizures
*c. dysrhythmias
d. confusion

[NP: IM, CL: CO]

Rationale: A common adverse effect related to amrinone therapy is dysrhythmias; therefore, cardiac monitoring during administration is indicated.

<u>Review Questions from Text</u>

1. As a class of drugs, the cardiac glycosides:
a. are produced from synthetic sources
b. increase the rate of ventricular ejection
c. are effective within a wide therapeutic range
*d. increase the force of cardiac contraction

[CL: KN}

Rationale: Cardiac glycosides are positive inotropic agents, increasing the force of contraction.

2. The overall effect of cardiac glycosides results in:
 a. increased diastolic volume
 b. increased systemic vascular resistance
 *c. reduced cardiac preload
 d. reduced sensitivity to acetylcholine

[CL: CO]

Rationale: Cardiac glycosides increase cardiac output, resulting in a secondary decrease in preload and diastolic volume.

3. The primary site of action by digitalis glycosides is the:
 *a. AV node
 b. SA node
 c. Bundle branches
 d. Purkinje fibers

[CL: KN]

Rationale: The primary site of action by the digitalis glycosides is the AV node.

4. Which of the following statements is correct regarding the effect of cardiac glycosides?
 a. These agents have an indirect effect on the cardiac conduction system.
 *b. Digitalis glycosides have a negative chronotropic effect on the cardiac muscle cells.
 c. The glycosides exert direct action on the heart through the autonomic nervous system.
 d. A greater magnitude of therapeutic effect is seen on the nonfailing heart than on the failing heart.

[CL: KN]

Rationale: By reducing heart rate, digitalis glycosides exert a negative chronotropic effect.

5. All of the following are outcomes associated with digoxin therapy except:
 *a. increased heart size
 b. increased urine output
 c. reduced afterload
 d. increased stroke volume

[CL: CO]

Rationale: In patients with cardiomegaly due to increased workload, digitalis preparations decrease heart size.

6. Which of the following dysrhythmias can be corrected with digitalis preparations?
 a. ventricular tachycardia
 b. sinus bradycardia
 c. first degree AV block
 *d. paroxysmal atrial tachycardia

[CL: KN]

Rationale: Digitalis glycosides slow the conduction through the AV node and are useful for atrial tachycardias such as paroxysmal atrial tachycardia.

7. Patients on concurrent phenobarbital and digitoxin therapy have the potential for:
 a. reduced phenobarbital levels
 b. elevated digitoxin levels
 *c. reduced digitoxin levels
 d. elevated phenobarbital levels

[CL: CO]

Rationale: Enzyme-inducing agents such as phenobarbital can potentially reduce digitoxin levels.

8. When given concurrently with digoxin, which drug will increase the digoxin concentration?
   a. bleomycin
   *b. nifedipine
   c. sulfasalazine
   d. procarbazine

   [CL: KN]

   Rationale: The calcium antagonist nifedipine (Procardia) increases digoxin concentration when given concurrently.

9. When adding quinidine therapy to patients who are on digoxin, the following may occur:
   *a. ventricular dysrhythmias
   b. reduced digoxin levels
   c. mental status changes
   d. elevated potassium levels

   [CL: CO]

   Rationale: The interaction of quinidine and digoxin produces a greater potential for ventricular dysrhythmias.

Additional Review Questions Not Presented in Text

1. The digitalis glycosides have the following effect on the action potential curve:
   a. prolonged phase 1
   *b. shortened phase 3
   c. shortened phase 4
   d. prolonged relative refractory period

   [CL: KN]

   Rationale: The digitalis glycosides shorten phase 3 of the action potential curve.

2. Which of the following statements is correct regarding Digoxin Immune Fab (Digibind)?
   a. This agent is derived from foxglove as an antidote for digoxin toxicity.
   b. Digibind is a cost effective agent which has a wide variety of side effects.
   c. A potentially dangerous side effect of this antidigoxin drug is hyperkalemia.
   *d. Derived from antidigoxin antibodies, this agent is used to treat emergency digoxin toxicities.

   [CL: KN]

   Rationale: Digoxin Immune Fab is derived from antidigoxin antibodies produced in sheep. This agent is expensive, and its use is limited to life-threatening digoxin toxicity. Hypokalemia may be a side effect of its use, as it allows potassium to move back into the cell.

3. Cardiac glycosides are administered for which of the following conditions?
   a. Wolff-Parkinson-White syndrome to increase heart rate
   *b. congestive heart failure to treat symptoms of low cardiac output
   c. acute myocardial infarction to increase myocardial oxygen consumption
   d. atrial dysrhythmias to increase conduction through the AV node

   [CL: CO]

   Rationale: Cardiac glycosides are used to treat congestive heart failure by increasing cardiac output and reducing symptoms.

4. Digitoxin is eliminated primarily by:

a. fecal excretion
b. plasma enzyme action
*c. hepatic mechanisms
d. renal excretion

[CL: KN]

Rationale: Digitoxin is eliminated from the body by hepatic mechanisms.

CHAPTER 29: DRUGS TO TREAT HYPERTENSION

Situations from Text

Situation 29-1

Justine Pack is a 50-year-old with essential hypertension diagnosed five years ago. She has been on a sodium restricted diet and hydrochlorothiazide (Hydro-Diuril). Her blood pressure has been recorded consistently around 160/94. Mrs. Pack is to be started on an additional antihypertensive agent.

1. The physician prescribes prazosin (Minipress) 1 mg po daily. When teaching the patient about this drug, the nurse will stress:
   a. taking the medication early in the day
   b. limiting fluid intake to 1000 cc per day
   c. taking the drug on an empty stomach
   *d. rising slowly from a supine position

   [NP: IM, CL: KN]

   Rationale: Initial therapy with prazosin tends to produce orthostatic hypotension; therefore, the patient should be taught to rise slowly from a supine position.

2. An important area of assessment pertaining to prazosin therapy includes noting evidence of the following:
   *a. hepatic disease
   b. kidney dysfunction
   c. severe depression
   d. moderate hypertension

   [NP: AS, CL: CO]

   Rationale: Prazosin is metabolized by the liver. The drug half-life is prolonged in patients with hepatic disease.

3. When planning for follow-up care for Mrs. Pack, the nurse is aware that:
   a. a majority of patients follow the treatment plan
   b. patients with hypertension have warning symptoms
   c. most patients understand the importance of compliance
   *d. patients actively involved in their care are more compliant

   [NP: PL, CL: CO]

   Rationale: Compliance can be improved by involving the patients in their own care, such as taking daily blood pressures.

4. Which of the following does <u>not</u> represent an expected patient outcome for Mrs. Pack?
   *a. maintenance of monthly blood pressure check-ups
   b. demonstration of ability to explain drug schedule
   c. evidence of systolic blood pressure <140 and >100 mmHg
   d. documentation that prescriptions have been filled

   [NP: EV, CL: AN]

   Rationale: Patients who are just being started on a new drug regime need close follow-up, preferably within five days of initial drug administration.

5. Mrs. Pack will be given dietary instructions by the nurse, which will include teaching her to avoid:
   a. fresh fruits
   b. bran fiber
   *c. chocolate

d. fluid intake

[NP: IM, CL: CO]

Rationale: Patients with hypertension should avoid caffeine-containing products which may potentially increase blood pressure.

6. Which of the following statements indicates an understanding of the hypertensive treatment regime?
   a. "If I miss a dose, I should take two at the next dosage time."
   b. "I should take the pills when I feel like my blood pressure is high."
   c. "For relaxation, I plan to soak in our hot tub every day."
   *d. "I am not supposed to stop taking the drug if I feel dizzy."

   [NP: EV, CL: AN]

   Rationale: Patients should be taught not to discontinue the medication. If the patient has adverse side effects, then she should contact the nurse or physician.

Situation 29-2

Paul Mathers, a 67-year-old, is admitted to the intensive care unit in hypertensive crisis. His blood pressure on admission is 230/150.

1. Mr. Mathers is to receive nitroprusside (Nipride) intravenously. The nurse will plan to infuse the drug within the following range:
   a. .02 to .5 mcg/kg/minute
   b. 10 to 20 mcg/kg/minute
   c. 5 to 15 mcg/kg/minute
   *d. .5 to 10 mcg/kg/minute

   [NP: PL, CL: KN]

   Rationale: The range of nitroprusside dosage is .5 to 10 mcg/kg/minute. Doses above 10 mcg/kg/minute should be administered only if necessary.

2. Pertaining to special nursing actions regarding nitroprusside administration, the following applies:
   a. The solution must be mixed in normal saline.
   *b. The IV bottle should be protected from light.
   c. Nitroprusside infusions can be maintained indefinitely.
   d. When properly mixed, the solution will be dark red.

   [NP: IM, CL: KN]

   Rationale: Nitroprusside solutions should be protected from light to prevent deterioration.

3. Should Mr. Mathers develop symptoms such as slurred speech, weakness, muscle twitching, and/or confusion, the following level should be checked:
   *a. thiocyanate
   b. potassium
   c. magnesium
   d. T_3, T_4

   [NP: PL, CL: KN]

   Rationale: Thiocyanate is a metabolite of nitroprusside which can be accumulate and cause adverse effects. Thiocyanate levels should be monitored in patients receiving intravenous nitroprusside longer than one to two days.

4. Which of the following nursing interventions would be most appropriate for Mr. Mathers?
   *a. lowering mean arterial blood pressure no more than 20 to 30 percent in the first 24 hours

b. teaching exercise and diet counseling along with stress reduction techniques
c. maintaining the nitroprusside infusion at a set rate regardless of the diastolic pressure
d. checking the blood pressure hourly while on nitroprusside infusion for accelerated hypertension

[NP: IM, CL: AP]

Rationale: Because of the potential for rapid reduction in blood pressure with intravenous nitroprusside, resulting in cerebral hypoperfusion, the mean arterial blood pressure should not be reduced more than 20 to 30 percent in the first 24 hours.

5. The nurse will expect the following outcome of nitroprusside therapy:
   a. reduced cardiac output
   b. increased preload
   *c. increased urine output
   d. increased afterload

   [NP: EV, CL: CO]

   Rationale: Nitroprusside reduces both preload and afterload, increasing cardiac output and renal blood flow. The expected outcome would be increased urine output.

6. When observing Mr. Mathers for side effects of nitroprusside therapy, which of the following apply?
   a. reflex tachycardia
   b. hyperthyroidism
   *c. chest pain
   d. difficulty voiding

   [NP: IM, CL: KN]

   Rationale: A reduction in diastolic pressure along with increased cardiac output can potentiate cardiac ischemia.

Additional Situation Not Presented in Text

Conrad Dyer is a 47-year-old with essential hypertension. When evaluated by the clinic nurse, his blood pressure is consistently around 160/95. Current medications include furosemide and verapamil. Mr. Dyer will be placed on a third drug, clonidine (Catapres).

1. When describing the classification of essential hypertension for Mr. Dyer, the nurse will use the following category:
   a. mild
   *b. moderate
   c. severe
   d. accelerated

   [NP: AS, CL: AP]

   Rationale: The patient demonstrates essential hypertension with a blood pressure of around 160/95.

2. Mr. Dyer is to be placed on clonidine .1 mg po bid. Prior to initiation of this drug, the nurse will assess for the following condition, which indicates cautious administration:
   a. migraine headache
   *b. mental depression
   c. open-angle glaucoma
   d. asthma

   [NP: AS, CL: KN]

   Rationale: Because of central nervous system side effects, clonidine should be used with caution in patients with mental depression.

3. When performing patient teaching for Mr. Dyer concerning clonidine therapy, the nurse will include:
   *a. avoiding the operation of heavy equipment or machinery
   b. discontinuing the drug immediately if sedation occurs
   c. taking the drug on an empty stomach to enhance absorption
   d. drinking 2 oz. of alcohol per day to enhance vasodilator effects

   [NP: IM, CL: KN]

   Rationale: Due to drowsiness, a common side effect of clonidine, the patient should avoid operating heavy equipment.

4. Mr. Dyer will be taught to be aware of the following side effect related to clonidine therapy:
   a. restlessness
   b. anxiety
   c. diarrhea
   *d. dry mouth

   [NP: IM, CL: KN]

   Rationale: Clonidine decreases salivary flow, causing a dry mouth.

5. Which of the following outcomes would be expected with the addition of clonidine therapy?
   a. increased cardiac output
   *b. decreased heart rate
   c. decreased need for diuretics
   d. increased standing blood pressure

   [NP: EV, CL: CO]

   Rationale: An action of clonidine is that of an increase in vagal activity, reducing the heart rate. Bradycardia may also contribute to the antihypertensive effects.

6. If, during a follow-up appointment, Mr. Dyer exhibits hypertension, agitation, and tachycardia, the nurse may suspect:
   a. a drug interaction
   b. clonidine toxicity
   c. an allergic reaction
   *d. clonidine withdrawal

   [NP: AS, CL: CO]

   Rationale: Patients who abruptly discontinue clonidine may exhibit symptoms of withdrawal, which include rebound hypertension, agitation, restlessness, and tachycardia.

Review Questions from Text

1. All of the following are sympathetic nervous system inhibitors except:
   a. clonidine hydrochloride
   b. methyldopa
   c. quanabenz
   *d. guanethidine sulfate

   [CL: CO]

   Rationale: Guanethidine exerts its action as an antihypertensive by neuroeffector blockade.

2. An antihypertensive drug which has been shown to be useful in opiate withdrawal is:
   a. reserpine
   b. propranolol
   *c. clonidine

d. hydralazine

[CL: KN]

Rationale: Clonidine hydrochloride is useful in the treatment of opiate withdrawal.

3. Diazoxide (Hyperstat) is a chlorothiazide derivative which:
 a. has a combined diuretic activity
 b. is used to treat mild hypertension
 c. is useful in ischemic heart disease
 *d. inhibits insulin release

[CL: CO]

Rationale: Diazoxide seems to inhibit insulin release from pancreatic islet cells and can cause hyperglycemia if used for several days.

4. Reserpine (Serpasil) is contraindicated in the following patient condition:
 *a. acute ulcerative colitis
 b. severe hypertension
 c. chronic pulmonary disease
 d. glaucoma

[CL: KN]

Rationale: Reserpine causes gastric and intestinal irritation, resulting in abdominal cramps and diarrhea.

5. Guanethidine sulfate (Ismelin) produces the following effect:
 a. increased cardiac output
 *b. decreased contractility
 c. increased venous return
 d. decreased sodium level

[CL: CO]

Rationale: Guanethidine has negative inotropic effects, resulting in reduced cardiac output and reduced venous return.

6. Minoxidil (Loniten) is a potent oral vasodilator which:
 *a. increases cardiac output
 b. reduces glomerular filtration rate
 c. causes reflex bradycardia
 d. reduces fluid retention

[CL: KN]

Rationale: Minoxidil causes increased cardiac output and reflex tachycardia.

7. Which of the following drugs is a ganglionic blocker?
 a. acebutolol hydrochloride
 b. prazosin
 *c. mecamylamine hydrochloride
 d. enalapril

[CL: KN]

Rationale: Mecamylamine hydrochloride is a ganglionic blocker which blocks transmission of the sympathetic and parasympathetic nerve impulses.

8. Which of the following is correct regarding methyldopa administration and other concurrent drug use?

a. The effects of methyldopa are increased when given with amphetamines.
*b. Verapamil may potentiate the effects of methyldopa.
c. A hyperglycemia effect is seen with methyldopa and Tolbutamide.
d. Use of methyldopa and propranolol results in paradoxic hypotension.

[CL: CO]

Rationale: Studies have shown that verapamil potentiates the effects of methyldopa (Aldomet).

9. Which of the following drugs is an alpha-adrenergic blocker?
a. diazoxide
*b. prazosin
c. hydralazine
d. diltiazem

[CL: KN]

Rationale: Prazosin (Minipress) relaxes smooth muscle by blocking $alpha_1$-adrenergic receptors, thereby reducing peripheral vascular resistance.

10. An example of an antihypertensive agent which competes with epinephrine for available beta-receptor sites is:
a. sodium nitroprusside
*b. atenolol
c. terazosin
d. hydralazine

[CL: CO]

Rationale: Atenolol (Tenormin) is an example of a beta-adrenergic blocking agent which competes with epinephrine for beta-receptor sites, inhibiting beta-adrenergic stimuli.

Additional Review Questions Not Presented in Text

1. Central acting $alpha_2$-adrenergic agonists stimulate receptors located in the:
*a. medulla oblongata
b. substantia nigra
c. cerebral cortex
d. reticular activating system

[CL: KN]

Rationale: The central acting alpha-adrenergic agonists stimulate receptors located in the medulla oblongata.

2. An example of a mixed arterial and venous dilator is:
a. hydralazine (Apresoline)
b. diazoxide (Hyperstat)
*c. nitroprusside (Nipride)
d. methyldopa (Aldomet)

[CL: KN]

Rationale: Nitroprusside (Nipride) acts directly to dilate arteries and veins for rapid reduction of blood pressure.

3. Which of the following is correct regarding angiotensin converting enzyme (ACE) inhibitors?
a. These drugs enhance degradation of bradykinin.
*b. ACE inhibitors do not cause reflex tachycardia.
c. The agents induce severe sodium and water retention.
d. ACE inhibitors prevent the urinary excretion of prostaglandins.

[CL: KN]

Rationale: ACE inhibitors do not cause reflex tachycardia as seen with direct vasodilators.

4. Hypertension of cardiac origin is best treated with:
   a. direct alpha antagonists
   b. direct-acting vasodilators
   *c. beta antagonists
   d. ganglionic blockers

[CL: KN]

Rationale: Hypertension of cardiac origin is dominated by beta adrenoreceptors, and therefore responds best to beta blockers.

5. Which of the following effects is seen with calcium-channel blockade?
   *a. relief of coronary spasm
   b. increased afterload
   c. stimulation of renin release
   d. promotion of reflex tachycardia

[CL: KN]

Rationale: Calcium-channel blockers relax regional smooth muscles and relieve coronary spasm and related angina.

CHAPTER 30: ANTIDYSRHYTHMIC MEDICATIONS

Situations from Text

Situation 30-1

Five days after a myocardial infarction, Velma Tidwell, a 58-year-old, develops atrial flutter with a ventricular response of around 100 beats per minute (bpm). Ms. Tidwell is currently on digoxin 0.125 mg po daily. She is on a cardiac monitor in the telemetry unit.

1. The physician orders quinidine sulfate 200 mg IM every 6 hours times 4 doses. The nurse will obtain the following baseline data prior to starting the medication:
   a. deep tendon reflexes
   b. abdominal girth
   *c. Q-T interval
   d. pupil size

   [NP: AS, CL: AP]

   Rationale: Quinidine action results in prolongation of the Q-T interval; therefore, baseline data documenting the Q-T interval are important.

2. The nurse will be aware of the following effect of combined digoxin and quinidine therapy:
   a. elevated quinidine levels
   b. reduced quinidine levels
   *c. elevated digoxin levels
   d. reduced digoxin levels

   [NP: AN, CL: CO]

   Rationale: Quinidine reacts with digoxin to increase serum digoxin levels.

3. After parenteral therapy, Ms. Tidwell is to begin quinidine 200 mg po every 6 hours. The nurse will be observant for the following common side effect associated with quinidine therapy:
   *a. diarrhea
   b. hypothermia
   c. seizures
   d. dysphagia

   [NP: IM, CL: KN]

   Rationale: The most common side effects related to quinidine therapy are gastrointestinal complaints, such as diarrhea.

4. Ms. Tidwell converts to sinus rhythm with a heart rate around 80 bpm. Patient teaching for Ms. Tidwell concerning quinidine therapy will include:
   a. crushing the sustained release tablets
   *b. taking the medication with meals
   c. increasing the intake of citrus fruit
   d. maintaining a high bran fiber diet

   [NP: IM, CL: KN]

   Rationale: Taking quinidine with meals may reduce gatrointestinal side effects.

5. As follow-up care, the nurse will monitor the following laboratory result, which can be altered by quinidine:
   a. lipid profile
   b. T_3, T_4

c. potassium
*d. platelet count

[NP: IM, CL: AP]

Rationale: Patients on quinidine therapy may develop thrombocytopenia, which is due to quinidine-platelet complexes, resulting in destruction of platelets.

6. Which of the following behaviors by Ms. Tidwell indicates successful patient teaching?
   a. neglecting to report symptoms such as nausea
   *b. reporting a weight gain of over 2 pounds per week
   c. taking the pulse rate once a week
   d. maintaining yearly blood pressure check-ups

[NP: EV, CL: AN]

Rationale: Evidence of increasing weight may indicate congestive heart failure and should be reported to the physician or nurse.

Situation 30-2

William Washington is a 71-year-old admitted to the emergency room with severe chest pain. He is diaphoretic and complaining of shortness of breath.

1. The nurse places Mr. Washington on a cardiac monitor, which shows sinus tachycardia and frequent premature ventricular complexes (PVC's). The patient is to receive an intravenous lidocaine bolus. The nurse is prepared to deliver the following dosage:
   *a. 1 mg/kg
   b. 0.5 mg/kg
   c. 2 mg/kg
   d. 4 mg/kg

[NP: PL, CL: KN]

Rationale: The standard IV bolus dose for lidocaine is 1 mg/kg.

2. After the loading (bolus) dose, Mr. Washington is to be placed on a lidocaine infusion. The following represents the standard range of drug dosage:
   a. 6 to 10 mg/minute
   b. .5 to 1 mcg/kg/minute
   c. 5 to 10 mcg/kg/minute
   *d. 1 to 4 mg/minute

[NP: PL, CL: KN]

Rationale: The standard dosage range for lidocaine infusion is 1 to 4 mg/minute.

3. The nurse will implement the following nursing interventions for Mr. Washington:
   a. Use only lidocaine with epinephrine for intravenous use.
   b. Use an infusion pump only for low dosage lidocaine.
   c. Maintain lidocaine infusion with macrodrip tubing.
   *d. Maintain lidocaine infusion separate from other drugs.

[NP: IM, CL: CO]

Rationale: Mixing lidocaine with other drugs may potentiate deterioration or precipitation.

4. The nurse will plan to observe for the following side effect of lidocaine therapy:
   *a. disorientation

b. photophobia
c. dry mouth
d. abdominal cramps

[NP: PL, CL: KN]

Rationale: Due to anesthetic properties and distribution into the central nervous system, side effects include disorientation, agitation, numbness, and more severe CNS effects.

5. Mr. Washington is cared for in the coronary care unit after a diagnosis of anterior myocardial infarction is made. The lidocaine drip is to be discontinued after several days. The nurse is aware that the half-life of lidocaine is:
 a. 30 minutes
 b. 10 hours
 *c. 4 to 5 hours
 d. 1 to 2 hours

[NP: AN, CL: KN]

Rationale: The half-life of lidocaine in patients with ischemic heart disease is 4 to 5 hours after discontinuation of infusions of 24 hours' duration.

6. Mr. Washington continues to have occasional to frequent PVC's. Tocainide is to be started orally. The nurse will teach Mr. Washington to report the following with regard to Tocainide:
 *a. excessive bruising
 b. difficulty voiding
 c. dry mouth
 d. photophobia

[NP: IM, CL: CO]

Rationale: Thrombocytopenia can occur with tocainide therapy; therefore, the patient should be alert to signs of increased bruising.

Additional Situation Not Presented in Text

Henry Kim, a 49-year-old, is recovering from coronary bypass surgery on the telemetry unit. He demonstrates episodes of frequent premature atrial and ventricular complexes, despite therapy with intravenous lidocaine, oral procainamide, and digoxin.

1. Mr. Kim is to begin treatment with flecainide (Tambocor). The nurse is aware that the usual oral adult dosage is:
 a. 600 to 800 mg daily
 *b. 100 to 200 mg q 12 hours
 c. 1 gm to 1.5 gm q 6 hours
 d. 250 to 500 mg q 12 hours

[NP: PL, CL: KN]

Rationale: The average adult dose of flecainide is 100 to 200 mg po q 12 hours.

2. Important laboratory baseline data which the nurse should obtain prior to administering flecainide include:
 *a. potassium level
 b. WBC count
 c. procainamide level
 d. platelet count

[NP: AS, CL: CO]

Rationale: Alteration in the potassium level may affect the action of flecainide; therefore, potassium levels should be normalized.

3. When monitoring Mr. Kim's EKG while on flecainide, the nurse will check for the following effect:
   a. shortened P-R interval
   b. presence of a u wave
   c. shortened Q-T interval
   *d. first degree AV block

   [NP: IM, CL: AP]

   Rationale: The effect of flecainide on the EKG may result in prolonged P-R interval. If a first degree AV block progresses to second or third degree block, the drug should be discontinued.

4. Mr. Kim is to be discharged on oral flecainide. The nurse will include the following in patient teaching:
   a. Drink plenty of cranberry juice.
   b. Report symptoms such as altered taste immediately.
   *c. Take the pulse daily and report irregularities.
   d. Take the medication with meals.

   [NP: IM, CL: AP]

   Rationale: Patients on antidysrhythmia agents should be taught to take their pulse daily and report a slow or irregular pulse rate.

5. An important aspect of evaluating effective teaching about flecainide therapy is:
   a. planning yearly check-ups
   b. reporting signs of dizziness
   *c. monitoring liver function
   d. maintaining sedentary lifestyle

   [NP: EV, CL: KN]

   Rationale: Antidysrhythmia drugs may adversely affect liver and kidney function; therefore, liver function studies should be performed at intervals.

6. The nurse will anticipate the following drug interaction effect when flecainide is added to Mr. Kim's current drug therapy:
   a. increased NAPA level
   b. reduced procainamide level
   c. enhanced inotropic effect
   *d. increased plasma digoxin

   [NP: AN, CL: AP]

   Rationale: Flecainide may increase plasma digoxin levels when given concurrently.

<u>Review Questions from Text</u>

1. Which of the following statements is <u>correct</u> regarding the use of antidysrhythmia agents?
   a. The new antidysrhythmia drugs have few side effects or toxic reactions.
   b. All of the antidysrhythmic medications act by similar mechanisms.
   *c. Atrial dysrhythmias are not life-threatening, but usually require therapy.
   d. Treatment of ventricular dysrhythmias does not affect mortality rate.

   [CL: KN]

   Rationale: Atrial dysrhythmias such as atrial fibrillation are not usually life-threatening, but require treatment whether or not they are symptomatic.

2. Group IV antidysrhythmia drugs act by the following mechanism:
   *a. depressing phase 4 depolarization and lengthening phases 1 and 2 of repolarization

b. stabilizing the cell membrane and depressing phase 0 of the action potential
c. prolonging refractoriness, slowing conduction, and decreasing membrane responsiveness
d. depressing phase 4 of depolarization and prolonging phase 3 of repolarization

[CL: KN]

Rationale: Group IV calcium-channel antagonists depress phase 4 of depolarization and prolong phases 1 and 2 of repolarization.

3. An example of a Group 1a antidysrhythmia drug is:
 a. amiodarone
 b. tocainide
 *c. disopryamide
 d. lidocaine

[CL: KN]

Rationale: Disopyramide (Norpace) is a Group 1a antidysrhythmia agent.

4. Procainamide (Pronestyl) is contraindicated in the following patient condition:
 a. Wolff-Parkinson-White syndrome
 *b. myasthenia gravis
 c. Parkinson's disease
 d. acute myocardial infarction

[CL: KN]

Rationale: Procainamide is contraindicated for use in patients with myasthenia gravis, due to its anticholinergic effects.

5. Which of the following statements is correct regarding verapamil, a Group IV antidysrhythmia drug?
 *a. It is used to treat supraventricular dysrhythmias.
 b. It increases conduction through the heart.
 c. It is used to treat AV nodal blocks.
 d. The drug can be given intravenously with propranolol.

[CL :KN]

Rationale: Verapamil is effective in treating supraventricular tachycardias, such as atrial fibrillation and atrial flutter.

6. An example of an antidysrhythmia drug which interferes with norepinephrine release from sympathetic nerve terminals is:
 *a. bretylium
 b. pindolol
 c. propafenone
 d. phenytoin

[CL: KN]

Rationale: Bretylium is an example of a Group III antidysrhythmia drug which interferes with norepinephrine, increasing the threshhold for developing ventricular fibrillation.

7. The Group II antidysrhythmia agents are useful in treating:
 a. re-entrant tachycardias involving AV node or accessory pathways
 b. life-threatening ventricular dysrhythmias resistant to lidocaine
 *c. ventricular dysrhythmias caused by exercise or excessive catecholamines
 d. ventricular dysrhythmias which arise from conduction delays

[CL: KN]

Rationale: Group II agents act by blocking sympathetic stimulation at the sinus node. These agents are useful in controlling ventricular dysrhythmias caused by exercise or excessive catecholamines.

8. Which of the following represents an investigational Group I drug?
   a. practolol
   b. sotalol
   c. bepridil
   *d. lorcainide

   [CL: KN]

   Rationale: Lorcainide is an investigational Group I drug which suppresses ventricular ectopic beats with minimal adverse side effects.

9. Torsade de Pointe can be treated with:
   a. lidocaine
   b. bretylium
   *c. propranolol
   d. quinidine

   [CL: CO]

   Rationale: Torsade de Pointe is a type of ventricular tachycardia associated with the presence of a prolonged Q-T interval. It is treated with beta blockers, isoproterenol, atropine, or by a cardiac pacemaker.

10. Mexiletine hydrochloride is structurally similar to which of the following drugs?
   a. quinidine
   *b. lidocaine
   c. propranolol
   d. bretylium

   [CL: KN]

   Rationale: Mexiletine hydrochloride is structurally similar to lidocaine in that it depresses automaticity.

Additional Review Questions Not Presented in Text

1. Which of the following blood concentrations would be considered therapeutic for procainamide?
   a. 0.5 to 2.0 mg/ml
   b. 10 to 30 mcg/ml
   c. 2 to 3.5 mg/ml
   *d. 4 to 8 mcg/ml

   [CL: KN]

   Rationale: Therapeutic blood concentrations for procainamide range between 4 and 8 mcg/ml.

2. Which of the following statements is correct regarding disopyramide (Norpace)?
   a. This drug causes peripheral vasodilation along with cholinergic effects.
   b. Norpace is indicated for treatment of AV blocks and various fasicular blocks.
   *c. Patients with atrial flutter should be digitalized prior to Norpace therapy.
   d. Norpace is useful for patients with poorly compensated congestive failure.

   [CL: KN]

   Rationale: Patients with atrial flutter or fibrillation should be digitalized prior to treatment with Norpace.

3. The following should be monitored for patients on procainamide therapy:
   *a. ANA titer

b. Epstein-Barr
c. indirect Combs
d. protein electrophoresis

[CL: CO]

Rationale: Procainamide potentiates development of a positive ANA titer and a syndrome similar to systemic lupus erythematosus (SLE).

4. Mexiletine hydrochloride (Mexitil) is useful in the treatment of ventricular dysrhythmias associated with:
   a. cardiogenic shock
   b. severe left ventricular failure
   c. bradycardia
   *d. digitalis toxicity

   [CL: KN]

   Rationale: Mexiletine hydrochloride is used for the treatment of ventricular tachydysrhythmias associated with digitalis toxicity, myocardial infarction, and prosthetic heart valves.

5. Which of the following statements is correct regarding phenytoin (Dilantin) administration as an antidysrhythmia agent?
   a. As a Group III drug, phenytoin depresses phase 4 depolarization.
   b. Phenytoin exerts a strong positive inotropic effect on the heart.
   *c. Phenytoin increases conduction time through the AV node.
   d. This agent prolongs the Q-T interval, potentiating Torsade de Pointe.

   [CL: KN]

   Rationale: Phenytoin prolongs the conduction time through the AV node, which is the reason that the drug is effective in digitalis toxicity.

CHAPTER 31: VASODILATORS/HEMORRHEOLOGIC AGENTS/SCLEROSING AGENTS

Situations from Text

Situation 31-1

Wayne Armstrong is a 74-year-old admitted to the coronary care unit with a diagnosis of unstable angina. He has a history of mild hypertension and is currently taking propranolol.

1. After 3 nitroglycerin tablets have not relieved his chest pain, Mr. Armstrong is to be started on a high dose nitroglycerin infusion. A nursing responsibility associated with this type of medication is:
   a. checking the blood pressure and pulse every hour
   *b. titrating the nitroglycerin by 20 to 50 mcg increments
   c. mixing nitroglycerin in normal saline only
   d. protecting the nitroglycerin infusion from light

   [NP: IM, CL: KN]

   Rationale: If high dose therapy is to be used, the infusion is titrated by 20 to 50 mcg increments. It is also important to monitor the blood pressure and pulse frequently, particularly with initial intravenous therapy.

2. When monitoring Mr. Armstrong's EKG, the following effect may be observed related to nitroglycerin therapy:
   a. rebound bradycardia
   b. widened Q-T interval
   c. shortened P-R interval
   *d. reflex tachycardia

   [NP: AS, CL: AP]

   Rationale: Nitrates can cause reflex tachycardia in patients with normal cardiac function.

3. Mr. Armstrong tells the nurse that he has a sudden pounding headache. The nurse is aware that this represents:
   a. an allergic reaction
   *b. an adverse effect
   c. a toxic effect
   d. an impending seizure

   [NP: AN, CL: CO]

   Rationale: A pounding headache represents an adverse side effect which is usually relieved by reducing the dosage or discontinuing the infusion.

4. After several days, the nitroglycerin infusion is discontinued. A transdermal nitroglycerin patch is to be applied in the morning and removed in the evening. The nurse is aware that this schedule of dosing reduces:
   a. nitrate dependence
   b. side effects
   c. toxic effects
   *d. nitrate tolerance

   Rationale: Altering nitrate levels by allowing nitrate-free periods reduces the development of nitrate tolerance.

5. When teaching Mr. Armstrong about administering nitroglycerin transdermal patches, the following information applies:
   a. taking off the patch when showering or swimming
   b. putting on an extra patch whenever chest pain occurs
   *c. applying the patch to any non-hairy area of the body
   d. replacing the transdermal patch every six hours

   [NP: IM, CL: CO]

Rationale: Transdermal nitroglycerin patches can be applied to any non-hairy area of the body.

6. In addition to the nitroglycerin patch, Mr. Armstrong will be advised to take sublingual nitroglycerin tablets as needed (prn) for chest pain. The nurse will teach that:
   a. if after eight consecutive doses the chest pain continues, he should notify the physician
   *b. to prevent angina, he should take a tablet before exertional exercise
   c. the nitroglycerin tablets should be replaced every year to maintain freshness
   d. the bottle of nitroglycerin tablets should be kept in a warm, moist environment

   [NP: IM, CL: KN]

   Rationale: Nitroglycerin tablets should be taken before any activity that is likely to induce angina, such as exercise or sexual activity.

Situation 31-2

Hazel Breaux is an 83-year-old with increasing episodes of angina with minimal exertion. She is admitted to the telemetry unit for close observation and medical management of chest pain.

1. Mrs. Breaux is to begin isosorbide dinitrate sustained-release 40 mg tablets. The nurse will instruct her to:
   a. take the dosage with milk to reduce gastric irritation
   b. allow the tablet to dissolve slowly under the tongue
   *c. swallow the tablet without chewing or crushing it
   d. place the tablet between the gum and upper lip

   [NP: IM, CL: KN]

   Rationale: Isosorbide dinitrate sustained-release tablets should not be chewed or crushed, as this would interfere with the sustained-release action.

2. In addition to the nitrate therapy, Mrs. Breaux is to begin nifedipine (Procardia) 10 mg po every 6 hours. When giving this medication along with nitrates the nurse will observe for:
   *a. hypotension
   b. tremor
   c. hyperkalemia
   d. tetany

   [NP: IM, CL: AP]

   Rationale: Nifedipine reduces peripheral vascular resistance and, along with concurrent use with nitrates, can cause hypotension with initial administration.

3. When establishing baseline data for Mrs. Breaux, which of the following conditions would indicate a need to administer nifedipine with caution?
   *a. kidney dysfunction
   b. migraine headaches
   c. sinus bradycardia
   d. Raynaud's syndrome

   [NP: AS, CL: KN]

   Rationale: The presence of kidney dysfunction may increase nifedipine levels and is important to note with assessment data.

4. An important area for assessment for patients on nifedipine is to be aware of the potential for:
   a. hallucinations
   *b. peripheral edema
   c. hyperglycemia
   d. photophobia

[NP: AN, CL: CO]

Rationale: Nifedipine can cause a noncardiac dependent peripheral edema, which can be treated with diuretics.

5. In order to reduce episodes of chest pain, Mrs. Breaux should be taught to avoid all of the following except:
   a. eating large meals
   b. smoking cigarettes
   *c. performing daily exercise
   d. going out into the cold

   [NP: IM, CL: CO]

   Rationale: The patient should avoid excessive strenuous exercise, but exercise activity which is tolerated without angina is acceptable.

6. Which of the following statements by Mrs. Breaux indicates adequate understanding concerning administration of coronary vasodilators?
   a. "I will only have to take these pills for a few weeks."
   b. "I can take the long-acting pill anytime during the day."
   c. "If I get a headache, I should stop taking the pills."
   *d. "The nitroglycerin is not habit-forming, so I can take as needed."

   [NP: EV, CL: AP]

   Rationale: Nitroglycerin tablets are not habit-forming and can be taken as needed. It should be stressed, however, that if chest pain becomes severe or is not relieved with nitroglycerin, the physician should be notified.

Additional Situation Not Presented in Text

Sherman Huff, a 66-year-old with peripheral vascular disease, is being treated as an outpatient for symptoms related to intermittent claudication. He has a history of hypertension and is currently taking methyldopa, furosemide, and a potassium supplement. After poor response to peripheral vasodilator agents, Mr. Huff is to begin treatment with pentoxifylline (Trental).

1. During the initial assessment, the nurse will check for the following sensitivity, which indicates a contraindication to therapy with pentoxifylline:
   a. pork
   *b. caffeine
   c. penicillin
   d. iodine

   [NP: AS, CL: CO]

   Rationale: Pentoxifylline is contraindicated in patients sensitive to xanthine products, such as caffeine.

2. Mr. Huff is to take pentoxifylline 400 mg po tid. When teaching him about taking the medication, the nurse will include:
   *a. taking the medication with meals
   b. combining the doses to take in the evening
   c. monitoring the pulse rate before taking
   d. avoiding a high protein diet

   [NP: IM, CL: KN]

   Rationale: Due to side effects related to gastrointestinal irritation, pentoxifylline is best taken with meals.

3. Because of the possible interaction between methyldopa and pentoxifylline, the nurse will schedule the following for Mr. Huff:
   a. monthly T_3, T_4 levels

b. daily blood sugars
c. monthly ECG's
*d. weekly blood pressure checks

[NP: PL, CL: CO]

Rationale: Concurrent use of antihypertensives and pentoxifylline may potentiate hypotension; therefore, periodic blood pressure checks are indicated.

4. Mr. Huff will be taught to report the following related to pentoxifylline therapy:
a. photophobia
b. tinnitis
*c. bruising
d. dysphagia

[NP: IM, CL: CO]

Rationale: Platelets are affected by pentoxifylline. Patients taking this drug need to be aware of the potential for bleeding.

5. Which of the following statements indicates successful teaching regarding Mr. Huff's medication regimen with pentoxifylline?
a. "For headaches or other aches, I can take aspirin products."
b. "The most common side effect of this drug is drowsiness."
*c. "It takes a couple of weeks to tell if this drug is going to be helpful."
d. "I should remain indoors and keep activities limited."

[NP: EV, CL: AN]

Rationale: Therapeutic effects do not occur with pentoxifylline for several weeks. Patients should not expect immediate results.

6. When Mr. Huff returns for follow-up care, which of the following laboratory results needs to be assessed relative to pentoxifylline therapy?
*a. fibrinogen
b. albumin
c. magnesium
d. phosphorus

[NP: EV, CL: AP]

Rationale: Pentoxifylline increases fibrinolytic activity which decreases fibrinogen concentration.

Review Questions from Text

1. As a class of drugs, nitrates have the following action:
a. constriction of collateral cardiac blood vessels
*b. reduction in systemic venous tone
c. relaxation of skeletal muscle tissue
d. constriction of cerebral blood vessels

[CL: CO]

Rationale: Nitrates produce pooling of blood in the peripheral veins, by reducing systemic venous tone.

2. Which of the following represents an outcome of high dose nitrate therapy?
a. increased left ventricular end-diastolic volume
*b. reduced ventricular outflow resistance
c. increased myocardial oxygen demand

d. reduced intracranial pressure

[CL: KN]

Rationale: Nitrates at high doses cause reduced peripheral vascular resistance and ventricular outflow resistance (afterload).

3. Which of the following descriptions is <u>correct</u> regarding the pharmacokinetics of nitroglycerin?
   a. readily absorbed via the oral route
   b. dependent on lipids for drug binding
   c. estimated half-life of two hours
   *d. extensive first-pass metabolism

[CL: KN]

Rationale: Nitroglycerin is metabolized extensively by the liver. This first-pass characteristic reduces the effectiveness of the oral route.

4. A drug which can act as a physiological antagonist to nitrates is:
   a. heparin
   b. verapamil
   *c. histamine
   d. diltiazem

[CL: KN]

Rationale: Agents such as histamine and norepinephrine act as a physiologic antagonist to nitrates.

5. When instructing the patient about use of nitroglycerin translingual (Nitrolingual) for relief of chest pain, the following is stressed:
   a. Inhale deeply after administration of translingual spray.
   b. Shake canister well before using translingual spray.
   c. Swallow immediately after administration of the spray.
   *d. Spray 1 or 2 metered doses into the oral mucosa.

[CL: AP]

Rationale: At the onset of chest pain, 1 or 2 metered doses of nitroglycerin translingual are sprayed into the oral mucosa.

6. An expected effect of the use of beta-adrenergic blockers to control angina is:
   a. increased heart rate
   *b. reduced force of contraction
   c. increased myocardial demand
   d. reduced tolerance to exercise

[CL: KN]

Rationale: Beta-adrenergic blockers decrease the force of cardiac contraction, thereby reducing myocardial oxygen demand.

7. Verapamil (Isoptin) is contraindicated in patients with the following condition:
   a. cerebral vascular spasm
   b. variant angina
   c. asthma
   *d. sick sinus syndrome

[CL: KN]

Rationale: Verapamil has a pronounced effect on AV node conduction and is contraindicated in patients with sick sinus syndrome who do not have a pacemaker.

8. An example of a beta-adrenergic stimulant is:
   a. phenoxybenzamine
   b. verapamil
   c. erythrityl tetranitrate
   *d. nylidrin hydrochloride

   [CL: KN]

   Rationale: Nylidrin hydrochloride, a beta-adrenergic stimulant, acts on $beta_2$ receptor cells in skeletal muscle to produce arteriole dilation.

9. Which of the following statements is <u>correct</u> regarding papaverine (Pavabid)?
   a. As an opium derivative, it is likely to cause habituation, tolerance, and analgesia.
   b. This drug acts directly on vascular smooth muscle to cause vasoconstriction.
   c. Papaverine has been shown to be very effective in treating peripheral vascular disease.
   *d. This drug is used primarily for treating peripheral ischemia associated with arterial spasm.

   [CL: KN]

   Rationale: Papaverine is a direct-acting vasodilator which has been used for relief of cerebral and peripheral ischemia related to arterial spasm and senile dementia.

Additional Review Questions Not Presented in Text

1. Peripheral vasodilators dilate blood vessels by the following mechanism:
   a. acting directly on the vascular smooth muscle causing constriction
   b. stimulating the sympathetic nervous system to reduce vasospasm
   *c. stimulating beta receptors, causing relaxation of vascular smooth muscle
   d. blocking alpha-adrenergic stimulation, causing profound vasodilation

   [CL: KN]

   Rationale: Beta-adrenergic stimulants cause vasodilation by relaxation of vascular smooth muscle.

2. Which of the following agents causes irritation of the lining of the vessel, forming a thrombus?
   *a. sodium morrhurate
   b. warfarin
   c. pentoxifylline
   d. nylidrin hydrochloride

   [CL :CO]

   Rationale: Sodium morrhurate is a sclerosing agent for use in obliterating veins. It works by producing a thrombus and development of fibrous tissue.

3. Which of the following drugs is most effective in treating Raynaud's disease?
   a. nylidrin hydrochloride
   *b. phenoxybenzamine
   c. pentoxifylline
   d. sodium tetradecyl sulfate

   [CL: CO]

   Rationale: Phenoxybenzamine is an example of an alpha-adrenergic blocking agent, which is most effective in treating Raynaud's disease.

4. After weaning a patient off of intravenous nitroglycerin, the effect will remain for:
   *a. 30 to 60 minutes

b. 24 hours
c. 2 to 4 hours
d. 12 hours

[CL: KN]

Rationale: Nitroglycerin will remain in the system for 30 to 60 minutes after discontinuation of the intravenous infusion.

CHAPTER 32: THERAPY FOR SPECIFIC DISORDERS OF THE CARDIOVASCULAR-HEMOTOLOGIC SYSTEM

Situations from Text

Situation 32-1

Tim Williams, a 56-year-old, has Type II hyperlipidemia uncontrolled with diet alone. He is to be managed as an outpatient through his physician's office.

1. The nurse will gather data pertinent to Mr. Williams. Which of the following items of patient information is of particular note related to hyperlipidemia?
   a. poor long-term memory
   *b. high stress position in a large accounting firm
   c. rheumatic heart disease as a child
   d. history of kidney stones as an adult

   [NP: AS, CL: AP]

   Rationale: Lifestyle patterns are important to note in patients with hyperlipidemia, especially the amount of stress which they may encounter.

2. Mr. Williams is to begin cholestyramine (Questran) 15 grams twice a day. The following represents a contraindication to the use of this drug:
   *a. evidence of triglyceride levels about 400 mg/dl
   b. presence of reduced VLDL levels
   c. history of narrow angle glaucoma
   d. presence of hyperthyroidism

   [NP: AS, CL: CO]

   Rationale: Cholestyramine, a bile sequestrant agent, may elevant triglyceride levels and should not be given to patients with triglyceride levels above 400 mg/dl.

3. When teaching Mr. Williams about taking cholestyramine at home, the nurse includes:
   a. using over-the-counter medications as needed
   b. eating a diet low in fiber
   c. taking the drug with antacids
   *d. mixing the drug with fluids before taking

   [NP: IM, CL: KN]

   Rationale: Cholestyramine should be mixed with fluids or high-moisture-content foods to disguise the taste and to dissolve the medication.

4. Because of mild hypertension, Mr. Williams has been taking a thiazide diuretic for many years. When adding cholestyramine to his drug regime, the nurse will instruct him to:
   a. monitor the blood pressure daily when taking the diuretic and cholestyramine
   b. eliminate milk products which may interfere with absorption of both drugs
   *c. take the diuretic 1 hour before or 6 hours after cholestyramine
   d. drink plenty of fluids after taking the diuretic and cholestyramine

   [NP: IM, CL: CO]

   Rationale: Cholestyramine may interfere with the absorption of thiazide diuretics; therefore, the diuretic should be taken within 1 hour before or 4 to 6 hours after cholestyramine.

5. When planning careful follow-up for Mr. Williams, the nurse will check the following laboratory result:
   *a. bleeding time

b. magnesium
c. calcium
d. T_3, T_4 levels

[NP: EV, CL: AP]

Rationale: Adverse effects related to cholestyramine therapy include bleeding tendencies. Patients taking this agent should be assessed for the potential for bleeding.

6. When Mr. Williams returns after one week for a check-up, which of the following represents successful therapy with cholestyramine?
*a. decrease in LDL levels
b. increase in IDL levels
c. increase in VLDL levels
d. decrease in HDL levels

[NP: EV, CL: KN]

Rationale: A fall in LDL levels is apparent within 4 to 7 days of treatment with cholestyramine.

Situation 32-2

Martha Hampton is a 37-year-old who is admitted to the medical floor for evaluation of fatigue and anorexia.

1. Initial laboratory data indicate a diagnosis of iron deficiency anemia. When checking the results of red blood cell appearance, the following is indicative of this type of anemia:
a. hyperchromic
b. macrocytic
*c. hypochromic
d. normocytic

[NP: AS, CL: KN]

Rationale: Red blood cells which appear hypochromic are characteristic of iron deficiency anemia.

2. Ms. Hamptom is to be started on ferrous sulfate orally. Prior to administering this drug, the nurse will check for the following condition which contraindicates its use:
a. acute glaucoma
b. tetracycline sensitivity
*c. peptic ulcer
d. pernicious anemia

[NP: AS, CL: CO]

Rationale: Oral iron is contraindicated in patients with peptic ulcer disease.

3. When planning Ms. Hampton's care, the nurse will include monitoring for the following side effect of oral iron:
a. clay-colored stools
b. hypotension
*c. constipation
d. hyperglycemia

[NP: PL, CL: AP]

Rationale: Constipation is a local effect of orally administered iron products.

4. The nurse will teach Ms. Hamptom to avoid eating the following food within an hour of taking the iron:
a. orange juice
*b. eggs

c. bran
d. mustard

[NP: IM, CL: CO]

Rationale: Eggs consumed with iron products can inhibit absorption.

5. Additional patient teaching for Ms. Hampton regarding oral iron administration includes:
   a. avoid products containing ascorbic acid
   b. take with antacids to reduce gastric irritation
   *c. avoid coffee and tea with meals
   d. take with meals to enhance absorption

   [NP: IM, CL: AP]

   Rationale: Coffee and tea consumed with meals can reduce iron absorption.

6. Which of the following outcomes would indicate successful treatment of anemia?
   a. elevated bleeding time
   *b. increased sense of well-being
   c. reduced anxiety level
   d. elevated bilirubin levels

   [NP: EV, CL: KN]

   Rationale: As the hemoglobin level rises due to iron therapy, the patient notes less fatigue and increased feelings of well-being.

<u>Additional Situation Not Presented in Text</u>

Bonita Huerta, a 49-year-old with Type IV hyperlipidemia, continues to have elevated cholesterol and triglyceride levels, despite dietary alterations. She is to be started on nicotinic acid and managed through the health clinic.

1. Nicotinic acid 1 gram po three times a day has been ordered for Ms. Huerta. The nurse will include the following in patient teaching:
   a. Take a forgotten dose whenever it is remembered.
   b. Avoid fat soluble vitamin supplements.
   c. Expect immediate beneficial effects.
   *d. Check with physician before taking other medications.

   [NP: IM, CL:CO]

   Rationale: Drug interactions may occur between antilipemic agents and other medications. The patient should check with the physician before additional medications are taken.

2. The nurse will inform Ms. Huerta about the following major side effect related to nicotinic acid:
   a. confusion
   b. fine motor tremor
   c. hypotension
   *d. intense flushing

   [NP: IM, CL: KN]

   Rationale: Intense flushing is a major side effect of nicotinic acid.

3. In order to reduce unwanted effects related to nicotinic acid therapy, the nurse will advise Ms. Huerta to take the following 30 minutes before each dose:
   a. scopolamine
   b. acetaminophen
   *c. aspirin

d. baking soda in water

[NP: IM, CL: KN]

Rationale: Adverse effects related to nicotinic acid therapy are thought to be related to prostaglandin medication; therefore, having the patient take aspirin prior to each dose is helpful.

4. Which of the following patient outcomes can be expected with this type of antilipemic therapy?
*a. reduction in LDL
b. elevation in triglycerides
c. reduction in HDL
d. elevation in plasma cholesterol

[NP: EV, CL: KN]

Rationale: Nicotinic acid reduces LDL levels by 15 to 35 percent.

5. In planning Ms. Huerta's medication regime, the nurse is aware that the maximum daily dose of nicotinic acid is:
a. 12 gm/day
b. 3 gm/day
*c. 8 gm/day
d. 6 gm/day

[NP: AN, CL: KN]

Rationale: The usual maximal dose of nicotinic acid is 8 gm/day.

6. Which of the following statements by Ms. Huerta indicates appropriate understanding concerning antilipemic therapy?
a. "Now that I take this drug, I can eat what I want."
*b. "I may have to take this medication all my life."
c. "I should expect dark-colored stools when taking this medicine."
d. "This drug will keep me from having a heart attack."

[NP: EV, CL: AP]

Rationale: Antilipid agents may have to be taken indefinitely. While lowering cholesterol and triglycerides reduces the risk of myocardial infarction, the medications do not prevent its occurrence.

Review Questions from Text

1. Which of the following compounds contains the largest proportion of lipids:
a. low-density lipoproteins (LDL)
b. high-density lipoproteins (HDL)
*c. very low-desity lipoproteins (VLDL)
d. intermediate-density lipoproteins (IDL)

[CL: CO]

Rationale: The greater the ratio of lipids to protein, the lower the density. Very low-density lipoproteins (VLDL) have larger amounts of lipids.

2. Normal iron loss through the bowel, skin, and genitourinary tract is:
a. 1.5 to 3.5 mg/day
b. 0.2 to 0.3 mg/day
c. 2 to 4.5 mg/day
*d. 0.5 to 1 mg/day

[CL: KN]

Rationale: Dietary iron, as well as oral preparations, are removed from the body via the loss of iron-containing cells from the bowel, skin, and genitourinary tract. Normal loss is 0.5 to 1 mg/day.

3. Which of the following drugs is a chelating agent with a specific affinity for ferric iron?
 a. hydroxocobalamin (Alpharedisol)
 b. ferrous fumarate (Ircon)
 *c. deferoxamine (Desferal)
 d. clofibrate (Atromid-S)

 [CL: KN]

 Rationale: Deferoxamine binds with ferric iron into a water-soluble chelate which is excreted by the kidneys.

4. An example of a simple lipid is:
 *a. triglyceride
 b. phospholipid
 c. lipoprotein
 d. cholesterol

 [CL: KN]

 Rationale: Triglyceride is an example of a simple lipid which consists of fatty acid and glycerol.

5. Type III hyperlipidemia can be treated with diet and:
 a. gemfibrozil
 *b. nicotinic acid
 c. lovastatin
 d. colestipol

 [CL: KN]

 Rationale: Type III hyperlipidemia is treated with diet alterations and nicotinic acid.

6. Which of the following drugs reduces serum triglycerides by up to 55 percent?
 a. colestipol
 b. probucol
 c. lovastatin
 *d. gemfibrozil

 [CL: CO]

 Rationale: Gemfrirozil decreases serum triglycerides by 40 to 55 percent and is used to treat patients with Type IV and V hyperlipidemia.

7. Development of cancer of the biliary tract is associated with high doses of which drug?
 *a. clofibrate
 b. gemfibrozil
 c. lovastatin
 d. deferoxamine

 [CL: KN]

 Rationale: Patients taking high doses of clofibrate are at risk for development of cancer of the biliary tract. The therapeutic use of this agent is limited.

8. An example of a megaloblastic type of anemia is:
 a. iron deficiency
 b. paroxysmal nocturnal hemoglobinuria
 *c. pernicious

d. aplastic

[CL: KN]

Rationale: Pernicious anemia is a type of megaloblastic anemia which is characterized by large germ cells in the bone marrow and by large immature red cells in the plasma.

9. Clofibrate (Atromid-S), an antilipemic medication, has the following action:
 a. inhibits lipolysis in adipose tissue
 b. decreases the hepatic synthesis of LDL
 *c. inhibits the hepatic synthesis of cholesterol
 d. decreases biliary excretion of triglycerides

[CL: KN]

Rationale: Clofibrate inhibits the synthesis of cholesterol.

Additional Review Questions Not Presented in Text

1. Which of the following lipid compounds contains the highest percentage of cholesterol?
 a. very low-density lipoproteins (VLDL)
 *b. low-density lipoproteins (LDL)
 c. intermediate-density lipoproteins (IDL)
 d. high-density lipoproteins (HDL)

[CL:KN]

Rationale: LDL contain a small portion of triglyceride and are 40 to 50 percent cholesterol.

2. A nursing responsibility associated with intravenous iron dextran administration is:
 *a. administer a test dose before starting infusion
 b. give the drug at a rate of 100 mg/minute
 c. reduce infusion rate if signs of allergy appear
 d. administer the drug undiluted to reduce phlebitis

[CL: KN]

Rationale: A test dose of iron dextran is given prior to intravenous use to reduce the chance of an anaphylactic reaction.

3. Cholestyramine (Questran) is a type of antihyperlipemic agent which:
 *a. combines with bile salts forming a complex that is excreted in the feces
 b. reduces triglyceride levels by inhibiting hepatic synthesis
 c. inhibits cholesterol biosynthesis, decreasing total plasma concentration
 d. reduces synthesis of VLDL and LDL and increases levels of HDL

[CL: CO]

Rationale: Cholestyramine is a bile acid sequestrant which exerts its action by combining with bile salts, forming a nonabsorbable complex that is excreted in the feces.

4. To administer iron dextran (Imferon) via the Z-track method, the nurse will:
 a. draw medication plus an additional .5 ml of air into the syringe
 *b. change needles after drawing up the medication into the syringe
 c. inject no more than 6 ml into the same injection site
 d. pull the skin to one side after injecting the needle deeply into muscle

[CL: KN]

Rationale: Iron dextran is irritating to surrounding tissue; therefore, the needle is changed before giving the drug intramuscularly.

CHAPTER 33: PROBLEMS OF COAGULATION

Situations from Text

Situation 33-1

Madeline Grabel, a 60-year-old, is admitted to the medical unit with complaints of severe calf pain. Her right lower leg is red, tender, and swollen.

1. Ms. Grabel is to be started on intravenous heparin therapy for thrombophlebitis of the right leg. If Ms. Grabel weighs 80 kg, the approximate initial dosage would be:
   a. 16,000 units
   *b. 8,000 units
   c. 800 units
   d. 1,600 units

   [NP: PL, CL: AP]

   Rationale: The adult intravenous bolus of heparin is approximately 100 units per kg of body weight.

2. After the bolus dose, Ms. Grabel is to begin an intravenous (IV) infusion of heparin at 1,000 units per hour. A nursing action related to this situation is to:
   a. monitor IV drip without infusion pump
   b. use macrotubing to regulate flow
   *c. avoid intramuscular injections
   d. protect tubing and bottle from light

   [NP: IM, CL: KN]

   Rationale: When patients are receiving heparin infusions, they should not be given intramuscular injections because of the increased risk of bleeding.

3. In planing nursing care for Ms. Grabel, the following drug should be available in case of heparin overdose:
   a. aminocaproic acid
   b. vitamin K
   *c. protamine sulfate
   d. tranexamic acid

   [NP: PL, CL: CO]

   Rationale: Protamine is a heparin antagonist which acts by neutralizing heparin.

4. To evaluate therapeutic effectiveness of heparin therapy, the nurse will note the following:
   a. fibrinogen
   b. prothrombin time (PT)
   *c. partial thromboplastin time (PTT)
   d. fibrin split products

   [NP: EV, CL: KN]

   Rationale: Partial thromboplastin time is monitored for evaluation of heparin therapy.

5. After four days of intravenous heparin therapy, Ms. Grabel is to be switched to subcutaneous heparin therapy. She is to receive 10,000 units every 12 hours. When giving heparin by this method, the nurse will:
   *a. apply pressure to site after injection
   b. withdraw plunger to check for flash-back of blood
   c. insert the needle at a 45-degree angle
   d. massage the site after injection of heparin

[NP: IM, CL: KN]

Rationale: After subcutaneous injection, pressure is applied at the site. However, the site should not be massaged.

6. Ms. Grabel complains of a headache and requests medication. Which of the following would be most appropriate for her?
   a. aspirin
   *b. acetaminophen
   c. ibuprofen
   d. indomethacin

[NP: AN, CL: CO]

Rationale: Due to increased potential for bleeding, the patient receiving heparin therapy should not take aspirin, ibuprofen, or indomethacin. Acetaminophen would be the most appropriate choice in this case.

Situation 33-2

Arnold Campbell, a 45-year-old, presents to the emergency room with severe crushing chest pain, unrelieved with nitroglycerin, which began 30 minutes earlier. A 12-lead ECG reveals elevated ST segments consistent with an acute anterior myocardial infarction.

1. Mr. Campbell is to receive streptokinase via peripheral infusion. The nurse is aware that the standard dosage is:
   a. 3 million units over 1 hour
   b. 50,000 units over 1 hour
   *c. 1.5 million units over 1 hour
   d. 20,000 units over 1 hour

[NP: PL, CL: KN]

Rationale: The peripheral intravenous dosage of streptokinase for occluded coronary arteries is 1.5 million units given over 1 hour.

2. During and after streptokinase infusion, the nurse will pay particular attention for signs of:
   a. peripheral edema
   b. dysphagia
   c. headache
   *d. urticaria

[NP: IM, CL: CO]

Rationale: Because streptokinase is a foreign protein, allergic reactions may be produced, as demonstrated by urticaria, warm flushed skin, or fever.

3. After successful treatment with streptokinase followed by heparinization, Mr. Campbell is started on coumadin 10 mg daily. The nurse will check the following laboratory data daily:
   *a. prothrombin time (PT)
   b. partial thromboplastin time (PTT)
   c. Lee-White clotting time (LWCT)
   d. activated clotting time (ACT)

[NP: EV, CL: AP]

Rationale: Initial coumadin therapy is based on daily prothrombin time.

4. Medical plans for Mr. Campbell include continuing daily coumadin (2.5 mg) after discharge from the hospital. The nurse will include the following in patient teaching:
   a. Take two pills in one day if a daily dose is missed.
   *b. Avoid drinking liquor, beer, or wine.

c. Eat a diet high in leafy green vegetables.
d. Take over-the-counter medications as needed.

[NP: IM, CL: AP]

Rationale: Drinking alcoholic beverages (especially in excess) may increase the potential for bleeding by affecting hepatic metabolism.

5. The nurse observes that Mr. Campbell has hematuria and gingival bleeding. After reporting these signs to the physician, the nurse will plan to administer:
   a. Dextran
   b. platelets
   c. protamine sulfate
   *d. vitamin K

   [NP: PL, CL: CO]

   Rationale: Vitamin K is the antagonist of coumadin and is the drug of choice when signs of hemorrhage are observed with coumadin therapy. The comadin dosage may also need to be held until bleeding subsides.

6. Which of the following statements by Mr. Campbell indicates successful patient teaching regarding coumadin therapy?
   a. "I need to include plenty of fish and cheese in my diet."
   *b. "It is better for me to use an electric razor for shaving."
   c. "If I notice any bruising, I should stop taking the pills."
   d. "I am taking this drug to dissolve the clots in my heart."

   [NP: EV, CL: AP]

   Rationale: Using an electric razor reduces the potential for bleeding related to shaving.

Additional Situation Not Presented in Text

Gatlin Lassalle is a 51-year-old admitted to the intensive care unit with symptoms of shortness of breath and chest pain on deep inspiraton. A lung scan confirms the diagnosis of pulmonary embolism.

1. Mr. Lassalle is to receive urokinase therapy. The nurse is aware that the usual intravenous infusion dosage is:
   a. 20 IU/kg/minute
   *b. 4,400 IU/kg/hour
   c. 1,000 IU/kg/minute
   d. 540 IU/kg/hour

   [NP: PL, CL: KN]

   Rationale: The usual dosage for urokinase infusion is 4,400 IU/kg/hour as treatment for pulmonary embolism.

2. The laboratory data which will be used to alter the urokinase as necessary is:
   a. fibrin split products
   b. partial thromboplastin time (PTT)
   c. prothrombin time (PT)
   *d. thrombin time (TT)

   [NP: EV, CL: CO]

   Rationale: Thrombin time (TT) should be obtained after initiation of treatment with urokinase, to determine adequate activation of the fibrinolytic system.

3. A nursing responsibility related to the care of Mr. Lassalle is:
   *a. avoid intravenous or intramuscular injections

b. monitor patient for anaphylactic shock
c. prepare to give penicillin if pulmonary infection arises
d. use macrodrip tubing with filter for administration

[NP: IM, CL: CO]

Rationale: Needle sticks should be avoided with patients receiving urokinase therapy, due to the risk of bleeding.

4. Mr. Lassalle begins to bleed from his IV sites, and his stools are positive for occult blood. Laboratory data reveal severely elevated bleeding times. The nurse will notify the physician and expect to:
a. reduce the dosage of urokinase and give vitamin K
b. stop the urokinase and give a protamine sulfate
c. reduce urokinase and put a topical hemostatic on IV sites
*d. stop the urokinase and give fresh-frozen plasma

[NP: IM, CL: AP]

Rationale: In the event of uncontrolled bleeding, the infusion of urokinase should be stopped. Whole blood products, fresh-frozen plasma, or cryoprecipitates may also be given.

5. Mr. Lassalle is to be started on aminocaproic acid (Amicar) to control bleeding related to urokinase therapy. The nurse is aware that the initial intravenous dosage is:
*a. 4 to 5 gms in 250 ml, infused over 1 hour
b. 2.5 gms per kg in 100 ml, infused over 2 hours
c. 10 to 15 gms in 500 ml, infused over 3 hours
d. 1.5 to 2 gms per kg in 100 ml, infused over 30 minutes

[NP: AN, CL: KN]

Rationale: The initial intravenous dose of aminocaproic acid is 4 to 5 gms in 250 ml of IV solution infused over 1 hour.

6. When administering aminocaproic acid to Mr. Lassalle, the nurse will observe for the following side effect:
a. agitation
b. peripheral edema
c. hypotension
*d. nausea

[NP: IM, CL: KN]

Rationale: An adverse side effect of aminocaproic acid is nausea. Other adverse side effects include diarrhea, dizziness, and malaise.

Review Questions from Text

1. In the clotting process, stage II is represented by:
a. resolution stage of clot formation
b. formation of active thromboplastin
c. conversion of fibrinogen to fibrin
*d. conversion of prothrombin to thrombin

[CL: KN]

Rationale: Stage II of the clotting process involves the conversion of prothrombin to thrombin by thromboplastin.

2. The intrinsic cascade is activated by:
*a. damage to the endothelium of blood vessels

b. presence of factors V, VII, and X
c. damage to surrounding tissue structures
d. presence of plasminogen and fibrinokinase

[CL: KN]

Rationale: The intrinsic cascade of the clotting system is activated when the endothelium lining the blood vessels is damaged.

3. The use of anticoagulant agents in the clinical setting is to:
 a. stimulate fibrinolysis
 b. dissolve existing clots
 *c. retard the clotting process
 d. dissolve clotting factors

[CL: KN]

Rationale: Anticoagulants do not dissolve existing clots; rather, they retard the clotting process at various stages.

4. In the human body, the highest concentration of heparin can be found in the:
 a. brain
 b. pancreas
 c. liver
 *d. lungs

[CL: CO]

Rationale: Heparin can be extracted from many cells, but highest concentrations are found in the lungs and intestines.

5. Oral anticoagulant agents are contraindicated in the following condition:
 a. subacute myocardial infarction
 b. pulmonary embolism
 c. transient ischemic attacks
 *d. precordial effusion

[CL: KN]

Rationale: Conditions such as precordial effusion may result in bleeding and represent contraindication to oral anticoagulant therapy.

6. Which of the following agents inhibits platelet aggregation?
 *a. dipyridamole (Persantine)
 b. dicumarol (Dicoumarin)
 c. anisindione (Miradon)
 d. negatol (Negatan)

[CL: KN]

Rationale: Dipyridamole blocks ADP-induced platelet aggregation and is classified as an antiplatelet agent.

7. Vitamin K-dependent clotting factors include which of the following?
 a. fibrinogen
 *b. prothrombin
 c. thromboplastin
 d. plasma thromboplastin antecedent (PTA)

[CL: CO]

Rationale: A blood clotting factor which is dependent on vitamin K is prothrombin. Synthesis of prothrombin is promoted by vitamin K in the liver.

8. Heparin exerts its therapeutic action by:
   a. antagonizing the production of factors V, VII, and XII
   b. deactivating calcium-dependent clotting factors
   c. blocking the action of plasminogen in stage IV
   *d. preventing formation of fibrin in stage III

   [CL: KN]

   Rationale: Heparin acts to inhibit the first stages of the clotting process by: preventing the formation of fibrin in stage III; reducing the amount of thromboplastin in stage I; and exerting an antiprothrombin action in stage II.

9. Agents such as streptokinase are contraindicated in the following situation/condition:
   a. arteriovenous cannulae occlusions
   b. chronic asthma
   c. thromboembolic disease
   *d. cerebrovascular disease

   [CL: KN]

   Rationale: Streptokinase is a thrombolytic agent which is contraindicated in patients with cerebrovascular accident due to the potential for intracerebral bleeding.

Additional Review Questions Not Presented in Text

1. Dihydroergotamine (DHE) exerts the following effect:
   a. prevention of thrombin formation
   *b. acceleration of venous blood return
   c. inhibition of intrinsic clotting factors
   d. stimulation of plasminogen production

   [CL: CO]

   Rationale: DHE, an alpha-adrenergic blocking agent, stimulates peripheral vascular smooth muscle, resulting in enhanced venous return. This action is particularly effective in the calf area, resulting in a thromboprophylactic effect.

2. Which of the following is correct regarding recombinant alteplase (Activase)?
   a. As a synthetic protein, it is associated with antibody formation and allergic reactions.
   *b. It is identical to natural activators, produced by vessel wall cells, which digest fibrin clots.
   c. This agent has a long half-life and is contraindicated in patients requiring immediate surgery.
   d. It is an inexpensive thrombolytic agent which is safer to use clinically than streptokinase.

   [CL: KN]

   Rationale: Activase is a protease enzyme identical to the activator produced by vessel wall cells which digest fibrin clots. It has a short half-life and is not associated with antibody formation.

3. Topical hemostatic agents are used to:
   a. stimulate platelet aggregation
   b. control arterial bleeding
   c. interfere in the clotting cascade
   *d. control capillary bleeding

   [CL: KN]

   Rationale: These topical agents are used to control bleeding from minute vessels during surgery or emergency situations.

4. An action of salicylates in anticoagulation is to decrease:
   *a. factor VII
   b. prothrombin
   c. kallikrein
   d. factor V

   [CL: KN]

   Rationale: Salicylates alter blood coagulability by decreasing factor VII in the clotting cascade.

5. Protamine sulfate is contraindicated in patients who are allergic to:
   a. penicillin
   b. aspirin
   c. citrus fruits
   *d. fish

   [CL: KN]

   Rationale: Protamine sulfate is derived from the sperm of salmon and other fish. It is contraindicated in patients allergic to fish.

CHAPTER 34: OVERVIEW OF FUNCTIONAL ANATOMY OF THE RESPIRATORY SYSTEM

Review Questions from Text

1. The upper airway is composed of the:
   a. trachea, bronchus, bronchiole
   b. throat, trachea, bronchus
   c. mouth, throat, trachea
   *d. nose, mouth, throat

   [CL: KN]

   Rationale: The upper airway is composed of the nose, mouth, and throat. The purpose of these structures is to warm and filter the inhaled air.

2. The larynx, which marks the transition of the upper airway to the lower airway, has the following function:
   *a. plays a role in airway clearance
   b. provides protection to the upper airway
   c. humidifies the inhaled air
   d. opens when food or liquid enters the oropharynx

   [CL: CO]

   Rationale: The larynx contains structures which protect the lower airway by playing a vital role in the coughing mechanism. The larynx closes tightly when food or liquid enters the oropharynx.

3. Which statement is correct regarding the operation of airway defense mechanisms?
   a. The mucociliary escalator traps and removes large particles of foreign matter from the alveoli.
   b. Alveolar macrophages are freely moving scavenger cells that regularly clean the tracheo-bronchial tree.
   *c. Mucus secreted by the bronchial epithelium holds particles and bacteria that come in contact with it.
   d. The tonsils and the adenoids prevent the aspiration of foreign matter and protect the lungs.

   [CL: CO]

   Ratoinale: The mucus secreted by the glands of the bronchial epithelium is sticky and traps most of the dust and bacteria which bypass the upper airway defense mechanisms.

4. Chemoreceptors, located in the arch of the aorta, are sensitive to changes in:
   a. posture
   b. blood pressure
   *c. pH levels
   d. temperature

   [CL: KN]

   Rationale: Specialized neurons, known as chemoreceptors, are sensitive to changes in blood pH and carbon dioxide levels.

5. Which statement is correct regarding neurological control of bronchial smooth muscle?
   a. Parasympathetic stimulation causes bronchial smooth muscle dilation.
   b. Sympathetic stimulation causes bronchial smooth muscle dilation.
   c. The autonomic nervous system stimulates release of Type II surfactant cells.
   *d. Humoral mediators released from mast cells cause bronchial constriction.

   [CL: CO]

   Rationale: Humoral mediators released from mast cells and basophils overstimulate the parasympathetic nervous system, causing bronchial constriction.

6. A cause of increased work of breathing is:
   a. increased elastic recoil
   b. increased lung compliance
   *c. muscular weakness
   d. decreased airway resistance

[CL: KN]

Rationale: The physiological work of breathing can be increased by any factor which weakens the muscles of respiration.

7. The most common cause of reduced lung compliance is:
   *a. infection
   b. cerebellar injury
   c. myasthenia gravis
   d. musculoskeletal blocking agents

[CL :KN]

Rationale: Infection is the most common cause of reduced lung compliance. Inflammatory exudate impedes lung expansion.

8. Which of the following statements is correct concerning airway resistance?
   a. When the lumen of the airway increases, airway resistance increases.
   *b. Airway resistance increases as a result of increased mucus production.
   c. Spasms of the bronchial smooth muscle reduce airway resistance.
   d. When airway resistance is high, air moves freely within the system.

[CL: CO]

Rationale: Excessive mucus production, a common feature of many lung diseases, partially obstructs the airway and results in increased airway resistance.

9. The specific autonomic receptors found in the bronchial smooth muscle are the:
   a. alpha
   b. muscarinic
   c. $beta_1$
   *d. $beta_2$

[CL: KN]

Rationale: Beta 2 are specific receptors of the sympathetic branch of the autonomic nervous system and are found in bronchial smooth muscle.

10. Of the following statements, which is correct concerning ventilation control mechanisms?
   a. Rhythmic impulses signaling the ventilatory muscles to contract and relax are found in the reticular activating center.
   b. Peripheral chemoreceptors located in the aortic arch are more sensitive to arterial oxygen levels than CO_2 levels.
   c. The medullary neurons are voluntary in nature and initiate the inhalation phase of ventilation.
   *d. Central chemoreceptors in the medulla are extremely sensitive to changes in arterial CO_2 levels.

[CL: CO]

Rationale: Chemoreceptors in the medulla are highly sensitive to changes in arterial carbon dioxide levels. A rise in carbon dioxide levels causes an increase in ventilation, which continues until the level of carbon dioxide returns to normal.

Additional Review Questions Not Presented in Text

1. The lowest portion of the pharynx is the laryngopharynx, which contains the:
   a. turbinates
   b. adenoids
   *c. epiglottis
   d. voice box

   [CL: KN]

   Rationale: The laryngopharynx contains the epiglottis, which protects the airway from aspiration of foreign matter.

2. The lower airway is composed of the following, in anatomical order:
   a. trachea, bronchioles, bronchi, carina, alveoli
   b. bronchus, trachea, bronchioles, carina, alveoli
   c. carina, trachea, bronchi, alveoli, bronchioles
   *d. trachea, carina, bronchi, bronchioles, alveoli

   [CL: KN]

   Rationale: The trachea branches at the carina into the bronchi. The bronchi continue to branch into bronchioles, which terminate in alveoli.

3. The alveolar space is kept open, in part, as a result of:
   a. atmospheric pressure
   *b. surfactant
   c. smooth muscle
   d. elastic recoil

   [CL: CO]

   Rationale: Surfactant, a phospholipid manufactured by the alveolar cells, prevents the collapse of the alveolar sacs. With surfactant lining the alveolar sacs, the subatmospheric pressure within the chest is sufficient to keep them open.

4. The primary muscle of respiration is the:
   a. external intercostal
   b. chest wall
   *c. diaphragm
   d. internal intercostal

   [CL: KN]

   Rationale: The primary muscle of respiration is the diaphragm, which drops downward during inspiration and allows air to enter the chest.

5. The accessory muscles of ventilation are:
   a. active in normal ventilation
   b. used before diaphragmatic movement
   *c. affected by skeletal muscle relaxants
   d. innervated by the autonomic nervous system

   [CL: KN]

   Rationale: All of the muscles used for breathing are striated and are affected by skeletal muscle relaxants.

CHAPTER 35: AGENTS USED TO TREAT BRONCHIAL OBSTRUCTION

Situations from Text

Situation 35-1

Teruyo Sakamoto, aged 45, has a history of asthma. He presents to the emergency department with shortness of breath.

1. An aminophylline infusion has been ordered for Mr. Sakamoto, and plans are to admit him to the medical unit. After a loading dose, the maintenance infusion dose of aminophylline should be:
   a. 10 to 20 μg/kg/hr
   *b. 0.2 to 0.9 mg/kg/hr
   c. .8 to 15 μg/kg/min
   d. 1.0 to 5.0 mg/kg/hr

   [NP: PL, CL: KN]

   Rationale: The maintenance intravenous dose for aminophylline is 0.2 to 0.9 mg/kg/hr, depending on serum levels.

2. Twenty-four hours later, Mr. Sakamoto is breathing easier. A serum theophylline level is drawn. Which of the following values represents a therapeutic level?
   *a. 18 μg/ml
   b. 25 μg/ml
   c. 4 μg/ml
   d. 30 μg/ml

   [NP: EV, CL: AP]

   Rationale: The therapeutic range for serum aminophylline is 10 to 20 μg/ml.

3. Mr. Sakamoto begins theophylline anhydrous and is weaned off of intravenous aminophylline. The nurse will be aware of the following precaution of oral theophylline:
   a. glaucoma
   b. pseudomembranous colitis
   *c. gastric bleeding
   d. photosensitivity

   [NP: IM, CL: AP]

   Rationale: Theophylline increases gastric acid secretion, aggravating gastric mucosa.

4. When administering oral theophylline, the nurse will observe Mr. Sakamoto for the following side effect:
   a. difficulty voiding
   b. drowsiness
   *c. palpitations
   d. confusion

   [NP: IM, CL: AP]

   Rationale: Side effects of theophylline frequently include palpitations, nervousness, insomnia, and frequent urination.

5. Mr. Sakamoto is to be discharged on Theodur 200 mg orally twice a day. Patient teaching for him will include the following information:
   *a. Limit intake of caffeine.
   b. Increase intake of high calcium foods.

c. Take only on an empty stomach.
d. Reduce oral fluid intake.

[NP: IM, CL: AP]

Rationale: Caffeine and caffeine-containing foods may accentuate some of the stimulating effects of theophylline.

6. The dosage of theophylline may need to be altered if Mr. Sakamoto:
   a. takes steroids
   b. operates machinery
   c. lifts weights
   *d. smokes cigarettes

[NP: AN, CL: CO]

Rationale: The metabolism of theophylline is accelerated by tobacco smoking; therefore, the dosage may need to be increased if the patient smokes cigarettes.

Situation 35-2

Pierre St. Phillip is a 62-year-old with chronic bronchitis, who has undergone a colon resection for cancer. Postoperatively he complains to the nurse of "tightness" in his chest.

1. When assessing Mr. St. Phillip for evidence of bronchial obstruction, the nurse would observe for:
   a. bronchial breath sounds
   *b. use of accessory muscles
   c. slowed pulse
   d. prolonged inspiration

[NP: AS, CL: AP]

Rationale: Signs of bronchial obstruction include the use of accessory muscles, wheezing on auscultation, increased heart rate, and/or mental status changes.

2. Mr. St. Phillip is to receive terbutaline sulfate inhaler 2 puffs every 4 to 6 hours. After administration of this drug, the nurse will monitor:
   a. muscle strength
   b. pupil reaction
   c. reflexes
   *d. heart rate

[NP: IM, CL: CO]

Rationale: Side effects of terbutaline therapy include tachycardia, dysrhythmias, and other cardiac complications. Patients receiving this drug should be monitored closely for evidence of cardiovascular effects.

3. Which of the following nursing interventions is most appropriate for Mr. St. Phillip concerning terbutaline therapy?
   a. Restrict oral fluids.
   *b. Monitor arterial blood gases.
   c. Measure abdominal girth.
   d. Check pupils every hour.

[NP: IM, CL: AP]

Rationale: Terbutaline has been known to cause paradoxical bronchospasm and reduced PaO_2 levels. Arterial blood gases should be monitored closely.

4. Bronchoconstriction improves, and two days later, Mr. St. Phillip is scheduled to receive beclomethasone

(Vanceril) 1 puff four times a day (qid). In order to safeguard against side effects of this drug, the nurse will instruct him to:
*a. rinse mouth after each dose
b. take benadryl before each dose
c. cough with force after using
d. avoid inhaling deeply after using

[NP: IM, CL: AP]

Rationale: Common side effects of inhaled steroid agents, such as beclomethasone, include hoarseness, sore throat, and sinusitis. These effects can be reduced by thoroughly rinsing the mouth after each dose.

5. When administering the inhalants to Mr. St. Phillip, the nurse will see that he:
a. lies in a semi-Fowler's position
b. holds chin in a downward position
*c. holds breath for several seconds after instilling medication
d. places nebulizer directly to lips and closes mouth tightly

[NP: AS, CL: CO]

Rationale: Patients using aerosol medication delivery systems should hold their breath for several seconds after instillation to allow for maximum absorption of the medication.

6. Which of the following statements by Mr. St. Phillip indicates the need for further teaching concerning the use of beclomethasone via metered-dose inhaler?
*a. "I should fully inhale before depressing the cartridge."
b. "I should wait 1 to 2 minutes before taking a second inhalation."
c. "It is best to use only one to two puffs at a dosage schedule."
d. "The nebulizer cartridge should be shaken well before using."

[NP: EV, CL: AN]

Rationale: The puff of medication must be delivered at the beginning of inhalation to ensure that the distal airways receive the dosage. The patient should begin a deep, slow inhalation through the mouth, while depressing the cartridge fully.

Additional Situation Not Presented in Text

Camille Oliver, aged 68 years, has a long history of emphysema, which has been difficult to treat because she continues to smoke 1/2 pack of cigarettes per day. She has demonstrated poor response to theophylline, and her physician plans to try aerosolized anticholinergic agents.

1. Before administering ipratroprium bromide (Atrovent), the nurse will assess Ms. Oliver for the following contraindication to its use:
a. Parkinson's disease
*b. narrow-angle glaucoma
c. gastric ulcers
d. hypothyroidism

[NP: AS, CL: AP]

Rationale: Ipratroprium causes many of the same effects as atropine sulfate and should not be used for patients with narrow-angle glaucoma. These agents dilate the pupil, increasing intraocular pressure.

2. After administration of Atrovent, the nurse will plan to monitor Ms. Oliver for:
a. seizures
b. restlessness
*c. palpitations
d. insomnia

[NP: PL, CL: CO]

Rationale: Like the sympathomimetics, anticholinergics may stimulate the heart, causing tachycardia and palpitations. Anticholinergics are not usually associated with CNS stimulation.

3. When planning care for Ms. Oliver, which of the following interventions is most appropriate related to anticholinergic therapy?
   a. Administer only for symptoms of bronchospasm.
   b. Restrict dietary fiber.
   *c. Maintain adequate oral intake.
   d. Measure abdominal girth.

   [NP: PL, CL: AP]

   Rationale: Anticholinergic agents tend to dry mucus gland secretions and, potentially, cause mucus plugging in the airways. Maintaining adequate fluid intake can eliminate this problem.

4. Because of a recent cold, Ms. Oliver complains of a "tight cough" which is not controlled with cough lozenges. Her physician orders an expectorant containing guaifenesin. The nurse will instruct her to:
   a. watch for tremors and nervous activity
   *b. withhold fluids for 30 minutes after taking
   c. chew capsules thoroughly before swallowing
   d. contact physician if cough persists longer than 3 weeks

   [NP: IM, CL: AP]

   Rationale: Withholding fluids for up to 30 minutes after administering guaifenesin promotes demulcent effects. The physician should be notified if the cough persists for a week or longer.

5. The nurse will be aware of the following side effects of guaifenesin when assessing Ms. Oliver:
   *a. nausea and vomiting
   b. dehydration and constipation
   c. nervousness and tremors
   d. chills and fever

   [NP: AS, CL: KN]

   Rationale: Nausea and vomiting are the major side effects of guaifenesin therapy.

6. When evaluating the effectiveness of expectorant therapy, the nurse will anticipate the following outcome:
   a. reduced breath sounds in all lung fields
   b. increase in rate and depth of respiration
   c. arterial blood pH remains between 7.46 and 7.50.
   *d. increased sputum clearance

   [NP: EV, CL: CO]

   Rationale: The use of expectorants should result in a more effective cough, increasing sputum clearance.

Review Questions from Text

1. The use of catecholamine compounds has declined due in part to:
   a. prolonged half-life
   b. reduction in bronchial diseases
   *c. short duration of action
   d. cost of production

   [CL: KN]

   Rationale: Catecholamine compounds are useful in controlling bronchospasm; however, their popularity has declined, due to short duration of action and cardiovascular side effects.

2. Drugs which reduce the effectiveness of sympathomimetics include:
   a. anticholinergics
   *b. beta-blocking agents
   c. hypoglycemics
   d. alpha-blocking agents

   [CL: CO]

   Rationale: Beta-blocking agents act as antagonists to sympathomimetics. Concomitant use of beta-blockers reduces the effectiveness of both agents.

3. Xanthine agents produce bronchial smooth muscle relaxation by:
   a. directly stimulating $Beta_1$ cells
   b. indirectly stimulating alpha receptor cells
   c. directly contributing to calcium blockade
   *d. indirectly contributing to cAMP production

   [CL: KN]

   Rationale: Xanthine agents such as theophylline have the ability to inhibit activity of the enzyme that inactivates cAMP. The effect is an indirect relaxation of bronchial smooth muscle.

4. An example of a drug which decreases the rate of metabolism of theophylline is:
   *a. cimetidine
   b. phenytoin
   c. carbamazepine
   d. furosemide

   [CL: KN]

   Rationale: Cimetidine is an example of a drug which decreases the rate of metabolism of theophylline, resulting in greater risk of toxicity.

5. Corticosteroids act to control bronchospasm by:
   a. direct relaxation of bronchial smooth muscle
   b. stimulation of parasympathetic nervous system
   c. inhibiting the sympathetic nervous system
   *d. counteracting bronchial inflammatory processes

   [CL: CO]

   Rationale: Corticosteroids are agents used to reduce bronchial inflammation, thereby reducing bronchial obstruction. They are thought to act by decreasing the release of inflammatory mediators from injured tissue.

6. The following drug is <u>not</u> indicated in an acute asthma attack:
   a. theophylline
   *b. cromolyn sodium
   c. atropine
   d. epinephrine

   [CL: CO]

   Rationale: Cromolyn sodium is an anti-inflammatory agent used to prevent asthma attacks. This drug is not a bronchodilator and can aggravate bronchospasm.

7. A side effect of ephedrine is:
   a. generalized vasodilation
   *b. premature atrial contractions

c. hyperglycemia
d. decreased blood pressure

[CL: CO]

Rationale: Major side effects of ephedrine involve cardiac irritability, such as premature atrial contractions.

8. Isoproterenol (Isuprel) has the following adverse effect:
*a. tremors
b. negative chronotropic effects
c. decreased myocardial oxygen demand
d. decreased cardiac contractility

[CL: KN]

Rationale: Adverse side effects of isoproterenol involve the central nervous system and include nervousness, tremors, and restlessness.

9. Anticholinergic bronchodilators exert their action through:
a. stimulating production of cAMP
b. stimulating the activity of acetylcholine
c. decreasing production of cAMP
*d. decreasing production of cGMP

[CL: CO]

Rationale: The effect of parasympathetic stimulation is release of a cyclic nucleotide (cGMP) which constricts bronchial smooth muscle. Anticholinergic bronchodilators act by decreasing production of cGMP, allowing cAMP to have greater influence and resulting in bronchial relaxation.

10. Which statement is correct regarding the signs and symptoms of bronchial obstruction?
a. Wheezing, audible with a stethoscope, is suggestive of mild bronchial obstruction.
*b. All breath sounds are greatly diminished with severe bronchial obstruction.
c. Evidence of central cyanosis is always present in partial bronchial obstruction.
d. Tachycardia and a bounding pulse are indicators of mild bronchial obstruction.

[CL: CO]

Rationale: In patients with severe bronchial obstruction, all breath sounds are greatly diminished due to the reduced volume of air passing into and out of the lungs.

Additional Review Questions Not Presented in Text

1. An advantage of aerosol medications is:
a. patient cooperation unnecessary
b. equipment economical to use
c. precise method of administration
*d. rapid onset of action

[CL: KN]

Rationale: The rapid onset of action is one major advantage of aerosol medications, making their use in acute episodes of bronchial obstruction quite helpful.

2. The most common side effect of iodide preparations is:
*a. GI upset
b. headache
c. laryngitis
d. fungal infection

[CL: KN]

Rationale: Gastrointestinal irritation is the most common side effect of iodide preparations. Therefore, the medication is best administered with fruit juice or milk.

3. Which of the following statements is correct regarding epinephrine (Adrenalin)?
   a. Intramuscular injections can be given in the gluteal muscle.
   *b. Some antihistamines may increase tachycardia and hypertensive effects.
   c. Antagonistic effects occur with concomitant theophylline therapy.
   d. Up to 25 mg can be given intravenously in a single dosage for asthma.

   [CL: KN]

   Rationale: Some antihistamines may increase the cardiovascular side effects of epinephrine, such as increased tachycardia and hypertension. Synergistic effects occur when theophylline and epinephrine are used concomitantly.

4. Side effects of theophylline levels of 30 μg/ml include:
   *a. ventricular dysrhythmias
   b. mild nausea
   c. jitteriness
   d. headache

   [CL: KN]

   Rationale: When serum theophylline levels rise above 30 μg/m, cardiovascular effects are likely, including ventricular dysrhythmias.

5. The expected outcome for patients on mucolytics such as acetylcysteine (Mucomyst) is:
   a. increased sputum viscosity
   b. increased force of cough
   *c. decreased sputum viscosity
   d. increased cough reflex

   [CL: CO]

   Rationale: Acetylcysteine loosens secretions by breaking bonds in the mucoprotein molecules. This results in a less viscous sputum, which eases removal via the coughing mechanism.

CHAPTER 36: MISCELLANEOUS RESPIRATORY AGENTS

Situation from Text

Situation 36-1

Clifford Sifert, a 72-year-old with chronic bronchitis, is admitted to the emergency department in mild respiratory distress. His PaO_2 is 50 mmHg.

1. The nurse will plan to monitor oxygen therapy. Which of the following oxygen concentrations would be most appropriate for Mr. Sifert?
   a. 100 percent per non-rebreather mask
   *b. 28 percent per Venturi mask
   c. 60 percent per aerosol mask
   d. 80 percent per reservoir mask

   [NP: PL; CL: AN]

   Rationale: Patients with chronic obstructive disease are at risk for oxygen-induced hypoventilation. Oxygen should be delivered at the lowest rate possible, while at the same time reducing the threat of hypoxemia.

2. An expected outcome of oxygen treatment for Mr. Sifert would be the following:
   a. PaO_2 of 96 mmHg
   b. PaO_2 of 86 mmHg
   *c. PaO_2 of 70 mmHg
   d. PaO_2 of 56 mmHg

   [NP: EV, CL: AP]

   Rationale: For patients with chronic obstructive pulmonary disease, a range of 60 to 70 mmHg is appropriate.

3. The nurse will monitor Mr. Sifert closely for the following:
   *a. lethargy
   b. pallor
   c. poor skin turgor
   d. sore throat

   [NP: IM, CL: AP]

   Rationale: Patients with chronic obstructive pulmonary disease are at risk for oxygen-induced hypoventilation. Signs of this condition include lethargy and decreasing respiratory rate and depth.

4. A nursing responsibility which applies in Mr. Sifert's case is:
   a. Teach him how to adjust the flow rate.
   *b. Ensure humidification of the oxygen delivered.
   c. Keep lips moistened with petroleum jelly.
   d. Change oxygen equipment every two days.

   [NP: IM, CL: KN]

   Rationale: Humidification reduces the drying effect of oxygen on mucous membranes.

5. Mr. Sifert tells the nurse that he is "breathing easier." Arterial blood gases reveal appropriate PaO_2 levels. Oxygen is ordered per nasal cannula at 24 percent. The nurse will set the flow rate of oxygen at:
   *a. 1 L/min
   b. 2 L/min
   c. 3 L/min
   d. .5 L/min

[NP: IM, CL: CO]

Rationale: To deliver 24 percent oxygen via nasal cannula, the flow meter should be set at one liter per minute.

6. When assessing Mr. Sifert, which of the following would indicate a sign of potential impaired gas exchange?
   a. photosensitivity
   b. warm flushed skin
   *c. wheezes
   d. unequal hand grips

   [NP: AS, CL: CO]

   Rationale: Adventitious breath sounds such as wheezes or rales indicate pulmonary problems which may alter the exchange of oxygen at the capillary level.

<u>**Additional Situation Not Presented in Text**</u>

Frank Bright is a 47-year-old recovering from pnenumonia. He is currently being treated with antibiotics and oxygen at 3 L/min via nasal cannula.

1. Mr. Bright complains of a persistent cough which disrupts his sleep. The nurse will perform the following assessment in relation to this complaint:
   a. determine need for pain medications
   b. count number of coughing spells
   c. ask him if he takes sleeping pills
   *d. observe for evidence of sputum

   [NP: AS, CL: CO]

   Rationale: It is important to determine if the cough is productive or non-productive.

2. Mr. Bright is to begin antitussive therapy with hydrocodone (Hycodan). In planning his care, the nurse will expect the duration of effect of this agent to be:
   a. 3 to 5 hours
   *b. 4 to 8 hours
   c. 8 to 10 hours
   d. 4 to 6 hours

   [NP: PL, CL: KN]

   Rationale: The expected duration of effect of hydrocodone is 4 to 8 hours.

3. A nursing responsibility for Mr. Bright includes:
   a. discourage him from resting during the day
   b. provide a stimulating environment
   *c. encourage oral fluid intake
   d. give 8 oz water after cough elixir

   [NP: IM, CL: KN]

   Rationale: Drinking fluids promotes thin, easily raised secretions.

4. The nurse will observe Mr. Bright for the following adverse reaction to treatment with hydrocodone:
   a. diarrhea
   *b. dry mouth
   c. agitation
   d. numbness in the chest

   [NP: IM, CL: KN]

Rationale: Drying of mucous membranes is a common adverse reaction associated with hydrocodone.

5. Which of the following potential nursing diagnostic categories is most appropriate to Mr. Bright's situation?
 a. Altered Comfort: chronic pain
 b. Ineffective Thermoregulation
 c. Impaired Physical Mobility
 *d. Alteration in Bowel Elimination: constipation

 [NP: AN, CL: AN]

 Rationale: Due to potential constipation with hydrocodone administration, the patient is at risk for Alteration in Bowel Elimination.

6. Which of the following statements by Mr. Bright indicates successful patient teaching concerning antitussive treatment?
 a. "Since the cough syrup is not addictive, I can take it frequently."
 b. "It is best to eat a little with the cough syrup to prevent an upset stomach."
 *c. "I should not drive or operate machinery when I take this medicine."
 d. "A little wine will help relieve the shakiness caused by the drug."

 [NP: EV, CL: AP]

 Rationale: Because of the tendency for hydrocodone to cause drowsiness, the patient should be advised to avoid driving or operating heavy equipment.

Review Questions from Text

1. Which of the following is an example of a respiratory stimulant?
 a. atropine
 *b. theophylline
 c. epinephrine
 d. dopamine

 [CL: KN]

 Rationale: Theophylline is an example of a respiratory stimulant which is particularly useful in treating apnea.

2. An early sign of oxygen toxicity is:
 a. tingling in extremities
 b. confusion
 c. cyanosis
 *d. cough

 [CL: KN]

 Rationale: Early signs of oxygen toxicity include cough, nasal congestion, sore throat, and increasing dyspnea.

3. As a narcotic antitussive agent, methadone (Dolophine) has the following characteristic:
 a. indicated for asthma
 b. low addictive potential
 c. safe for head trauma
 *d. rapid onset of action

 [CL: KN]

 Rationale: Methadone has a rapid onset of action and long duration of effect. This agent has high addiction potential.

4. Carbon dioxide acts to increase breathing by:
 *a. stimulation of chemoreceptors

b. stimulation of central nervous system
c. activation of diaphragm muscles
d. elevation of the blood pH

[CL: KN]

Rationale: Carbon dioxide increases ventilation by stimulating the chemoreceptors which signal the respiratory center to increase rate and depth of ventilation.

5. Medroxyprogesterone acetate (Provera) exerts its action on respirations by:
a. influencing the pons and medulla oblongata to increase ventilation
*b. increasing responsiveness of respiratory center to carbon dioxide
c. reducing the level of oxygen, thereby stimulating chemoreceptors
d. stimulating the chemoreceptors directly, affecting respiratory drive

[CL: CO]

Rationale: This hormone increases responsiveness of the respiratory center to carbon dioxide and decreases the center's excitatory threshhold.

6. The optimum oxygen range for PaO_2 in premature infants is:
a. 80 to 100 mmHg
b. 70 to 90 mmHg
c. 40 to 60 mmHg
*d. 50 to 80 mmHg

[CL: KN]

Rationale: Oxygen should be administered to premature infants at a sufficient level to prevent hypoxemia. These patients are best maintained below 80 mmHg. A range of 50 to 80 mmHg for the PaO_2 is generally acceptable.

7. An oxygen concentration of 35 percent is best delivered by the following device:
a. nasal cannula
*b. Venturi mask
c. simple oxygen mask
d. rservoir mask

[CL: CO]

Rationale: Very precise oxygen concentrations, such as 35 percent, are delivered by Venturi mask devices.

8. Which of the following statements is correct regarding oxygen therapy?
a. It is administered in concentrations of 10 percent for therapeutic effectiveness.
*b. High concentrations can cause toxicity and lung damage when given for long periods of time.
c. A nasal cannula is the delivery system of choice for patients requiring high concentrations.
d. Oxygen concentrations of 60 percent are administered to patients with unresponsive respiratory centers.

[CL: KN]

Rationale: Oxygen toxicity can occur if high oxygen concentrations are given over long periods of time.

9. The amount of air moved with each breath is known as the:
*a. tidal volume
b. minute volume
c. vital capacity
d. exhaled volume

[CL: KN]

Rationale: Tidal volume is the amount of air that is inhaled and exhaled with each breath.

Additional Review Questions Not Presented in Text

1. Carbon dioxide should not be used in the following case:
   a. post-anesthesia hypoventilation
   b. severe anxiety reaction
   *c. oxygen-induced hypoventilation
   d. hiccoughs

   [CL: KN]

   Rationale: Carbon dioxide should not be used in patients with oxygen-induced hypoventilation because they become sensitized to the carbon dioxide as a breathing stimulus.

2. An example of a non-analeptic respiratory stimulant is:
   a. nikithamide
   b. doxapram
   *c. carbon dioxide
   d. caffeine

   [CL: KN]

   Rationale: Carbon dioxide is a non-analeptic respiratory stimulant which is useful in selective cases.

3. Which of the following statements is <u>correct</u> regarding hypoxemia?
   a. It is represented by a PaO_2 concentration of 83 mmHg.
   b. Hypoxemia cannot be corrected by oxygen therapy alone.
   c. It is represented by tissue oxygen deprivation.
   *d. Hypoxemia can result from thickened alveolar tissue.

   [CL: KN]

   Rationale: Conditions which alter the ability of oxygen to easily pass into the blood stream, such as thickened alveolar tissues, can cause hypoxemia.

4. Cyanosis, a bluish coloration of the skin, is:
   *a. assessed by examining the lips and conjunctiva
   b. present in all cases of hypoxemia
   c. absent in mild cases of hypoxemia
   d. thought to be indicative of an anemic state

   [CL: CO]

   Rationale: Assessment of mucous membranes is a valuable method of determining the presence of cyanosis. The presence of cyanosis may or may not indicate hypoxemia/hypoxia. Patients who are anemic may not demonstrate cyanosis.

CHAPTER 37: ANATOMY AND PHYSIOLOGY OF THE URINARY SYSTEM

Review Questions from Text

1. The process of excreting waste products as urine occurs in the following sequence:
 a. collecting ducts, glomerulus, proximal tubule, loop of Henle
 b. glomerulus, loop of Henle, proximal tubule, collecting ducts
 c. proximal tubule, glomerulus, loop of Henle, collecting ducts
 *d. glomerulus, proximal tubule, loop of Henle, collecting ducts

 [CL: CO]

 Rationale: The filtration of blood occurs in the glomerulus, forming glomerular filtrate. The proximal tubule then reabsorbs 70 yo 80 percent of the filtrate and returns it to the systemic circulation. Fluid leaving the proximal tubule enters the loop of Henle and then moves into the collecting ducts, where the filtrate is either concentrated or diluted prior to excretion as urine.

2. The kidney maintains acid-base homeostasis by:
 a. keeping extracellular pH within the range of 7.0 to 7.70
 *b. controlling bicarbonate concentration by renal H^+ excretion
 c. forming ammonia in the cells of the proximal tubule
 d. secreting H^+ ions into the proximal tubule in exchange for ammonium ions

 [CL: KN]

 Rationale: The kidney maintains acid-base regulation by generation of HCO_3^- through H^+ excretion.

3. Parathyroid hormone (PTH) elevates plasma calcium by working with Vitamin D to decrease:
 a. bone resorption
 b. intestinal calcium absorption
 *c. renal calcium excretion
 d. renal elimination of phosphate

 [CL: KN]

 Rationale: Parathyroid hormone (PTH) is secreted by the parathyroid glands when the plasma calcium is low. This hormone elevates plasma calcium by decreasing renal calcium excretion, increasing bone resorption, and increasing intestinal calcium absorption.

4. Antidiuretic hormone (ADH) acts on the following renal structure:
 *a. collecting ducts
 b. proximal tubule
 c. loop of Henle
 d. glomerulus

 [CL: KN]

 Rationale: ADH acts on the cortical and medullary collecting ducts of the kidney to alter water permeability.

5. The exchange of sodium for potassium in the distal convoluted tubule is regulated by:
 a. active chloride pump
 *b. aldosterone
 c. posterior pituitary gland
 d. antidiuretic hormone

 [CL: KN]

 Rationale: Aldosterone mediates the exchange of sodium for potassium in the distal convoluted tubule.

6. Vitamin D (cholecalciferol) is synthesized in the:
   a. large intestine
   b. stomach
   c. pancreas
   *d. skin

   [CL: KN]

   Rationale: Vitamin D which is ingested through the diet is synthesized in the skin.

7. The kidney produces a substance in response to hypoxia which increases red blood cell levels. This substance is known as:
   a. renin
   *b. erythropoietin
   c. prostaglandin
   d. angiotensin

   [CL: KN]

   Rationale: Erythropoietin, produced by the liver in response to hypoxia or other factors, stimulates erythrocyte production in the liver.

8. Patients with renal disease and diabetes mellitus may require:
   a. additional insulin
   *b. less insulin
   c. longer-acting insulin
   d. no insulin

   [CL: KN]

   Rationale: As much as 20 percent of insulin produced by the pancreas is degraded in the renal tubular cells. Therefore, diabetic patients with renal disease may require less insulin.

9. The primary site of actions for the triazide diuretics is the:
   a. loop of Henle
   b. proximal tubule
   c. collecting ducts
   *d. distal convoluted tubule

   [CL: CO]

   Rationale: The distal convoluted tubule is impermeable to water and urea, but contains a sodium pumping mechanism which is the site of action for thiazide diuretics.

10. One method of elimination of acid by the kidneys is accomplished by combining H^+ with:
   *a. ammonia
   b. chloride
   c. magnesium
   d. urea

   [CL: CO]

   Rationale: Ammonia (NH_3) diffuses into the lumen, combining with H^+ to form ammonium (NH_4), which is eliminated through the urine. This results in a reduction of H^+.

Additional Review Qustions Not Presented in Text

1. The thin segment of the loop of Henle is permeable to:
   a. water
   *b. urea

c. potassium
d. ammonium

[CL: KN]

Ratioale: The thin segment of the loop of Henle is impermeable to water, but allows NaCl and urea to pass out into the medullary interstitium.

2. The portion of the kidney which contains 6 to 12 cone-shaped masses is the:
*a. medulla
b. hilus
c. cortex
d. calyces

[CL: CO]

Rationale: The medulla is the inner portion of the kidney which contains cone-shaped masses called renal pyramids.

3. Which of the following renal structures is the primary site of "loop diuretics"?
a. thin segment of the loop of Henle
b. distal portion of convoluted tubule
c. proximal tubule
*d. thick segment of the loop of Henle

[CL: KN]

Rationale: The thick segment of the loop of Henle contains an active chloride pump which is the primary site of "loop diuretics."

4. The filtrate which leaves the proximal tubule has the following osmolarity:
a. hyperosmolar
b. hypertonic
*c. isotonic
d. hypotonic

[CL: CO]

Rationale: Fluid which leaves the proximal tubule has approximately the same osmolarity as plasma, which is isotonic.

5. When the H^+ decreases, the body attempts to correct the situation by:
a. increasing ventilation
*b. decreasing ventilation
c. reabsorption of HCO_3^-
d. increasing urine output

[CL: KN]

Rationale: As the H^+ concentration decreases, ventilation decreases in an attempt to retain acid (CO_2).

CHAPTER 38: DIURETICS

Situations from Text

Situation 38-1

Duncan McKeough is admitted to the medical-surgical unit with symptoms of shortness of breath and peripheral edema. Mr. McKeough is 52 years old and has a history of ETOH abuse and recurrent congestive heart failure.

1. An IV is started, and Mr. McKeough is to receive furosemide (Lasix) 40 mg IV. Because of his history, the nurse will assess the following with regard to diuretic therapy:
   a. T_3, T_4
   b. 12-lead EKG
   *c. albumin levels
   d. neurological status

   [NP: AS, CL: AN]

   Rationale: Because of the patient's history of ETOH abuse and potential for hepatic dysfunction, albumin levels should be noted. Patients with hypoalbuminemia may need protein replacement as well as diuretic therapy.

2. The nurse will observe for the following side effect of intravenous furosemide by assessing for:
   a. blurred vision
   b. rhinitis
   c. drowsiness
   *d. hearing loss

   [NP: IM, CL: CO]

   Rationale: Ototoxicity has been associated with loop diuretics such as furosemide. This may occur, in particular, with patients receiving large doses by intravenous infusion.

3. Mr. McKeough is started on oral furosemide 40 mg twice a day. The nurse will check lab values daily because of the potential for:
   *a. hyponatremia
   b. hyperchloremia
   c. hypermagnesemia
   d. hypophosphatemia

   [NP: IM, CL: KN]

   Rationale: Furosemide potentiates the exretion of sodium, causing hyponatremia.

4. Mr. McKeough is to continue furosemide (Lasix) 20 mg daily after discharge. The nurse will teach him to:
   a. take the medication on an empty stomach
   b. eat foods high in calcium
   *c. weigh daily and report rapid changes
   d. take medication in the evening

   [NP: IM, CL: KN]

   Rationale: Due to the diuretic effect, patients should weigh daily and report any rapid changes in weight. Rapid weight loss can cause dehydration and hypotension.

5. The nurse will teach Mr. McKeough to include the following in his daily diet while taking furosemide:
   a. milk
   b. red meats
   *c. dried fruits

d. grains

[NP: IM, CL: CO]

Rationale: Due to potassium depletion with diuretics, patients should include foods high in potassium, such as dried fruits.

6. When evaluating Mr. McKeough for the effects of diuretics, which of the following factors might be noted:
   *a. elevated clotting time
   b. reduced BUN levels
   c. acidosis
   d. hypoglycemia

[NP: EV, CL: AP]

Rationale: Patients on diuretic therapy should be observed for evidence of altered coagulation.

Situation 38-2

Margaret Roberts, aged 47 years, is recovering from a craniotomy. The nurse monitors the intracranial pressure (ICP) and reports an elevated reading.

1. The physician orders mannitol (Osmitrol) to be given via intravenous infusion. The nurse is aware that the usual dosage for a 25 percent solution would be:
   a. 5 to 6 gms per kg
   b. 600 to 1,000 mg per kg
   c. 200 to 300 mg per kg
   *d. 1.5 to 2.0 gms per kg

[NP: PL, CL: KN]

Rationale: To reduce intracranial pressure, the usual dosage for a 15 to 25 percent solution is 1.5 to 2.0 gms per kg.

2. The nurse will expect to observe Ms. Roberts for a reduction in the ICP within:
   a. 2 hours
   b. 5 minutes
   *c. 15 minutes
   d. 1 hour

[NP: PL, CL: KN]

Rationale: In general, a reduction in the ICP will be noted within 15 minutes of starting the infusion of mannitol.

3. A nursing responsibility associated with administration of mannitol to Ms. Roberts is to:
   a. discard the solution if crystals are present
   b. use only specially prepared tubing for administration
   *c. rewarm the solution if crystals are present
   d. cover the solution with foil to prevent deterioration

[NP: IM, CL: KN]

Rationale: Mannitol solutions frequently crystalize, but may be rewarmed gently to dissolve formed crystals.

4. Which of the following nursing diagnostic categories is <u>most</u> applicable to Ms. Roberts' situation in relation to mannitol therapy?
   *a. Alteration in Oral Mucous Membrane
   b. Alteration in Bowel Elimination: constipation

c. Sleep Pattern Disturbance
d. Hypothermia

[NP: AN, CL: AP]

Rationale: Dry mucous membranes are a common adverse effect of mannitol therapy; therefore, Alteration in Oral Mucous Membranes is an appropriate nursing diagnostic category.

5. When planning Ms. Roberts' care, the following interventions apply regarding mannitol therapy:
   a. weigh every third day
   b. give with blood products if necessary
   c. use a 21-gauge needle for infusion
   *d. use an inline IV filter

   [NP: PL, CL: KN]

   Rationale: It is recommended that mannitol be infused with an inline IV filter to prevent infusion of microcrystals.

6. Which of the following outcomes <u>best</u> represents therapeutic effects of mannitol therapy for Ms. Roberts?
   *a. improved neurological status
   b. increased intracranial pressure
   c. decreased peripheral edema
   d. enhanced creatinine clearance

   [NP: EV, CL: AN]

   Rationale: A therapeutic outcome of mannitol therapy for patients with increased intracranial pressure would be best demonstrated by improved neurological status.

Additional Situation Not Presented in Text

Sam Weiss is being treated as an outpatient for mild hypertension. He is a 60-year-old with a history of adult onset diabetes mellitus.

1. Mr. Weiss is to begin treatment with chlorothiazide (Diuril) 500 mg orally daily. The nurse will note the following as important assessment data prior to administration with chlorothiazide:
   a. T_3, T_4 levels
   b. serum gastrin levels
   c. protein electrophoresis
   *d. creatinine clearance

   [NP: AS, CL: AP]

   Rationale: Diminished renal function reduces the efficacy of thiazide diuretics. When the creatinine clearance is less than 40 to 50 ml/minute, the patient becomes unresponsive to this type of diuretic.

2. The nurse will plan to teach Mr. Weiss about the side effects of chlorothiazide, which include:
   a. angina-like pain
   *b. gastric irritation
   c. photosensitivity
   d. reduced hearing

   [NP: PL, CL: KN]

   Rationale: A common side effect of which patients need to be aware is gastric irritation, including nausea and vomiting.

3. When instructing Mr. Weiss about home management with chlorothiazide, the following is included:

a. Stop the medication if weakness is noted.
b. Take nonprescription drugs as needed.
c. Maintain a high sodium diet
*d. Change body positions slowly.

[NP: IM, CL: KN]

Rationale: Due to the potential for dizziness and orthostatic hypotension associated with chlorothiazide, patients should be taught to change positions slowly.

4. Five days after starting diuretic therapy, Mr. Weiss calls to tell the nurse that he is having "palpitations" and "skipped heart beats." The nurse informs the physician and is aware that these symptoms may relate to:
*a. hypokalemia
b. hypermagnesemia
c. hyperglycemia
d. hyponatremia

[NP: IM, CL: AP]

Rationale: The nurse should be alert for symptoms related to hypokalemia in patients on thiazide diuretics. Cardiac arrhythmias may be associated with hypokalemia.

5. Mr. Weiss has been taking chlorpropamide (Diabinese) 250 mg per day. The nurse is aware that potential interaction of this anti-hyperglycemic agent with chlorothiazide may result in:
a. increased diuresis
b. reduced diuresis
c. hypoglycemia
*d. hyperglycemia

[NP: PL, CL: KN]

Rationale: Patients taking oral hypoglycemic agents may demonstrate elevated blood sugars when thiazide diuretics are added to the medication regime.

6. When evaluating Mr. Weiss for effective therapy with chlorothiazide, it will be important for the nurse to consider that therapeutic antihypertensive effect may take:
a. 2 months
b. 2 weeks
*c. 4 weeks
d. 5 days

[NP: EV, CL: CO]

Rationale: The full therapeutic antihypertensive effect of thiazide diuretics may take up to one month.

Review Questions from Text

1. Carbonic anhydrate inhibitors:
a. create an osmotic gradient
b. result in acidic diuresis
c. decrease potassium excretion
*d. lead to systemic acidosis

[CL: KN]

Rationale: Carbonic anhydrase inhibitors block the formation of carbonic acid, resulting in excretion of Na^+ and HCO_3^- in the urine. This creates a state of systemic hyperchloremic acidosis.

2. Aldosterone antagonists:

a. produce a potent diuretic action
*b. inhibit the exchange of sodium for potassium
c. produce severe hypokalemia
d. have a rapid onset of action

[CL: KN]

Rationale: These diuretic agents compete with aldosterone and prevent the reabsorption of sodium (in exchange for potassium) in the distal tubules.

3. The pressure generated by contraction of the heart is referred to as:
*a. hydrostatic
b. nephrotic
c. oncotic
d. osmotic

[CL: KN]

Rationale: Hydrostatic pressure is that which is created by the contraction of the heart.

4. Fluid accumulates in the interstitial space when there exists:
a. increased intravascular oncotic pressure
b. decreased intravascular hydrostatic pressure
*c. altered capillary permeability
d. reduced volume of sodium in third space

[CL: KN]

Rationale: Fluid accumulates within the interstitial space when there exists an alteration in capillary permeability, an increase in intravascular hydrostatic pressure, or a decrease in intravascular oncotic pressure.

5. Angiotensin I is converted to angiotension II in the:
a. liver
b. adrenal glands
*c. lungs
d. kidneys

[CL: KN]

Rationale: Angiotensin I is converted to angiotension II in the lungs.

6. When treating patients who have ascites but no evidence of peripheral edema, the maximum extra diuresis that should be induced is:
*a. 900 ml/day
b. 2,000 ml/day
c. 1,500 ml/day
d. 1,200 ml/day

[CL: KN]

Rationale: Overdiuresis of patients with ascites results in depletion of intravascular volume. Peripheral edema fluid is mobilized faster than ascitic fluid. Patients without peripheral edema should not diurese over 900 ml/day.

7. Carbonic anhydrase inhibitors are contraindicated in the following patient situation:
a. open-angle glaucoma
*b. pulmonary obstruction
c. drug-induced edema
d. absence seizures

[CL: KN]

Rationale: Carbonic anhydrase inhibitors should not be used in situations, such as pulmonary obstruction, in which the resulting acidotic state would increase the respiratory rate.

8. Which of the following is an example of an osmotic diuretic?
   a. ethacrynic acid (Edecrin)
   b. bumefanide (Bumex)
   c. quinethazone (Hydromox)
   *d. urea (Ureaphil)

   [CL: KN]

   Rationale: Urea (Ureaphil) is an osmotic diuretic which is used to reduce intracranial and intraocular pressure.

9. Patients taking triamterene (Dyrenium) should not be given:
   a. aspirin
   b. calcium salts
   c. warfarin
   *d. potassium supplements

   [CL: AP]

   Rationale: Triamterene is a potassium-sparing agent with mild diuretic action. Patients taking this drug should not be given potassium supplements.

10. Edema which is generalized in all body tissue is known as:
   a. ascites
   *b. anasarca
   c. pitting edema
   d. peripheral edema

   [CL: KN]

   Rationale: Anasarca is a term referring to severe generalized edema.

<u>**Additional Review Questions Not Presented in Text**</u>

1. Thiazide-like diuretics acting in the distal tubule:
   a. inhibit potassium and chloride transport
   b. actively pump chloride out of the filtrate
   *c. work primarily in the cortical diluting segment
   d. inhibit the action of carbonic anhydrase

   [CL: KN]

   Rationale: Thiazide-like diuretics have as their primary site of action the cortical diluting segment of the nephron.

2. Osmotic diuretics have which of the following characteristics?
   a. high-molecular-weight
   b. hypo-osmolar
   c. pharmacologically active
   *d. limited reabsorption

   [CL: CO]

   Rationale: Osmotic diuretics are low-molecular-weight agents which are relatively inert and remain in high concentration in the renal tubules. Diuresis is caused by increased osmolarity of the glomerular filtrate, inhibiting the reabsorption of water. Their reabsorption by the renal tubule is limited.

3. Spironolactone (Aldactone) is a diuretic which is contraindicated in the following patient condition:
*a. hyperkalemia
b. hypomagnesemia
c. diabetes mellitus
d. secondary aldosteronism

[CL: KN]

Rationale: Spironolactone is a potassium-sparing diuretic which is contraindicated in patients who have hyperkalemia, due to potential for toxicity.

4. Which of the following is an example of a nonprescription diuretic?
a. amiloride
*b. pamabrom
c. metolazone
d. glycerin

[CL: KN]

Rationale: Pamabrom is a nonprescription diuretic which is used to alleviate premenstrual discomfort associated with fluid retention.

5. Carbonic anhydrase inhibitors (CAI) act at the following site:
*a. proximal tubule
b. Bowman's capsule
c. loop of Henle
d. distal convoluted tubule

[CL: KN]

Rationale: CAI's bind to carbonic anhydrase, which is found in the brush border of the proximal tubule.

CHAPTER 39: DRUG THERAPY FOR THE PATIENT WITH RENAL DISEASE

Situations from Text

Maude McKeever is a 49-year-old, transferred to the intensive care unit for management of acute tubular necrosis (ATN) related to hypovolemia secondary to an anaphylactic reaction.

1. Ms. McKeever is to be started on a continuous furosemide (Lasix) infusion. The nurse will expect to infuse the drug at a rate no greater than:
   a. 5 mg/min
   b. 2 mg/min
   c. 6 mg/min
   *d. 4 mg/min

   [NP: PL, CL: KN]

   Rationale: Due to the potential for ototoxicity, the furosemide infusion rate should not exceed 4 mg/minute.

2. The nurse will check Ms. McKeever's urine for specific gravity every eight hours. Which of the following values corresponds with a diagnosis of ATN?
   *a. 1.011
   b. 1.001
   c. 1.009
   d. 1.003

   [NP: IM, CL: CO]

   Rationale: In diseases such as ATN, the kidneys lose the ability to concentrate urine. A specific gravity of greater than 1.010 reflects impaired renal concentration.

3. Ms. McKeever has a urine output of 22 cc/hour on the furosemide infusion. In addition, the physician orders a dopamine drip at renal (dopaminergic) dosage. The nurse will begin the infusion at the following rate:
   a. 8 μg/kg/min
   b. 10 μg/kg/min
   *c. 2 μg/kg/min
   d. 15 μg/kg/min

   [NP: IM, CL: KN]

   Rationale: For stimulation of dopaminergic sites and dilation of renal and mesenteric arteries, the dopamine infusion should be between 1 and 5 μg/kg/min for optimum glomerular filtration rate.

4. Ms. McKeever is taking calcium channel blockers for management of elevated blood pressure. In addition, the nurse will expect to:
   *a. restrict dietary sodium
   b. encourage high protein diet
   c. restrict fluid intake
   d. encourage high fat intake

   [NP: PL, CL: AP]

   Rationale: Restricting dietary sodium may be an important aspect of management of hypertension related to acute renal failure.

5. Ms. McKeever's serum potassium is reported to be 7.0 mEq/L. A sodium polystyrene sulfonate (Kayexalate) enema is ordered to be given. The nurse will mix the drug with sorbitol for administration. The nurse is aware that the sorbitol reduces the potential for:
   a. Kayexalate tolerance

b. allergic reaction
c. diarrhea
*d. intestinal obstruction

[NP: AN, CL: KN]

Rationale: Sorbitol is an osmotic laxative which reduces the potential for constipation and prevents intestinal obstruction.

6. An expected outcome for Ms. McKeever following two Kayexalate enemas would be a serum potassium of:
*a. 5.5 mEq/L
b. 4.5 mEq/L
c. 4.0 mEq/L
d. 3.5 mEq/L

[NP: EV, CL: AP]

Rationale: Maximal results from one Kayexalate enema may lower the serum potassium by .5 to 1.0 mEq/L. In this case, a reduction of the serum potassium from 7.0 to 5.5 mEq/L is an appropriate outcome.

Situation 39-2

Hung Vu is a 52-year-old with chronic renal failure, admitted for placement of an A-V fistula for the purpose of hemodialysis. In addition to hemodialysis, he is to be managed medically for renal dysfunction-related problems and congestive heart failure.

1. Mr. Vu is to take an aluminum-containing antacid (Basagel) three times a day. The nurse is aware that the purpose of this antacid is to correct:
*a. hyperphosphatemia
b. hypokalemia
c. hypomagnesemia
d. hypercalcemia

[NP: AN, CL: CO]

Rationale: Aluminum-containing antacids bind with phosphate, reducing absorption of phosphate in the gastrointestinal tract.

2. The nurse will plan to administer the Basagel to Mr. Vu at the following times:
a. between meals
*b. with meals
c. an hour before meals
d. an hour after meals

[NP: PL, CL: KN]

Rationale: The phosphate binding effect is greater when Basagel is given with meals.

3. Mr. Vu is currently taking Schol's solution (Bicitra) daily. An adverse effect of this agent may be demonstrated by:
a. acidosis
*b. fluid excess
c. sedation
d. reduced urine output

Rationale: Patients with a secondary cardiac condition may demonstrate fluid volume excess related to Bicitra administration, which provides increased sodium in the form of $NaHCO_3$.

4. Mr. Vu complains of pain in the right big toe. It is red, swollen, and warm to touch. He is to be started on allopurinol (Zyloprim) 600 mg daily for three days. When evaluating benefit of this therapy, the nurse will

assess which laboratory value?
 a. ammonia
 b. calcium
 c. BUN
*d. uric acid

[NP: EV, CL: AP]

Rationale: Allopurinol is a xanthine oxidase inhibitor which decreases the production of uric acid. Hyperuricemia (gout) is a common result of renal failure.

5. The nurse reports that Mr. Vu is pale and complains of weakness. His hematocrit is 22.8. The nurse is aware that, when assessing anemia in the renal failure patient, the following must be taken into account:
 a. iron intake
 b. kidney size
*c. dilutional factors
 d. activity level

[NP: AS, CL: KN]

Rationale: The dilutional phenomena of renal failure must be considered when assessing for anemia in patients with renal failure.

6. Mr. Vu is to begin treatment with rHU-EPO (recombinant human erythropoietin) following hemodialysis three times weekly. An outcome of this type of therapy would be:
 a. decreased BUN levels
 b. elevated platelet count
 c. redued creatinine levels
*d. elevated red blood cell count

[NP: EV, CL: AP]

Rationale: Recombinant human erythropoietin has been shown to increase the erythrocyte count in 7 to 14 days following intravenous injection. This polypeptide acts on the bone marrow to accelerate maturation of red blood cells.

<u>Additional Situation Not Presented in Text</u>

Martin Winslow, aged 60 years, is being treated for congestive heart failure related to end stage renal disease (ESRD). He is to be dialyzed every day until fluid volume status is stable.

1. During the nursing assessment phase, Mr. Winslow complains of pruritis. In examining his skin, the nurse notes yellow-white crystals on the skin surface. The nurse is aware that this is related to:
 a. excess sodium in the diet
 b. Vitamin D deficiency
*c. excess urea in the sweat
 d. fatty acid deficiency

[NP: AS, CL: KN]

Rationale: The presence of yellow-white crystals on the skin surface is a result of excess urea in the sweat. This condition is called uremic frost.

2. Mr. Winslow is taking digoxin 0.125 mg po daily. In planning for administration of dialysis days, the nurse knows that hemodialysis has the following effect on digoxin levels:
*a. no effect on digoxin levels
 b. reduction in serum digoxin
 c. elevation in serum digoxin
 d. total elimination of digoxin

[NP: PL, CL: CO]

Rationale: Digoxin is not removed during hemodialysis.

3. Which of the following represents the best criterion for evaluating digoxin therapy for Mr. Vu?
   *a. serum digoxin
   b. heart rate
   c. blood pressure lying
   d. serum potassium

   [NP: EV, CL: KN]

   Rationale: Due to renal failure, digoxin toxicity represents a potential patient problem. Serum digoxin levels should be used to determine dosage.

4. When teaching Mr. Vu about dietary restrictions, the nurse will include the following food as one to be limited:
   a. grains
   b. fats
   *c. proteins
   d. sugars

   [NP: PL, CL: CO]

   Rationale: Patients in severe renal failure need to limit dietary protein. Protein metabolism adds to the total nitrogen excess already present.

5. Mr. Vu is weighed daily. He denies excessive fluid intake, but his weight is up 2 kgs from the previous day. The nurse is aware that this represents:
   a. 1 liter of fluid
   b. .5 liter of fluid
   c. 4 liters of fluid
   *d. 2 liters of fluid

   [NP: AS, CL :CO]

   Rationale: Weight gain may be the first sign of fluid retention. One kg of body weight equals about 1 liter of fluid.

6. The following nursing intervention will be included in the plan of care for Mr. Vu:
   *a. Record blood pressure lying and standing.
   b. Encouage intake of high potassium foods.
   c. Instruct him to swallow antacid tablets with water.
   d. Adjust salt intake according to serum osmolarity.

   [NP: IM, CL: KN]

   Rationale: In patients with renal dysfunction, the blood pressure should be recorded in both lying and standing positions. Patients with extra fluid on board exhibit an increase in blood pressure in a supine position.

Review Questions from Text

1. Patients with chronic renal failure may also exhibit the following condition:
   a. Addison's disease
   b. hyponatremia
   c. hypomagnesemia
   *d. Vitamin D deficiency

   [CL: CO]

   Rationale: Vitamin D metabolism is suppressed in patients with chronic renal failure. This results in altered absorption of calcium from the gastrointestinal system.

2. The body responds to metabolic acidosis (a decrease in arterial pH) by:
   a. decreasing renal ammonia production
   *b. increasing ventilation
   c. excreting large amounts of potassium
   d. retaining carbon dioxide

   [CL: CO]

   Rationale: In response to a decrease in arterial pH in metabolic acidosis, the body attempts to compensate by increasing the rate and depth of respirations, blowing off carbon dioxide.

3. Metabolic alkalosis is associated with:
   a. decreased arterial pH
   *b. increased plasma HCO_3^-
   c. increased ventilation
   d. decreased PCO_2

   [CL: KN]

   Rationale: Metabolic alkalosis is characterized by elevated plasma concentrations of bicarbonate (HCO_3^-), causing elevated pH levels.

4. A patient is said to be oliguric when the urine output is:
   *a. less than 20 ml/hour
   b. greater than 30 ml/hour
   c. less than 10 ml/hour
   d. greater than 200 ml/hour

   [CL: KN]

   Rationale: Oliguria is defined as urine output which is less than 20 ml/hour or 500 ml/day.

5. In a patient's chronic renal failure, the regulation serum calcium and phosphate are altered. A result of this dysfunction leads to:
   a. hypothyroidism
   b. hypoparathyroidism
   *c. secondary hyperparathyroidism
   d. primary hyperthyroidism

   [CL: KN]

   Rationale: Reduced calcium levels stimulate the production of parathormone from the parathyroid gland. As renal failure progresses, a condition of hyperparathyroidism develops.

6. For a serum potassium of 2.8 mEq/L, the intravenous potassium supplement flow rate is:
   a. $\leq$ 40 mEq/hour
   b. $\leq$ 20 mEq/hour
   *c. $\leq$10 mEq/hour
   d. $\leq$5 mEq/hour

   [CL: AP]

   Rationale: For moderate potassium deficits (not below 2.5 mEq/L), the intravenous potassium concentrations should not exceed 30 mEq/L, and the flow rate should be $\leq$10 mEq/hour.

7. Proximal renal tubular acidosis results in:
   a. impaired acidification of buffers

b. decreased formation of bicarbonate
*c. increased excretion of bicarbonate
d. increased formation of ammonia

[CL: CO]

Rationale: Proximal renal tubular acidosis is caused by altered bicarbonate reabsorption. This results in increased excretion of bicarbonate.

8. A creatinine clearance of 30 ml/min is classified as:
   a. normal renal function
   *b. moderate renal failure
   c. mild renal failure
   d. severe renal failure

   [CL: KN]

   Rationale: A creatinine clearance of 30 ml/minute is classified as moderate renal failure.

9. Elevation in the blood urea nitrogen (BUN) greater than the rise in serum creatinine early in the oliguric patient is termed:
   a. severe renal failure
   b. osteitis fibrosa
   c. uremic poisoning
   *d. pre-renal axotemia

   [CL:KN]

   Rationale: Pre-renal axotemia is said to exist in the oliguric patient when an elevation in the BUN is greater than the rise in the serum creatinine.

Additional Review Questions Not Presented in Text

1. In peritoneal dialysis, excess urea and waste products can be removed by:
   *a. increasing the concentration of glucose in dialysate
   b. decreasing the concentration of sodium in dialysate
   c. adding potassium to the peritoneal dialysate
   d. decreasing the nitrogen-containing products in dialysate

   [CL: KN]

   Rationale: By increasing the glucose concentrate in the dialysate, a greater osmotic gradient is created and more waste products are removed.

2. Which of the following is the most valid indicator of renal status?
   a. BUN
   b. sodium levels
   c. potassium levels
   *d. creatinine clearance

   [CL: KN]

   Rationale: Creatinine clearance, which reflects glomerular filtration, is the most valuable indicator of renal status. BUN is less sensitive and may not be abnormal until creatinine clearance is moderately abnormal.

3. Which of the following drugs is lost through hemodialysis?
   a. phenytoin
   b. furosemide
   *c. phenobarbital

d. diazepam

[CL: KN]

Rationale: Phenobarbital is extracted from the system via hemodialysis. In cases of severe phenobarbital overdose, hemodialysis may be one aspect of treatment.

4. Of the following values, which represents a normal creatinine clearance for females?
   a. 140 ml/min
   b. 86 ml/min
   *c. 102 ml/min
   d. 167 ml/min

[CL: CO]

Rationale: Normal creatinine clearance values for females are 112 ± 20 ml/minute.

CHAPTER 40: OVERVIEW OF ANATOMY AND PHYSIOLOGY OF THE ENDOCRINE SYSTEM

Review Questions from Text

1. Of the following glands, which one is not a part of the endocrine system?
   *a. thymus
   b. pancreas
   c. parathyroid
   d. pituitary

   [CL: CO]

   Rationale: The function of the thymus involves the immune system, particularly in the newborn. The pancrease, parathyroid, and pituitary are all part of the endocrine system.

2. A polypeptide hormone synthesized by the anterior pituitary gland is:
   a. oxytocin
   b. thyrotropin
   *c. prolactin
   d. melanocyte-stimulating hormone

   [CL: KN]

   Rationale: The polypeptide hormones secreted by the anterior pituitary include growth hormone, prolactin, and corticotropin.

3. Which statement is correct regarding the neuroregulation of the endocrine system?
   a. Neuroregulation operates on a positive feedback principle.
   b. Endocrine glands secrete a limited amount of hormone when stimulated.
   *c. When the target organ responds strongly, endocrine activity is suppressed.
   d. The main factor in neuroregulation is the strength of the regulating hormone.

   [CL: CO]

   Rationale: Regulation of hormonal activity is by negative feedback mechanisms. The endocrine gland will continue to excrete hormone until the target organ responds appropriately. When the target organ's response is strong, hormonal activity is suppressed.

4. Which of the following hormones is secreted by the thyroid gland?
   a. thyrotropin
   *b. calcitonin
   c. chymotrypsin
   d. growth hormone

   [CL: KN]

   Rationale: Calcitonin is secreted by the thyroid gland and functions to regulate calcium and phosphorus levels.

5. Somatostatin, secreted by the delta cells of the pancreas, has the following action:
   *a. inhibition of insulin secretion
   b. stimulation of glucagon synthesis
   c. inhibition of growth hormone
   d. stimulation of nutrient assimilation

   [CL: KN]

   Rationale: Somatostatin, a hormone secreted by the delta cells of the pancreas, depresses insulin and glucagon secretion.

6. Which of the following hormones is secreted by the adrenal cortex?
   a. progesterone
   b. trypsin
   c. epinephrine
   *d. aldosterone

   [CL: KN]

   Rationale: Aldosterone is the major mineralocorticoid produced by the adrenal cortex. This hormone functions to stimulate reabsorption of sodium and chloride in the renal distal tubule.

7. Which of the following hormones acts to increase serum calcium levels?
   a. calcitonin
   b. oxytocin
   *c. parathormone
   d. somatatropin

   [CL: CO]

   Rationale: Parathormone, released by the parathyroid gland, increases serum calcium levels.

8. The estrogen hormones have the following action:
   *a. increase osteoblastic activity
   b. decrease fat deposits in the breast
   c. increase sodium and water excretion
   d. inhibit endometrial proliferation

   [CL: KN]

   Rationale: Estrogens increase osteoblastic activity which is concerned with the formation of bone tissue.

9. Cortisol is a hormone which:
   *a. stimulates gluconeogenesis in the liver
   b. increases the rate of glucose utilization
   c. increases the rate of protein anabolism
   d. inhibits fat storage in breast tissue

   [CL: KN]

   Rationale: By stimulating gluconeogenesis in the liver, cortisol maintains serum blood levels.

10. Which of the following hormones requires a protein carrier for transport?
   a. glucagon
   b. insulin
   *c. testosterone
   d. antidiuretic hormone

   [CL: KN]

   Rationale: Testosterone is an example of a more insoluble hormone which requires a protein carrier.

<u>Additional Review Questions Not Presented in Text</u>

1. Endocrine secretions are:
   a. secreted via ducts to an epithelial surface
   b. metabolized in the target organs
   *c. structured as a protein or steroid
   d. excreted via the liver ducts

   [CL: CO]

Rationale: Endocrine secretions, called hormones, are structurally either steroids or proteins.

2. Which statement is correct regarding the endocrine system?
   a. The anterior lobe of the pituitary gland is referred to as the neurohypophysis.
   b. Thyrotropin has as its target organ the parathyroid gland.
   *c. The anterior pituitary secretes hormones in response to the hypothalamus.
   d. Adrenocorticotropic hormone (ACTH) has as its target organ the adrenal medulla.

   [CL: CO]

   Rationale: The anterior pituitary (or adrenohypophysis) secretes hormones in response to releasing or inhibiting factors from the hypothalamus.

3. Antidiuretic hormone (ADH) or vasopressin is released from the posterior pituitary in response to:
   *a. decreased blood pressure
   b. expansion of atrial stretch receptors
   c. decreased osmotic pressure
   d. increased blood volume

   [CL: KN]

   Rationale: A decrease in blood pressure influences ADH release, inhibiting the excretion of water by the kidneys.

4. Which of the following statements is correct regarding the function of pancreatic digestive enzymes?
   a. Trypsin aids in fat digestion.
   *b. Amylase aids carbohydrate digestion.
   c. Lipase aids in protein digestion.
   d. Chymotrypsin aids fat digestion.

   [CL: KN]

   Rationale: Pancreatic amylase aids in the digestion of carbohydrates.

5. Oversecretion of thyroxine results in:
   a. cretinism
   b. Addison's disease
   c. Cushing's disease
   *d. Graves' disease

   [CL: KN]

   Rationale: Hypersecretion of thyroxine results in hyperthyroidism or Graves' disease.

CHAPTER 41: PITUITARY DRUGS

Situation from Text

Situation 41-1

Inez Greenberg, aged 47 years, is admitted to the intensive care unit after a craniotomy for removal of a pituitary tumor.

1. On the second postoperative day, the nurse notes that Ms. Greenberg's urine output for 3 consecutive hours is >300 cc per hour. The nurse informs the physician and is aware that this sign is related to:
   a. diabetes mellitus
   b. acute renal failure
   c. nephrogenic diabetes insipidus
   *d. hypothalamic diabetes insipidus

   [NP: AS, CL: AP]

   Rationale: Due to removal of pituitary tumor, this patient is at risk for development of hypothalamic diabetes insipidus. This condition exists due to the reduced release of antidiuretic hormone.

2. The nurse is to administer vasopressin tannate to Ms. Greenberg. The expected route of administration of this drug is:
   a. oral
   *b. intramuscular
   c. intravenous
   d. intranasal

   [NP: PL, CL: KN]

   Rationale: Vasopressin tannate is given intramuscularly. It is not to be used intravenously. Vasopressin is destroyed by digestive enzymes and cannot be given orally.

3. A nursing action associated with vasopressin tannate therapy for Ms. Greenberg includes:
   a. taking the blood pressure before administration
   b. keeping the patient on bed rest
   *c. shaking the medication to mix well
   d. storing the medication away from light

   [NP: IM, CL: KN]

   Rationale: Vasopressin tannate is an oil suspension which must be thoroughly mixed to ensure that all the particles are included in the suspension.

4. Two hours after administration of vasopressin, Ms. Greenberg complains of a throbbing headache. This symptom most probably relates to:
   a. subtherapeutic dose of vasopressin
   *b. adverse effects of vasopressin
   c. allergic reaction to vasopressin
   d. toxic effects of vasopressin

   [NP: AN, CL: AP]

   Rationale: Adverse effects of vasopressin tannate include pounding in the head, pallor, and sweating.

5. An expected outcome for Ms. Greenberg would be a urine output of:
   *a. 1.5 to 2 liters per day
   b. 200 cc/hour for 24 hours

c. 3 to 3.5 liters per day
d. 150 cc/hour for 24 hours

[NP: PL, CL: CO]

Rationale: Patients on antidiuretic therapy should have the medication adjusted to maintain a urine output of 1.5 to 2 liters per day.

6. In monitoring Ms. Greenberg, the nurse will report the following subjective symptom:
   a. tremors
   b. nasal congestion
   c. sore throat
   *d. thirst

   [NP: IM, CL: KN]

   Rationale: Signs of dehydration, such as thirst, should be reported promptly because they indicate a need for alteration of the dosage.

<u>Additional Situation Not Presented in Text</u>

Connie Gagnard is a 6-year-old with a deficiency of endogenous growth hormone. She is being evaluated for therapy with growth hormone.

1. Connie receives an injection of arginine for the purpose of a stimulation test. An outcome which is consistent with her diagnosis would be:
   a. increased muscle strength
   b. elevated somatotropin levels
   c. no increase in muscle strength
   *d. no elevation in somatotropin

   [NP: AS, CL: AP]

   Rationale: In patients with growth hormone deficiency, a stimulation test with arginine will show no inrease in somatotropin levels.

2. During the assessment, which of the following items of information elicited from the parents about Connie is of concern related to growth hormone therapy?
   a. refusal to drink milk
   *b. loss of vision
   c. dry mucous membranes
   d. display of sibling rivalry

   [NP: AS, CL: CO]

   Rationale: When assessing patients for growth hormone therapy, the nurse should be in tune to signs of craniopharyngioma, which include headache, nausea, and/or loss of vision. The presence of craniopharyngioma is a contraindication to therapy.

3. Before administration of somatotropin to Connie, the nurse will check documentation of:
   a. ability to understand treatment
   *b. evidence of open bone epiphyses
   c. retarded growth rate
   d. adequate urine output

   [NP: PL, CL: AP]

   Rationale: Somatotropin should be administered to children prior to closure of the bone epiphyses. This assures best results of hormonal therapy.

4. The nurse will teach Connie's parents about growth hormone therapy and their role in Connie's care. This includes to:
   a. test the urine specific gravity daily
   b. administer the drug daily with meals
   *c. record the child's height and weight regularly.
   d. restrict oral fluids in order to prevent overhydration

   [NP: IM, CL: CO]

   Rationale: Somatotropin is administered by the physician, but the parents should be involved in monitoring the child's growth and development.

5. During Connie's follow-up visits, the nurse will check the following laboratory value in relation to somatotropin therapy:
   a. white blood cells
   b. platelets
   *c. glucose
   d. creatinine

   [NP: EV, CL: KN]

   Rationale: Blood glucose levels should be monitored in patients receiving growth hormone because this drug may cause insulin resistance.

6. An anticipated growth rate for Connie would be:
   *a. 7 cm per year
   b. 2.5 cm per year
   c. 3 cm per year
   d. 1 cm per month

   [NP: EV, CL: KN]

   Rationale: Growth rates in children on growth hormone should average about 7 cm per year.

Review Questions from Text

1. Somatotropin hormone produces which of the following effects?
   *a. produces a positive nitrogen balance
   b. increases cell size in specific organs
   c. inhibits protein synthesis within the cell
   d. increases glucose transport into the cell

   [CL: CO]

   Rationale: Somatotropin (growth hormone) stimulates a protein-building cycle, increasing the nitrogen balance. This hormone has no specific target organ; instead, generalized tissue growth occurs.

2. The lipolytic effect of growth hormone leads to:
   a. excess low-density lipids in the plasma
   b. reduction of fat storage in the liver
   *c. conversion of fatty acids to ketone bodies
   d. decreased availability of fatty acids for energy

   [CL: KN]

   Rationale: The lipolytic or ketogenic effect of growth hormone results in increased fat stores in the liver and leads to the conversion of fatty acids to ketone bodies.

3. Certain drugs may stimulate vasopressin release, including:

a. caffeine
b. insulin
*c. nicotine
d. levodopa

[CL: KN]

Rationale: Drugs such as nicotine and chlorpropamide (Diabinese) stimulate vasopressin release.

4. In large doses, the following effect may occur with vasopressin therapy:
   a. inhibition of peristaltic activity in the large bowel
   b. dilation of the superior mesenteric artery
   c. increased blood flow to the splanchnic system
   *d. contraction of smooth muscle in arterioles

   [CL: KN]

   Rationale: In larger doses, vasopressin stimulates smooth muscle contraction, which is particularly evident in small arterioles.

5. The agent of choice in maintaining hemostasis during surgery in patients with Von Willebrand's disease is:
   a. posterior pituitary injection
   *b. desmopressin
   c. lypressin
   d. vasopressin

   [CL: KN]

   Rationale: Desmopressin increases factor VIII levels and is used to maintain hemostasis during and after surgery in patients with Von Willebrand's disease.

6. Vasopressin is produced by the:
   a. posterior pituitary
   b. anterior pituitary
   *c. hypothalamus
   d. thymus

   [CL: KN]

   Rationale: Vasopressin is produced in the hypothalamus and stored in the posterior pituitary, to be released as needed by the body.

7. A major disadvantage of somatotropin (Humatrope) therapy is:
   *a. cost
   b. side effects
   c. antibody production
   d. contamination

   [CL: CO]

   Rationale: Somatotropin therapy is quite expensive, costing around $5,000 to $25,000 per year.

8. The secretion of growth hormone is suppressed by:
   a. stress
   b. emotional excitement
   c. hypoglycemic agents
   *d. glucocorticoid drugs

   [CL: KN]

Rationale: Secretion of growth hormone is suppressed by glucocorticoid drugs.

9. Drugs which inhibit vasopressin release inclue:
   a. tricyclic antidepressants
   *b. alcohol
   c. caffeine
   d. barbiturates

   [CL: KN]

   Rationale: Alcohol inhibits vasopressin release. Other agents which depress vasopressin release include phenytoin and chlorpromazide.

Review Questions Not Presented in Text

1. When giving vasopressin, the nurse is aware that this drug is:
   a. contraindicated in massive gastrointestinal bleeding
   b. recommended for long-term treatment of diabetes mellitus
   *c. followed with 1 to 2 glasses of water to reduce adverse effects
   d. used to decrease the permeability of the distal tubules to water

   [CL: KN]

   Rationale: After vasopressin administration, the patient is encouraged to drink 1 to 2 glasses of water in order to minimize side effects.

2. Regarding dosage and administration of antidiuretic drugs, which of the following is correct?
   a. Lypressin (Diapid) is administered as a nasal spray once a day.
   *b. Desmopressin (Stimate) is given intravenously 0.3 μg/kg diluted in normal saline.
   c. The usual dosage of lypressin (Diapid) is 1 to 4 ml per day in divided doses.
   d. Desmopressin (Stimate) may be administered subcutaneously 4 to 40 mEq per day.

   [CL: CO]

   Rationale: In certain situations, desmopressin (Stimate) may be administered intravenously. The dosage is 0.3 mcg/kg diluted in normal saline and infused over 15 to 30 minutes.

3. In patients with upper respiratory infections, the current dosage of lypressin may need to be:
   *a. increased
   b. withheld
   c. reduced
   d. continued

   [CL: AP]

   Rationale: For patients who have upper respiratory disease causing nasal congestion, the dosage of lypressin may need to be increased.

4. The expected duration of vasopressin (Pitressin) injection is:
   a. 48 to 96 hours
   b. one week
   c. 24 hours
   *d. 2 to 8 hours

   [CL: KN]

   Rationale: Vasopressin injection has a relatively short duration of action, approximately 2 to 8 hours.

CHAPTER 42: ADRENAL CORTICAL DRUGS

Situations from Text

Situation 42-1

Mac Rubin is a 55-year-old undergoing diagnotic testing for suspected Addison's disease. He is being cared for on a medical floor.

1. After obtaining baseline 24-hour urine samples for 17-KS, 17-KSG, and 17-OHCS, the nurse administers dexamethasone and ACTH as ordered. A second 24-hour urine specimen is obtained for the same values. The nurse is aware that the following results correlate with a diagnosis of primary adrenal insufficiency:
   a. increase in urinary steroid levels threefold
   b. decrease in urinary steroid levels threefold
   *c. no increase in urinary steroid levels
   d. increase in urinary steroid levels tenfold

   [NP: AS, CL: KN]

   Rationale: In patients with primary adrenal insufficiency, the second 24-hour urine after ACTH stimulation will reveal no increase in urinary steroid levels. In the normal individual, urinary steroid levels will increase threefold to fivefold after ACTH stimulation.

2. Mr. Rubin is to receive desoxycorticosterone acetate (DOCA) 5 mg intramuscularly. After giving the drug, the nurse will monitor the following:
   a. attention span
   b. fine mtor movement
   c. deep tendon reflexes
   *d. blood pressure

   [NP: IM, CL: CO]

   Rationale: A major adverse effect of mineralocorticoids is sodium and water retention, increasing blood volume. This can lead to increased blood pressure in some cases.

3. In planning care for Mr. Rubin after initiating therapy DOCA, the nurse will include the following nursing measure:
   a. Maintain the patient NPO until two days past first dose.
   b. Force oral fluids at 73000 cc per day.
   c. Reduce protein and sodium intake.
   *d. Encourage a diet high in potassium.

   [NP: IM, CL: KN]

   Rationale: Reduced potassium levels are associated with mineralocorticoid therapy, and patients should be encouraged to increase dietary intake of potassium-rich foods.

4. For discharge, Mr. Rubin is to begin cortisone acetate (Cortone) 25 mg orally three times a day. Patient teaching should focus on:
   a. taking the drug on an empty stomach
   b. stopping the medication if drowsiness occurs
   c. using aspirin-containing products as needed
   *d. avoiding excessive intake of coffee and alcohol

   [NP: IM, CL: CO]

   Rationale: Due to the high potential for gastric irritation with adrenal cortical drugs, patients should avoid excessive intake of coffee and alcoholic beverages.

5. An anticipated outcome of therapy for Mr. Rubin would be:
   *a. less fatigue
   b. increased cardiac output
   c. increased urine output
   d. altered consciousness

   [NP: PL, CL: AP]

   Rationale: An oucome or goal which indicates appropriate therapy for Addison's disease would be increased energy resulting in less fatigue.

6. When providing follow-up care for Mr. Rubin, the nurse will check the following laboratory result, which tends to elevate due to steroid therapy:
   *a. cholesterol
   b. T_3
   c. potassium
   d. T_4

   [NP: EV, CL: KN]

   Rationale: Cholesterol and triglyceride levels increase as a result of steroid therapy.

Situation 42-2

Ralph Kuper is a 62-year-old admitted to the emergency room in acute respiratory distress related to status asthmaticus.

1. In addition to respiratory inhalation treatments, Mr. Kuper is to receive methylprednisolone sodium succinate (Solu-Medrol) intravenously. Prior to administering this drug, the nurse will assess for the following condition, which represents the need for cautious administration:
   a. coronary artery disease
   b. chronic lung disease
   *c. peptic ulcer disease
   d. urinary retention

   [NP: AS, CL: KN]

   Rationale: Peptic ulcer disease represents a condition in which steroids should be given cautiously, due to exacerbation of the disease and gastrointestinal bleeding.

2. When administering 1 gram of Solu-Medrol should be given over 10 to 20 minutes.

3. After initial emergency treatment, Mr. Kuper is transferred to a telemetry unit. A nursing history reveals that he has adult onset diabetes which is controlled by oral medication. Because he is receiving glucocorticoids, the nurse is aware of the potential for:
   a. reduced blood glucose levels
   b. increased effect of hypoglycemic agents
   c. reduced effectiveness of Solu-Medrol
   *d. increased blood glucose levels

   [NP: AN, CL: AP]

   Rationale: Glucocorticoids increase blood sugar levels, particularly in those patients with diabetes mellitus who are taking hypoglycemic agents.

4. Before Mr. Rubin begins long-term therapy with steroids as anti-inflammatory agents, the nurse will anticipate the following test:
   a. Tensilon
   *b. tuberculosis

c. ACTH stimulation
d. creatinine clearance

[NP: PL, CL: KN]

Rationale: Prior to long-term therapy with glucocorticoids, patients should be tested for the presence of active or arrested tuberculosis. If this condition exists, careful monitoring is indicated, as well as prophylactic INH therapy.

5. Mr. Rubin is to use a becomethasone (Vanceril) inhaler prn for asthma attacks. Which statement indicates adequate understanding of its use?
 a. "Since it is habit forming, I shouldn't use it every day."
 *b. "If I have to use the drug more often than prescribed, I will call the doctor."
 c. "Nausea and vomiting are side effects to be expected with this drug."
 d. "I should keep the inhaler in a dry, warm place when it is not in use."

[NP: EV, CL: CO]

Rationale: Although there are fewer side effects with a steroidal inhaler (local appliation) than with the systemic route, overuse or abuse can lead to hypothalamic-pituitary-adrenal (HPA) suppression.

6. Mr. Rubin will be discharged on prednisone 5 mg po qid. The nurse will plan the following goal for him:
 *a. maintenance on short-term therapy at lowest dose possible
 b. elimination of all symptoms associated with asthma
 c. maintenance on long-term glucocorticoid therapy
 d. elimination of all side effects associated with prednisone

[NP: PL, CL: CO]

Rationale: For patients on glucocorticoids for anti-inflammatory purposes, maintenance on the smallest dose possible for the shortest period of time reduces the potential for serious side effects.

Additional Situation Not Presented in Text

Dorothy Appleton is a 38-year-old with systemic lupus. She has been on long-term steroid therapy and is admitted for exacerbation of the disease.

1. During assessment of Ms. Appleton, which one of the following objective signs relates to chronic steroid use?
 a. dry flaky skin
 *b. thin, easily damaged skin
 c. muscle wasting in torso
 d. limited night vision

[NP: AS, CL: AP]

Rationale: Patients who are on long-term glucocorticoid therapy exhibit thin, delicate skin, which may bruise or tear easily. This adverse effect is related to altered protein metabolism due to steroid therapy.

2. Ms. Appleton is currently on prednisone 20 mg twice a day. She is scheduled for an arthroscopy for the next morning and is to be NPO past midnight. The nurse will anticipate the following:
 a. reduction in steroid dosage before surgery
 b. discontinuation of steroids until after surgery
 *c. maintenance on IV steroids during surgery
 d. elevation of dosages needed for pain relief

[NP: PL, CL:CO]

Rationale: Ptients who have been on long-term steroid therapy should receive intravenous steroids if they are unable to take the medication by mouth. In addition, surgery represents a stressful situation which may require increased steroid therapy.

3. Which of the following nursing diagnostic categories would be most applicable to Ms. Appleton's situation?
   *a. Potential for Infection
   b. Decreased Cardiac Output
   c. Ineffective Airway Clearance
   d. Alteration in Temperature Regulation

   [NP: AN, CL: AP]

   Rationale: Due to the effect of steroid use on the immune system, patients on steroid therapy are prone to infection.

4. In planning for care of Ms. Appleton postoperatively, the nurse will include the following nursing measure:
   a. Withhold steroid if nauseated.
   b. Force oral fluids
   c. Reduce protein intake.
   *d. Check stools for occult blood.

   [NP: IM, CL: KN]

   Rationale: Gastrointestinal bleeding is a possible side effect of steroid therapy; therefore, checking all stools for occult blood is an appropriate nursing measure.

5. When evaluating Ms. Appleton's CBC results, the nurse is aware that the following is most likely related to steroid therapy:
   *a. elevated WBC's
   b. elevated platelets
   c. reduced RBC's
   d. reduced RBC size

   [NP: EV, CL: KN]

   Rationale: Neutrophils have been shown to be modestly high in relation to steroid therapy. A WBC count of 10,000 to 15,000 may result from steroids rather than an infectious process.

6. To discharge home, Ms. Appleton is instructed to take the prednisone every other day. The nurse explains that the purpose of this is to:
   a. eliminate unwanted side effects
   b. prolong therapeutic effects
   c. maintain steroid tolerance
   *d. reduce adverse systemic effects

   [NP: IM, CL: KN]

   Rationale: Alternate-day therapy may be helpful in reducing adrenocortical suppression and related side effects of long-term steroid therapy.

Review Questions from Text

1. A sign related to adrenal cortex hypofunction is:
   a. hyperglycemia
   *b. electrolyte imbalances
   c. muscle wasting
   d. increased stress response

   [CL: KN]

   Rationale: Common signs of adrenal cortex hypofunction (as in Addison's disease) include fluid and electrolyte imbalances resulting in water and sodium loss and potassium retention.

2. Aldosterone secretion is controlled by potassium and:

a. antidiuretic hormone
b. serum osmolality
c. sodium levels
*d. angiotensin

[CL: KN]

Rationale: Angiotensin stimulates the release of aldosterone from the adrenal cortex.

3. An agent used for maintenance therapy for patients with salt-losing adrenogenital syndrome is:
*a. desoxycorticosterone pivalate
b. paramethasone acetate
c. dexamethasone
d. beclomethasone dipropionate

[CL: KN]

Rationale: Desoxycorticosterone pivalate (Pivalate) is a mineralocorticoid used to provide maintenance therapy for patients with salt-losing adrenogenital syndrome and adrenocortical insufficiency.

4. Glucocorticoid regulation is mediated by:
a. somatotropin
b. renin
c. sodium levels
*d. corticotropin

[CL: KN]

Rationale: Corticotropin (ACTH) secreted by the anterior pituitary gland controls the release of glucocorticoids from the adrenal cortex.

5. The effect of glucocorticoids in protein metabolism results in:
a. greater coordination, particularly hand-eye coordination
*b. muscular weakness, particularly lower extremities
c. massive muscular bulk without concomitant strength
d. marked growth in height and weight in children

[CL: KN]

Rationale: The effect of glucocorticoids on protein metabolism leads to muscle weakness in all extremities, especially the lower extremities.

6. Which statement regarding glucocorticoid drugs is correct?
a. Physiologic doses usually cause the adverse effects of therapy.
b. These drugs are most often used for their anti-stress effects.
*c. Therapy is adjusted to mimic the normal diurnal pattern of cortisol.
d. All glucocorticoids are effective when given by the oral route.

[CL: CO]

Rationale: In some cases, glucocorticoid drugs are adjusted to mimic the normal diurnal pattern of cortisol excretion.

7. Patients who are on long-term glucocorticoid therapy may take on the cushingoid appearance, typified by the following characteristic:
a. fat deposits in extremities
*b. cervicodorsal fat pad
c. clubbing of fingernails
d. exophthalamos

[CL: CO]

Rationale: Redistribution of fat stores is associated with glucocorticoid therapy, resulting in a cervicodorsal fat pad or buffalo hump.

8. When patients are abruptly withdrawn from long-term glucocorticoid therapy, acute adrenal insufficiency may occur. An indicator of this life-threatening complication is:
*a. syncope
b. palpitations
c. hypertension
d. shortness of breath

[CL: KN]

Rationale: Abrupt withdrawal of long-term glucocorticoid therapy may result in syncope, muscular weakness, nausea, anorexia, and hypotension.

9. Which statement is correct regarding adrenal drugs as a group?
a. Maintenance doses should be at the high end of the usual adult dosage.
b. All adrenal cortex agents are among the safest drugs on the market.
*c. The synthetic steroids are more potent than naturally-occurring agents.
d. The sodium-retaining potential is enhanced in synthetic corticosteroids.

[CL: KN]

Rationale: The synthetic corticosteroids are more potent than cortisone and hydrocortisone, which are natural products. Additionally, the sodium-retaining potential is greatly decreased or eliminated in synthetic products.

Additional Review Questions Not Presented in Text

1. Mineralocorticoid is the term applied to those corticosteroids that:
a. are indicated in patients with hypertension
b. act directly on protein and carbohydrate metabolism
c. enhance sodium and chloride excretion in the urine
*d. affect electrolyte and water balance in the body

[CL: KN]

Rationale: Mineralocorticoids are those steroids which exert major effects on water and electrolyte balance.

2. In terms of carbohydrate metabolism, the glucocorticoids:
*a. promote glucose storage
b. promote protein anabolism
c. increase glucose utilization
d. inhibit gluconeogenesis

[CL: CO]

Rationale: Glucocorticoids promote glucose storage in the form of glycogen and stimulate gluconeogenesis.

3. Glucocorticoids exert an anti-inflammatory response by:
a. increasing capillary permeability and dilation
b. stimulating fibroblast proliferation
*c. preventing the release of bradykinins and prostaglandins
d. promoting movement of neutrophils to the site of injury

[CL: KN]

Rationale: Glucocorticoids reduce the signs of inflammation by preventing the release or synthesis of vasodilator substances such as bradykinins, prostaglandins, and histamines.

4. Of the following drug interactions, which one correctly describes the effect of corticosteroids and other agents?
   a. Glucocorticoids increase salicylate levels.
   *b. Phenytoin increases glucocorticoid metabolism.
   c. Rifampin reduces glucocorticoid metabolism.
   d. Glucocorticoids increase the response of anticoagulants.

   [CL: CO]

   Rationale: The use of phenytoin (Dilantin) increases glucocorticoid metabolism.

CHAPTER 43: HORMONES: MALE AND FEMALE

Situations from Text

Situation 43-1

Jonathan Stance, an 18-year-old, has been evaluated for hypogonadism and is to be treated through the health clinic.

1. During the nursing assessment, the nurse will check Jonathan for:
   *a. excessive growth of long bones
   b. decreased subcutaneous fat
   c. heavy growth of facial hair
   d. increased muscle strength

   [NP: AS, CL: CO]

   Rationale: Assessment of the patient in his late teens with hypogonadism will reveal excessive growth of long bones, absence of male pattern hair growth, and small exteral genitalia.

2. Jonathan is to begin treatment with testosterone cypionate (Depo-testosterone). The nurse will expect that this drug will be given by the following route:
   a. intravenous
   b. subcutaneous
   *c. intramuscular
   d. buccal

   [NP: PL, CL: KN]

   Rationale: Testosterone cypionate is an androgen which is administered intramuscularly on a regular schedule until sexual characteristics have developed. Oral agents are less effective initially, due to high first-pass effect.

3. The nurse will plan for Jonathan's medication schedule of testosterone cypionate based on the following length of drug effectiveness:
   a. 2 months
   *b. 2 to 4 weeks
   c. 5 days
   d. 24 to 48 hours

   [NP: PL, CL: KN]

   Rationale: Testosterone cypionate, a long-acting androgen, lasts approximately 2 to 4 weeks.

4. The nurse will teach Jonathan about side effects related to testosterone therapy. The following side effect is included:
   *a. insomnia
   b. high-pitched voice
   c. weakness
   d. photosensitivity

   [NP: IM, CL: KN]

   Rationale: A side effect related to testosterone therapy is sleeplessness. Other nervous system effects are excitation and changes in libido.

5. On a follow-up visit, Jonathan is to begin oral therapy with fluoxymesterone (Halotestin) after evidence of sexual characteristics develops. The nurse will instruct him to:
   a. use antacids regularly
   b. force oral fluids

c. reduce protein intake
*d. take the drug with meals

[NP: IM, CL: KN]

Rationale: Common side effects of oral testosterone therapy are nausea, vomiting, and diarrhea. Taking the drug with meals will reduce these effects.

6. When evaluating Jonathan, an important aspect to monitor would be:
 a. tuberculin skin test
 *b. liver function tests
 c. creatinine clearance
 d. cardiac enzyme levels

[NP: EV, CL: CO]

Rationale: Hepatic function can be altered by testosterone therapy. Liver function tests should be monitored at regular intervals.

Situation 43-2

Lauren Mann, aged 46, presents to the health clinic with symptoms of postmenopausal syndrome. She complains of excessive perspiration, hot flashes, and fatigue.

1. Ms. Mann will be placed on 1 mg of conjugated estrogens (Premarin). The nurse will anticipate the following schedule of administration of Premarin:
 a. every other day
 b. every third day
 c. fourteen days on/fourteen days off
 *d. three weeks on/one week off

[NP: PL, CL: KN]

Rationale: Conjugated estrogens optimally should be administered in a cyclic fashion, three weeks on and one week off.

2. When taking Ms. Mann's history, the nurse will report the following, which represents a contraindication to estrogen therapy:
 a. osteoporosis
 b. chronic asthma
 c. coronary artery disease
 *d. liver disease

[NP: AS, CL: CO]

Rationale: Estrogen therapy is contraindicated in patients with liver dysfunction. Estrogens are metabolized extensively by the liver.

3. The nurse will include the following in a teaching session with Ms. Mann:
 a. avoid strenuous activity
 *b. check weight regularly
 c. report any nausea imediately
 d. take as needed for hot flashes

[NP: IM, CL: CO]

Rationale: Sodium and water retention have been associated with estrogen therapy. Patients should be taught to weigh regularly and to report sudden weight gain.

4. Which of the following activities reported by Ms. Mann warrants immediate attention by the nurse?

a. voracious reading
b. gourmet cooking
c. jogging
*d. cigarette smoking

[NP: AS, CL: KN]

Rationale: Patients taking estrogen should be encouraged to reduce or eliminate cigarette smoking due to the link with increased risk of vascular disease.

5. Additional teaching information relative to Ms. Mann's care would include:
   a. reducing intake of citrus juices
   b. avoiding large meals
   *c. taking medication after meals
   d. preventing excess sun exposure

   [NP: IM, CL: AP]

   Rationale: The side effect of nausea and vomiting may be reduced by taking estrogen agents on a full stomach.

6. The nurse takes a diet history of Ms. Man and will encourage a high dietary intake of:
   a. potassium
   b. sodium
   *c. calcium
   d. Vitamin C

   [NP: IM, CL: AP]

   Rationale: Postmenopausal women should increase their dietary intake of calcium in order to prevent osteoporosis.

Additional Situation Not Presented in Text

Phoebe Walden is a 29-year-old desiring to have a family. She has not been able to conceive since stopping oral contraceptives two years ago. She is seen in the fertility clinic for medical treatment of infertility.

1. Ms. Walden is to begin treatment with clomiphene (Clomid) 50 mg for five days. The nurse will teach her to begin taking this agent on the:
   a. first day of the menstrual cycle
   b. day that ovulation is determined
   c. last day of the menstrual cycle
   *d. fifth day of the menstrual cycle

   [NP: PL, CL: KN]

   Rationale: The patient will start taking clomiphene on the second or fifth day of the menstrual cycle and continue for five days.

2. When Ms. Walden returns to the clinic for follow-up, the nurse will question her about the presence of any:
   a. tingling in the extremities
   b. feelings of paranoia
   c. urinary urgency
   *d. unilateral pelvic pain

   [NP: AS, CL: AP]

   Rationale: Patients on fertility drugs should be evaluated for the presence of pain related to ovarian enlargement, which may indicate the presence of ovarian cysts.

3. After two unsuccessful courses of clomiphene, Ms. Walden returns to the clinic for additional drug therapy.

Clomiphene will be combined with human chorionic gonadotropin (HCG) during the next cycle. The nurse will teach Ms. Walden the following schedule for administration of HCG:
a. take orally along with clomiphene
*b. inject intramuscularly midcycle
c. take orally at midcycle
d. inject intramuscularly second day of cycle

[NP: IM, CL: KN]

Rationale: HCG is given intramuscularly at midcycle in conjunction with the clomiphene as ordered.

4. The nurse will instruct Ms. Walden about side effects related to HCG therapy. The following effect is included:
a. rhinitis
b. drowsiness
*c. headache
d. diarrhea

[NP: IM, CL: KN]

Rationale: Side effects related to HCG therapy include headache and nausea and vomiting.

5. In order to assure successful conception, Ms. Walden will be taught to have intercourse within:
a. 2 hours after HCG administration
b. 12 hours after clomiphene administration
c. 16 hours after clomiphene administration
*d. 12 hours after HCG administration

[NP: PL, CL: AP]

Rationale: The couple should be directed to have intercourse within 12 to 18 hours following HCG administration and daily for the next two days.

6. Which of the following signs/symptoms reported to the nurse by Ms. Walden would indicate that the physician should be notified immediately?
*a. abdominal distention
b. photophobia
c. restlessness
d. weight loss

[NP: PL, CL: KN]

Rationale: Signs and symptoms of ovarian enlargement and/or rupture of ovarian cysts, such as abdominal distention and/or unilateral pelvic pain aggravated by walking, should be reported to the physician immediately.

Review Questions from Text

1. Testosterone has anabolic activity and produces:
a. negative nitrogen balance
b. decreased red blood cell production
*c. increased musculature
d. decreased bone thickness

[CL: KN]

Rationale: Testosterone, the male sex hormone, produces a positive nitrogen balance and increase in musculature as a result of its anabolic activity.

2. Androgen therapy is contraindicated in the following condition:
a. postpartum breast engorgement

b. endometriosis
*c. cancer of the prostate gland
d. metastatic breast cancer

[CL: KN]

Rationale: Certain carcinomas (prostate and male breast) may be exacerbated by the use of male hormone therapy.

3. Which of the following hormonal agents is classified as an anabolic steroid?
*a. ethylestrenol (Maxibolin)
b. testolactone (Teslac)
c. estradiol vallerate (Delestrogen)
d. norethindrone (Nurlutin)

[CL: KN]

Rationale: Ethylestrenol (Maxibolin) is an anabolic steroid which promotes weight gain and bodybuilding processes.

4. Estrogen preparations increase the effect of the following drug when used in combination:
*a. hydrocortisone
b. phenytoin
c. tetracycline
d. rifampin

[CL: KN]

Rationale: Estrogen increases the effects of hydrocortisone by potentiating the anti-inflammatory effect.

5. Patients who are taking androgens along with coumadin should be observed for:
a. elevated clotting time
b. elevated ptt levels
*c. subtherapeutic pt levels
d. reduced white blood cells

[CL: AP]

Rationale: Androgens decrease the effect of oral anticoagulants, which, in the case of coumadin therapy, would be seen in subtherapeutic prothrombin times.

6. Which of the following signs would indicate the need to discontinue oral contraceptives?
a. nausea and vomiting
b. upper quadrant abdominal pain
c. headache with eyestrain
*d. pain and tenderness in the calf

[CL: KN]

Rationale: Oral contraceptives are contraindicated in patients with thrombophlebitis. When signs of calf pain and tenderness are reported, these agents should be discontinued.

7. An advantage of triphasic oral contraceptive products is:
a. reduced risk of vascular effects
*b. reduced breakthrough bleeding
c. increased protection in the early cycle
d. increased resistance to infection

[CL: KN]

Rationale: The triphasic pill provides greater protection at midcycle, reducing the occurrence of breakthrough bleeding.

8. The following is correct regarding the use of spermicidal creams:
   a. Spotting or bleeding is a common side effect.
   *b. Douching is avoided for 6 to 8 hours after use.
   c. Contracting the HIV virus is increased with use.
   d. Applying the product two hours before coitus is suggested.

   [CL: KN]

   Rationale: Patients using spermicidal creams should not douche for 6 to 8 hours after use, in order to maintain protection against pregnancy.

9. At times, a patient may need to change from one estrogen product to another. One milligram of diethylstilbesterol equals:
   a. 1.5 mg conjugated estrogen
   b. 10 mg Estrone
   c. 5 mg mestranol
   *d. 0.5 mg estradiol

   [CL: KN]

   Rationale: One milligram of diethylstilbesterol equals 0.5 mg of estradiol, 5 mg of conjugated estrogen, and 0.8 mg of mestranol.

Additional Review Questions Not Presented in Text

1. A major contribution to noncompliance in both men and women taking androgenic drugs is:
   a. cost of the drug
   b. frequent dosage schedule
   *c. change in body image
   d. lack of reported benefit

   [CL: CO]

   Rationale: Changes in body image in both men and women may contribute to noncompliance.

2. During the luteal phase of the menstrual cycle:
   a. progesterone is converted to cholesterol
   b. reduced estrogen signals menses
   *c. progesterone levels are increased
   d. estrogen secretion is inhibited

   [CL: CO]

   Rationale: During the luteal phase of the menstrual cycle, 10 to 20 mg of progesterone are secreted daily. The declining levels of progesterone signal the onset of menses.

3. Progestin-only agents used for contraception are referred to as "mini-pills." The progestins exert their contraceptive action by:
   *a. altering cervical mucus
   b. causing delayed ovulation
   c. blocking ovulation
   d. interfering with androstenedione

   [CL: KN]

   Rationale: Progestins, used as contraceptives, exert their action by altering the endometrium and cervical mucus, creating unfavorable conditions for sperm transport and implantation.

4. Women taking androgenic therapy for cancer of the breast should be observed for signs of:
   *a. hypercalcemia
   b. hypokalemia
   c. hyponatremia
   d. hypermagnesemia

   [CL: CO]

   Rationale: Women who are taking androgenic drugs should be monitored for signs of hypercalcemia. This is particularly true of women with cancer metastasis to the bone.

CHAPTER 44: AGENTS TO TREAT DIABETES MELLITUS

Situations from Text

Situation 44-1

Karen, a six-year-old, has just been diagnosed with Type I diabetes (IDDM). She is being cared for on the pediatric unit.

1. Karen is to receive Regular Humulin Insulin 10 units and NPH Humulin Insulin 30 units subcutaneously before breakfast (7:30 AM). The nurse will anticipate the onset of insulin action in approximately:
   a. three hours
   *b. 30 minutes
   c. 1 1/2 hours
   d. two hours

   [NP: PL, CL: CO]

   Rationale: The onset of action of regular insulin is 15 minutes to 1 hour. Regular Humulin Insulin has an even more rapid onset.

2. At what time of the day would the nurse be alert to the potential for a hypoglycemic reaction?
   a. after breakfast
   b. at midnight
   c. before bedtime
   *d. before supper

   [NP: AN, CL: AP]

   Rationale: The most likely time for an insulin reaction to occur in a patient who takes an intermediate-acting insulin in the morning is prior to supper.

3. When teaching Karen's mother about signs and symptoms of hypoglycemia, the nurse will include the following sign:
   *a. sweating
   b. polyuria
   c. polydipsia
   d. "fruity" breath

   [NP: IM, CL: AP]

   Rationale: Sweating is an early sign of hypoglycemia and is related to the release of epinephrine as a compensatory response.

4. The nurse will teach Karen's mother to administer insulin. The following information should be included:
   a. Intermediate-acting insulins should be clear in color.
   b. The vial of insulin should be shaken well before drawing up the dose.
   *c. Regular insulin is drawn up before NPH insulin in the same syringe.
   d. An air bubble should remain in the syringe for proper injection.

   [NP: IM, CL: KN]

   Rationale: Regular insulin should be drawn up first if mixed with an intermediate-acting insulin such as NPH. If NPH is drawn up first, it may contaminate the vial of regular insulin.

5. A potential nursing diagnosis category which <u>best</u> fits Karen's situation would be:
   *a. Alteration in Growth and Development
   b. Self Care Deficit

c. Anxiety
d. Sleep Pattern Disturbance

[NP: AN, CL: AN]

Rationale: Children with diabetes mellitus are at risk for Altered Growth and Development related to the effects of impaired glucose regulation.

6. Which of the following statements by Karen's mother indicates a need for further education?
a. "It is important to accurately prepare the dosages of insulin."
b. "The insulin should be injected at a 90-degree angle."
c. "Some kind of sugar should always be available in case of a reaction."
*d. "Periods of increased exercise will mean Karen will need more insulin."

[NP: EV, CL: AN]

Rationale: periods of increased exercise may require a reduced insulin dosage because exercise increases glucose utilization.

Situation 44-2

Bernard Wallace is a 50-year-old with a history of obesity and congestive heart failure. His blood sugars have not been well controlled by diet, and he is to begin therapy with an oral hypoglycemia agent.

1. Before starting treatment with chlorpropamide (Diabinese), Mr. Wallace will have complete blood work and assessment performed. The nurse will be aware that the following result indicates a contraindication to treatment with this drug:
a. elevated prothrombin time
b. low hemoglobin
*c. elevated creatinine
d. reduced calcium

[NP: AS, CL: AP]

Rationale: Chlorpropamide is a long-acting first generation agent which is not recommended for the diabetic with renal failure (as evidenced by elevated creatinine) because hypoglycemia may last for several days.

2. Additional data which is important to assess prior to beginning therapy with chlorpropamide is that of allergy history. Mr. Wallace should not take this agent if he is allergic to:
a. iodine
b. insulin
*c. sulfa
d. caffeine

[NP: AS, CL: CO]

Rationale: Cross sensitivity may occur in patients taking chlorpropamide (a sulfonylurea) who are allergic to sulfa medications.

3. Laboratory data are within normal limits, and Mr. Wallace is started on 250 mg of chlorpropamide (Diabinese) daily. Patient teaching about this agent will include the following information:
*a. Report headache and feelings of lethargy promptly.
b. Take the medication with an antacid.
c. Sporadic mealtimes are allowed with this agent.
d. Avoid exercising, since this can potentiate the drug's effect.

[NP: IM, CL: AP]

Rationale: Patients taking chlorpropamide are prone to inappropriate antidiuretic hormone secretion. Symptoms related to this condition correspond to hyponatremia. The patient should report headache/lethargy and signs of swelling promptly.

4. Additional patient teaching regarding chlorpropamide should include listing medication which should be avoided while taking this drug. An example would be:
   a. cimetidine
   b. prednisone
   c. penicillin
   *d. aspirin

   [NP: IM, CL: CO]

   Rationale: Salicylates may displace sulfonylureas from protein binding sites, resulting in enhanced hypoglycemic activity.

5. Mr. Wallace has been taking digoxin 0.25 mg po daily. Aware of the interaction between chlorpropamide and digoxin, the nurse will observe for signs of:
   a. hyperglyceima
   b. digoxin toxicity
   c. hypoglycemia
   *d. subtherapeutic digoxin levels

   [NP: EV, CL: CO]

   Rationale: Oral hypoglycemic agents may enhance the metabolism of digoxin by microsomal enzyme induction.

6. If Mr. Wallace takes chlorpropamide at 8:00 AM, he should expect the drug's peak activity to be at:
   a. 12:00 midnight
   *b. 8:00 PM
   c. 4:00 PM
   d. 10:00 PM

   [NP: PL, CL: AP]

   Rationale: Chlorpropamide is a long-acting agent which begins activity one hour after administration and peaks 12 hours later.

<u>**Additional Situation Not Presented in Text**</u>

Constance Rodriguez is a 36-year-old with a history of type I diabetes (IDDM), who is to begin insulin pump therapy to better control blood sugars.

1. Prior to beginning intensified insulin therapy, the nurse must <u>first</u> assess:
   a. financial status
   b. intellectual ability
   *c. willingness to adhere to schedule
   d. lifestyle factors

   [NP: AS, CL :KN]

   Rationale: Patients who will be on intensified insulin therapy must first demonstrate ability and willingness to adhere to the regimen.

2. Mr. Rodriguez will be instructed to use the following type of insulin in the pump:
   a. Humulin NPN
   b. regular pork insulin
   *c. Humulin BR
   d. Semilente

   [NP: IM, CL: KN]

Rationale: Humulin BR (buffered human insulin) has been developed for use in insulin pumps. It is a regular or short-acting insulin.

3. It will be important for Mr. Rodriguez to check her blood sugar at least:
   a. once daily
   b. weekly
   c. twice a day
   *d. four times a day

   [NP: PL, CL: AP]

   Rationale: Patients on intensified insulin therapy usually check blood sugars at least four times a day.

4. The nurse will include the following in patient teaching:
   *a. Report signs of infection at insertion site.
   b. Administer bolus regardless of planned activity.
   c. Change the administration set once a week.
   d. Refrigerate the insulin when not in use.

   [NP: IM, CL: AP]

   Rationale: A complication of insulin pump therapy is infection at the insertion site. Patients should be instructed to report signs of redness, swelling, or drainage promptly.

5. Ms. Rodriguez will be using a home blood glucose testing product for blood sugar monitoring. It will be most important for her to:
   a. check urine for acetone
   b. check urine for glucose
   c. clean set after use
   *d. record results daily

   [NP: IM, CL: AP]

   Rationale: It is important for the patient to record blood glucose results in order for the nurse to evaluate daily blood sugar trends.

6. In order to evaluate Ms. Rodriguez for compliance with medication, diet, and insulin pump use, the nurse will check lab values on a routine basis. Which of the following represents the best indicator of compliance?
   a. serum blood sugar
   b. urine acetone
   c. serum acetone
   *d. glycosylated hemoglobin

   [NP: EV, CL: AP]

   Rationale: Glycosylated hemoglobin is useful in evaluating diabetic control over a period of time, reflecting the mean glucose level over 3 to 8 weeks. The normal glycosylated hemoglobin level for the well-controlled patient is 8 percent or less.

Review Questions from Text

1. In the absence of insulin:
   a. glucose is readily transported into cells
   b. amino acids are converted to protein
   c. gluconeogenesis is inhibited
   *d. free fatty acids are converted to ketone bodies

   [CL: KN]

   Rationale: The fragments of fatty acid metabolism, which occurs in the absence of insulin, are referred to as ketone bodies. The presence of excess ketone bodies is termed ketosis.

2. Individuals with diabetes are at risk for artherosclerosis because of:
   *a. increased conversion of fatty acids to cholesterol in the absence of insulin
   b. increased cell metabolism of proteins important for maintaining vascular wall structure
   c. reduced ability of the liver to break down cholesterol which is consumed in excess
   d. decreased triglycerides in the liver as a result of ketoacidosis

   [CL: CO]

   Rationale: A reduction in insulin availability results in increased triglycerides and increased conversion of fatty acids into phoshpolipids and cholesterol. This results in a greater risk for the development of atherosclerosis.

3. Insulin can be made to be longer acting by the addition of:
   a. lipid
   *b. zin
   c. iron
   d. copper

   [CL: KN]

   Rationale: An insulin compound with longer action can be made by adding zinc, protamine, or globin.

4. An example of an individual who would benefit from human insulin administration would be:
   *a. a gestational diabetic
   b. an older adult with Type I diabetes
   c. the patient without dietary restrictions
   d. a chronic diabetic on pork insulin

   [CL: CO]

   Rationale: Humulin insulin is recommended for those individuals who will be on insulin therapy intermittently, such as the gestational diabetic or the nondiabetic receiving parenteral nutrition.

5. Which of the following is true of long-acting insulins?
   a. These insulin agents are frequently used alone for chronic diabetics.
   b. Insulin reactions may occur at night since they peak in four to nine hours.
   c. An example of a long-acting insulin is NPH, which peaks in 24 hours.
   *d. At low doses, they suppress glucogenolysis and gluconeogenesis.

   [CL: CO]

   Rationale: Long-acting insulins are usually given with a short-acting insulin. In low doses, they suppress gluconeolysis and gluconeogenesis, mimicking physiologic insulin release.

6. Which of the following individuals would benefit from a single dose of intermediate-acting insulin per day?
   a. gestational diabetic over 18 years old
   b. Type I newly diagnosed
   *c. Type II diabetic over 60 years old
   d. Type I diabetic less than 60 years old

   [CL: KN]

   Rationale: Generally, a single dose of intermediate-acting insulin does not maintain adequate glucose control 24 hours a day. This method of treatment is often limited to the type II diabetic over 60 years old. Strict control is not as urgent in these patients.

7. The plasma half-life of insulin injected intravenously is usually less than:
   *a. 9 minutes

b. 2 minutes
c. 90 seconds
d. 60 seconds

[CL: KN]

Rationale: Concerning the biotransformation of insulin, the plasma half-life of insulin injected intravenously is less than 9 minutes. Antibody formation may extend the half-life up to 13 hours.

8. Late symptoms of hypoglycemia inclue:
a. tachyardia
b. hunger
*c. blurred vision
d. headache

[CL: KN]

Rationale: Late symptoms of hypoglyemia include blurred vision and disorientation.

9. A medication which antagonizes the effect of insulin is:
a. fenfluramine
*b. epinephrine
c. alcohol
d. acetohexamide

[CL: KN]

Rationale: Epinephrine antagonizes the effect of insulin by mobilizing glycogen to increase the blood glucose.

10. Which of the following hypoglycemia agents is best taken on an empty stomach:
a. tolzamide
*b. glipizide
c. chlorpropamide
d. orinase

[CL: KN]

Rationale: The presence of food delays absorption of glipizide (Glucotrol); therefore it must be taken on an empty stomach.

Additional Review Questions Not Presented in Text

1. Which of the following statements is correct regarding types of insulin?
a. Most insulin used today is a combination regarding types of insulin?
b. Beef insulin differs from human insulin by one amino acid.
c. Human insulin is produced from proinsulin.
*d. Beef and pork insulin may induce antibody formation.

[CL: CO]

Rationale: Because beef and pork insulin differ structurally from human insulin, antibodies may be produced in response to their use as therapeutic agents.

2. The majority of the body's cells require insulin for glucose entry. The exception is:
*a. brain cells
b. lung cells
c. muscle cells
d. vascular epithelium

[CL: KN]

Rationale: Brain cells do not require insulin for transport of glucose into the cell.

3. In the liver, insulin functions in the following manner:
   a. increases gluconeogenesis
   *b. decreases the rate of gluconeogenesis
   c. inhibits formation of free fatty acids
   d. facilitates production of adipocyte cells

   [CL: KN]

   Rationale: In the liver, the presence of insulin decreases the rate of gluconeogenesis.

4. Oral hypoglycemia agents:
   a. stimulate the alpha cells in the pancreas
   b. decrease the number of insulin receptors
   c. decrease the peripheral uptake of glucose
   *d. suppress hepatic glucose production

   [CL: KN]

   Rationale: The exact mechanism of oral hypoglycemics is not fully understood. These agents have been found to stimulate beta cells of the pancreas and to suppress hepatic glucose production.

5. An example of a rapid-acting insulin is:
   a. lente
   *b. semilente
   c. Isophane Insulin Suspension
   d. ultralente

   [CL: KN]

   Rationale: Semilente (prompt insulin zinc suspension) begins to act in one to four hours after administration.

CHAPTER 45: THYROID AND PARATHYROID DRUGS

Situations from Text

Mr. Emile Haus is a 50-year-old admitted to the Medical Unit with a history of weight loss, nervousness, and insomnia. A diagnosis of hyperthyroidism is made.

1. The nurse may note the following sign of hyperthyroidism when assessing Mr. Haus:
   a. constipation
   b. anorexia
   c. dry skin
   *d. exophthalmos

   [NP: AS, CL: KN]

   Rationale: Patients with hyperthyroidism may exhibit exophthalmos, which is an abnormal protrusion of the eyeball.

2. Mr. Haus' blood pressure elevates to 210/150, and heart rate increases to 150 beats per minute. He is transferred to the Intensive Care Unit for management of athyrotoxic crisis. Propylthiouracil (PTU) 30 mg has been ordered. The nurse will expect to give this drug by the following route:
   a. intramuscularly
   *b. orally
   c. subcutaneously
   d. intravenously

   [NP: PL, CL: KN]

   Rationale: Propylthiouracil is effectively absorbed via the gastrointestinal tract and is not available in parenteral forms.

3. A drug of choice for Mr. Haus' cardiac symptoms related to thyroid crisis would be:
   a. atropine
   b. digoxin
   c. epinephrine
   *d. propranolol

   [NP: AN, CL: AP]

   Rationale: Thyroid crisis can be fatal because of excessive cardiac stimulation. As a beta blocker, propranolol can protect the heart from life-threatening tachycardia, a manifestation of catecholamine release.

4. In addition to PTU administration, Mr. Haus will receive sodium iodide 2 gms IV. The nurse will monitor him for the following side effects of iodide therapy:
   *a. increased salivation
   b. urinary hesitancy
   c. dizziness
   d. tinnitis

   [NP: AS, CL: AP]

   Rationale: Side effects of sodium iodide include those related to iodism: increased salivation, burning sensations in the mouth and throat, and gingival soreness.

5. After successful treatment of thyroid crisis, Mr. Haus is transferred back to the Medical Unit. He is to be discharged on PTU 50 mg per day and Lugol's solution .3 ml tid. Which of the following foods should be eliminated from his diet?
   *a. seafood

b. alcohol
c. green vegetables
d. citrus fruits

[NP: IM, C: AP]

Rationale: Patients on antithyroid medication should be taught to limit iodine-rich foods such as seafood.

6. Mr. Haus will need to be monitored regularly for effects of PTU therapy. This includes checking:
*a. prothrombin time
b. serum protein electrophoresis
c. serum calcium levels
d. 2-hour urine amylase

[NP: EV, CL: KN]

Rationale: Bleeding related to thrombocytopenia may occur with antithyroid therapy; therefore, prothrombin times and cell counts should be evaluated on a routine basis.

<u>**Additional Situation Not Presented in Text**</u>

1. The nurse assessing Mr. Williams will be alert to the following sign of hypocalcemia:
*a. tetany
b. lethargy
c. polyuria
d. flank pain

[NP: AS, CL: AP]

Rationale: Calcium is necessary for proper muscular functioning. Hypocalcemic manifestations include tetany, laryngospasm, and/or other muscular spasms.

2. Mr. Williams is to receive calcitriol (Rocaltrol) 1 μg orally per day. The nurse will plan to teach him about the following side effect of calcitriol:
a. diarrhea
b. hyperactive reflexes
*c. constipation
d. tacycardia

[NP: PL, CL: KN]

Rationale: The side effects of calcitriol reflect those of hypercalcemia. The most common gastrointestinal effects are anorexia, nausea, vomiting, constipation, and abdominal pain.

3. Which of the following statements by Mr. Williams indicates a need for further teaching?
*a. "Lethargy and confusion are common side effects of treatment."
b. "I will need to take this drug for the rest of my life."
c. "I need to know about the effects of hypercalcemia."
d. "Regular check-ups are an important part of treatment."

[NP: EV, CL: AN]

Rationale: The patient should be aware of and report both hypofunction and hyperfunction of the parathyroid. Central nervous system effects of hypercalcemia, such as lethargy and confusion, should be reported immediately.

4. Mr. Williams will be taught to avoid the following while on calcitriol:
a. high fiber
*b. mineral oil

c. seafood
d. caffeine

[NP: IM, CL: AP]

Rationale: Mineral oil will decrease the absorption of calcitriol, which is a synthetic form of Vitamin D.

5. 5. During follow-up visits, the nurse will assess for signs of hypocalcemia, which include:
a. Chadwick's sign
b. altered stereognosis
*c. Chvostek's sign
d. pulsus paradoxus

[NP: AS, CL: AP]

Rationale: The presence of Chvostek's sign indicates hypocalcemia. This sign, indicative of tetany, is a spasm of muscles following a tap on one side of the face over the area of the facial nerve.

6. As a result of routine laboratory tests, which would signal a need to alter therapy with calcitriol?
*a. azotemia
b. hypokalemia
c. hypermagnesemia
d. hyponatremia

[NP: EV, CL: CO]

Rationale: Azotemia is indicative of renal dysfunction which may be related to hypercalcemia as a result of calcitriol therapy.

<u>Review Questions from Text</u>

1. The ratio of T_4 to T_3 is:
a. 1:1
*b. 4:1
c. 2:1
d. 20:1

[CL: KN]

Rationale: The ratio of T_4 to T_3 is 4:1. Decreased serum levels of T_3 and T_4 stimulate the pituitary gland to secrete TSH, which controls the release of thyroid hormones.

2. A function of the thyroid hormones (T_3 and T_4) is to:
a. decelerate chemical reactions
*b. increase oxygen consumption
c. impede heat production
d. act as enzymes

[CL: KN]

Rationale: T_3 and T_4 function as regulators of metabolic rate and cell growth. They accelerate chemical reactions, oxygen consumption, and heat production.

3. The ratio between thyroid gland iodine and serum iodine (T/S ratio) is normally:
*a. 20:1
b. 4:1
c. 2:1
d. 10:1

[CL: KN]

Rationale: The normal T/S ratio is 20:1. Hyperactivity or hypoactivity is reflected in this ratio.

4. Thyrocalcitonin is released from the thyroid gland in response to:
   a. low serum phosphorus
   b. low serum calcium
   *c. high serum calcium
   d. high serum phosphorus

   [CL: KN]

   Rationale: Thyrocalcitonin is released in response to high serum calcium. It acts to decrease calcium absorption in the gut and to prevent resorption of calcium in the bone.

5. Parathormone acts on various organs to produce the following:
   a. increasing excretion of calcium
   b. reducing calcium absorption
   c. decreasing excretion of phosphorus
   *d. enhancing bone resorption

   [CL: CO]

   Rationale: Parathormone affects bone, causing calcium resorption.

6. The thyroid hormones:
   *a. strengthen rate and force of cardiac contraction
   b. reduce protein synthesis
   c. regulate growth in the adult
   d. increase cholesterol concentration

   [CL: KN]

   Rationale: Thyroid hormones strengthen the rate and force of cardiac contraction, thereby increasing cardiac output to the tissues.

7. Iodides are used as antithyroid drugs by:
   a. increasing the vascularity of the thyroid gland
   b. decreasing the quantity of bound thyroid
   *c. inhibiting the release of T_3 and T_4 into circulation
   d. binding with TSH for thyroid inhibition

   [CL: CO]

   Rationale: Iodides act as antithyroid drugs by inhibiting the release of hormones into circulation, increasing the quantity of bound (inactive) hormone, and reducing the vascularity of the thyroid gland.

8. An action of the antithyroid medication propylthiouracil (PTU) is to:
   a. block TSH production
   b. reduce serum calcitonin levels
   *c. inhibit peripheral conversion of T_4 and T_3
   d. block release of TRH

   [CL: KN]

   Rationale: In addition to inhibition of the synthesis of thyroid hormones, propylthiouracil partially inhibits the peripheral conversion of T_4 to T_3.

9. Vitamin D derivatives elevate serum calcium by:
   a. stimulating the kidney to reduce excretion
   b. inducing parathyroid hormone production
   *c. stimulating calcium absorption in the intestine

d. inducing the production of calcitonin by the thyroid

[CL: KN]

Rationale: Vitamin D agents elevate serum calcium levels by stimulation of calcium absorption in the intestine and mobilization of calcium absorption in the intestine and mobilization of calcium from bones.

10. The most common side effects of antithyroid drugs are:
 a. nausea and vomiting
 *b. pruritus and urticaria
 c. diarrhea and weakness
 d. tremor and restlessness

Rationale: Pruritus and urticaria are the most common adverse effects of antithyroid medications.

Additional Review Questions Not Presented in Text

1. Which of the following statements is correct concerning signs and symptoms of hypothyroidism?
 *a. They often appear insidiously and over a long period of time.
 b. Symptoms follow a predictable pattern in every individual.
 c. Weight is not directly affected by thyroid dysfunction.
 d. Signs and symptoms are related to low iodine levels.

[CL: KN]

Rationale: Signs and symptoms of hypothyroidism usually occur slowly over a period of time. Patients do not necessarily demonstrate a predictable pattern of symptoms, making the disease difficult to diagnose.

2. Most of the thyroid hormones in circulation are found:
 a. in the liver
 b. stored in the thymus
 *c. bound to protein
 d. bound to phospholipid

[CL: KN]

Rationale: A high percentage (99.94 percent) of thyroid hormone is bound to protein, particularly thyroxine-binding globulin (TBG).

3. Thyroid hormones are contraindicated for individuals with:
 *a. adrenal insufficiency
 b. lithium therapy
 c. lymphocytic thyroiditis
 d. metastatic cancer

[CL: KN]

Rationale: Thyroid hormone increases the tissue demand for adrenal hormones, creating adrenal crisis for patients with adrenal insufficiency.

4. The following is correct regarding thyroid drugs:
 a. Thyroglobulin (Proloid) is obtained from beef sources.
 b. Thyroid USP (Thyroid) may be given intravenously for myxedema.
 *c. Liotrix (Thyrolar) may produce bronchial asthma.
 d. Liothyronine sodium (Cytomel) is obtained from pork souces.

[CL: KN]

Rationale: Liotrix contains tartrazine yellow dye, which may produce bronchial asthma in susceptible persons.

5. A symptom of myxedema is:
   a. weight loss
   b. photosensitivity
   c. palmar erythema
   *d. facial edema

   [CL: KN]

   Rationale: Facial edema is a symptom of myxedema or hypothyroidism.

CHAPTER 46: ANTI-INFECTIVES

Situations from Text

Leonard Olds is a 34-year-old who is admitted to the medical unit with episodes of fever, night sweats, and a persistent cough. The preliminary diagnosis is respiratory tuberculosis.

1. Mr. Olds is to begin isoniazide (INH) orally 350 mg per day. The nurse will be alert to adverse side effects of the drug, such as:
   a. photosensitivity
   b. crystalluria
   *c. muscle twitching
   d. pseudomembranous colitis

   [NP: IM, CL: AP]

   Rationale: Neuroloical side effects are common with INH therapy. These include muscle twitching, peripheral neuritis, and paresthesias.

2. Due to INH therapy, the nurse will expect to administer the following nutritional supplement:
   *a. B6 (pyridoxine)
   b. Vitamin C
   c. Vitamin A
   d. folic acid

   [NP: IM, CL: CO]

   Rationale: INH interferes with the normal action of pyridoxine, Vitamin B6, which is an essential component in nerve conduction. Supplementing pyridoxine can help to alleviate neurotoxicities.

3. Along with INH therapy, Mr. Olds is to take rifampin 600 mg orally daily. Assessment of Mr. Olds may reveal the following in relation to rifampin therapy:
   a. "butterfly" rash
   b. discoloration of teeth
   c. cherry red lips
   *d. reddish-orange urine

   [NP: AS, CL: KN]

   Rationale: Rifampin may produce a reddish-orange discoloration of urine, sweat, or tears.

4. When teaching Mr. Olds about his drug regimen, the nurse will plan to include the following information:
   *a. Rifampin should be taken on an empty stomach.
   b. INH therapy is usually 2 weeks in length.
   c. Rifampin interacts with milk and should only be taken with water.
   d. The drugs may be discontinued when symptoms subside.

   [NP: PL, CL: CO]

   Rationale: Food may delay absorption of rifampin; therefore, it should be taken on an empty stomach.

5. The nurse will monitor the following lab values while caring for Mr. Olds:
   a. magnesium level
   b. urinary amylase
   *c. liver enzymes
   d. urine osmolarity

   [NP: EV, CL: AP]

Rationale: Liver damage may occur due to concomitant use of INH and rifampin. Liver enzymes should be monitored on a routine basis.

6. The nurse performs discharge teaching for Mr. Olds and his wife. Which of the following statements by Mrs. Olds indicates successful teaching?
   a. "If one dose is missed, he should take two doses the next day."
   *b. "I should report mental changes promptly."
   c. "Hearing loss is expected with this medication."
   d. "He must measure his urine output daily."

   [NP: EV, CL: AN]

   Rationale: Mental status changes may occur in patients taking INH. The family should be aware of this and report signs of psychosis promptly.

Situation 46-2

Mary Greco is a 57-year-old who suffered a ruptured appendix. Following surgery, she has been admitted to the surgical unit with orders including gentamycin (Garamycin) 80 mg IVPB every 8 hours.

1. While caring for Ms. Greco, the nurse will carefully monitor the following lab value relative to therapy with gentamycin:
   a. urinary amylase
   *b. creatinine
   c. serum albumin
   d. phosphorus

   [NP: AS, CL: AP]

   Rationale: Patients on aminoglycoside therapy should be monitored for the development of nephrotoxicity, which is indicated by an elevation in serum creatinine levels.

2. After the third IV dose of gentamycin, Ms. Greco is to have a serum peak level drawn. Which of the following results indicates a therapeutic gentamycin peak level?
   *a. 8 μg/ml
   b. 3 μg/ml
   c. 12 μg/ml
   d. 20 μg/ml

   [NP: EV, CL: AP]

   Rationale: Peak serum concentrations of gentamycin should range between 4 and 10 μg/ml.

3. On the third post-operative day, Ms. Greco's chest x-ray shows consolidation of the left lower lobe, conistent with pneumonia. An additional antibiotic, ticarcillin/clavulanic acid(Timentin) 3.1 grams is started IVPB every 12 hours. The nurse will include the following intervention:
   a. Infuse the two antibiotics together in the same IV solution.
   b. Discontinue the gentamycine befroe starting the penicillin agent.
   *c. Monitor white blood cell (WBC) count daily.
   d. Obtain sputum cultures after two doses of Timentin are given.

   [NP: IM, CL: CO]

   Rationale: Patients on antibiotic therapy should be monitored for elevated or depressed WBC levels. Elevated WBCs indicate continuing infection, while very low levels may indicate depressed bone marrow funtion as a result of antibiotic therapy.

4. Which of the following nursing diagnostic categories applies to Ms. Greco?
   a. Noncompliance
   *b. Potential for Injury: Bleeding

c. Alteration in Cardiac Output
d. Fluid Volume Excess

[NP: AN, CL: AN]

Rationale: Timentin may inhibit platelet aggregation, resulting in a prolonged bleeding time and potential for injury due to coagulation abnormalities.

5. Considering penicillin therapy, which of the following electrolytes may need to be supplemented:
a. calcium
b. chloride
c. sodium
*d. potassium

[NP: PL, CL: CO]

Rationale: Penicillins may induce hypokalemia due to enhanced renal distal tubular secretion of potassium.

6. Because of aminoglycoside therapy, the nurse will assess Ms. Greco daily for the presence of:
a. crystalluria
*b. hearing loss
c. diarrhea
d. tetany

[NP: AS, CL: AP]

Rationale: A common side effect of aminoglycoside therapy is ototoxicity; therefore, patients should be monitored closely for evidence of hearing disturbances.

<u>**Additional Situation Not Presented in Text**</u>

Ken Combes, a 68-year-old diabetic, has undergone coronary artery bypass surgery and has been admitted to the Surgical Intensive Care Unit. Post-operative orders include cefazolin (Ancef) 1 gram IVPB every 6 hours.

1. When administering the first dose of cefazolin, the nurse will monitor Mr. Combes closely for a cross-sensitivity reaction if he has an allergy to:
*a. penicllin
b. streptomycin
c. sulfa
d. tetracycline

[NP: IM, CL: AP]

Rationale: Some patients who are allergic to penicillin will be cross-sensitive to cefazolin, a cephalosporin.

2. Should Mr. Combes develop antibiotic-associated colitis, the expected treatment of choice would be to discontinue the cephalosporin and administer:
a. metronidazole intravenously
b. gentamycin intravenously
*c. vancomycin orally
d. penicillin orally

[NP: PL, CL: AP]

Rationale: A complication of cephalosporins is pseudomembranous colitis. This may be life-threatening. Antibiotic therapy should be discontinued (or changed) and oral vancomycin administered.

3. The nurse should monitor the following value in relation to therapy with cefazolin:
a. blood sugar

b. sodium
*c. bleeding time
d. potassium

[NP: EV, CL: CO]

Rationale: Cephalosporins may inhibit normal platelet function and the synthesis of prothrombin, resulting in a prolonged bleeding time.

4. On the fifth post-operative day, Mr. Combes complains of frequent burning urination. A urine culture is positive for E. coli, and he is to begin therapy with trimethoprim/sulfamethoxazole (Bactrim) 160 mg orally BID. An important nursing measure for Mr. Combes would be to:
   a. administer with antacids only
   *b. maintain adequate fluid intake
   c. restrict fluid intake
   d. administer with folic acid

5. Mr. Combes is also taking chlorpropamide for control of hyperglycemia. The nurse will monitor Mr. Combes for the effects of drug interaction which may result in:
   a. hyperglycemia
   b. hypokalemia
   c. hyperkalemia
   *d. hypoglycemia

   [NP: EV, CL: AP]

   Rationale: The combination of sulfonamides and oral hypoglycemic agents may lead to episodes of hypoglycemia.

6. The nurse will monitor Mr. Combes for side effects of Bactrin, which include:
   a. chest pain
   *b. arthritis
   c. spastic colitis
   d. hypotension

   [NP: IM, CL: AP]

   Rationale: Joint pain/arthritis may be related to sulfonamide therapy.

Review Quetions from Text

1. "Normal flora," microorganisms inhibiting the internal and external surfaces of healthy human beings, are found in the:
   a. upper genitourinary tract
   b. lymphatic fluid
   c. liver
   *d. skin

   [CL: CO]

   Rationale: Areas of the body where various bacteria, fungi, and protozoa exist include the skin, intestine, oropharynx, conjunctiva, and lower genitourinary tract.

2. A factor to consider in selection of appropriate antibiotic therapy is:
   a. duration of infection
   b. status of the host's gastrointestinal functioning
   *c. sensitivity of the organism to selected antibiotics
   d. presence of a secondary bacterial "superinfection"

   [CL: KN]

Rationale: An important factor to be considered when selecting an antibiotic for therapy is the sensitivity of the organism to antibiotics.

3. Which of the following statements is correct regarding the absorption of various forms of penicillin?
   a. Penicillin G has a highly stable absorption pattern following oral administration.
   *b. Ampicillin is well absorbed following oral ingestion.
   c. Intramuscular injections of procaine penicillin G last up to 26 days.
   d. Pencillin G benzathine is rapidly absorbed, providing short-acting effect.

   [CL: CO]

   Rationale: Ampicillin is stable in gastric contents and is well absorbed following oral administration.

4. An antimicrobial agent for which no reduction in dosage is necessary for patients with renal insufficiency is:
   a. gentamycin
   *b. clindamycin
   c. penicillin
   d. tobramycin

   [CL: KN]

   Rationale: While most antibiotics must be reduced or the interval increased in patients with renal insufficiency, some agents require no reduction in dosage. An example is clindamycin.

5. The addition of clavulanic acid to selected broad-spectrum penicillins has the following effect:
   *a. beta-lactamase inhibition
   b. inhibition of plasmid transfer
   c. enhancement of bacterial cell wall destruction
   d. prolongation of penicillin half-life

   [CL: CO]

   Rationale: The addition of clavulanic acid, which is a beta-lactamase inhibitor, broadens the penicillin activity to include penicillinase-producing organisms.

6. The spectrum of antibiotic activity of aztreonam includes:
   a. fungal microorganisms
   b. aerobic gram-positive coci
   *c. aerobic gram-negative rods
   d. anaerobic microorganisms

   [CL: KN]

   Rationale: Aztreonam, a monocyclic antibiotic, has an antibiotic activity which is limited to aerobic gram-negative rods.

7. The action of cilastatin, which is given with imipenem in the form of Primaxin, is to:
   a. inhibit the growth of anaerobic organisms
   *b. inhibit dihydropeptidase enzymes
   c. interfere with the action of penicillinase
   d. augment the action of imipenem

   [CL: KN]

   Rationale: Cilastatin inhibits dehydropeptidase in the proximal tubules. This enzyme inactivates imipenem. Cilastatin has no antibacterial activity.

8. Sulfonamides act to suppress bacterial growth by:
   *a. interfering with folic acid synthesis

b. inhibiting cell wall structure
c. translocating the DNA structure
d. inhibiting beta-lactamase

[CL: CO]

Rationale: Sulfonamides compete for the enzyme which synthesizes folic acid in bacterial cells. The effect is suppression of purine and DNA synthesis, resulting in cell death.

9. Which of the following statements is correct regarding erythromycin drug interactions?
   a. Subtherapeutic digoxin levels may occur with erythromycin.
   b. Erythromycin enhances phenytoin activity.
   c. Corticosteroids enhance erythromycin activity.
   *d. Erythromycin inhibits the metabolism of theophylline.

[CL: KN]

Rationale: Erythromycin inhibits the metabolism of theophylline and may precipitate signs of theophylline toxicity.

10. The most notable side effect of clindamycin is:
   a. hearing loss
   b. nausea
   *c. diarrhea
   d. rash

[CL: KN]

Rationale: The most common side effect of clindamycin therapy is diarrhea. If significant diarrhea occurs, the antibiotic should be discontinued.

Additional Review Questions Not Presented in Text

1. Bacterial cell wall synthesis:
   *a. provides a supportive architecture for the organism and protects the cell membrane
   b. is dependent on strands of complex fat molecules cross-linked by carbohydrate chains
   c. is dependent on plasmids to facilitate membrane permeability, permitting antibiotics to enter the cell
   d. is dependent on chromosomal mutation to decrease bacterial resistance to antibiotics

[CL: KN]

Rationale: The bacterial wall provides a supportive architecture for the organism and is composed of strands of complex sugar molecules cross-linked by peptide chains.

2. Which of the following statements is correct concerning the penicillins and their spectrum of activity?
   a. Natural agents are active against gram-negative bacillary infections.
   b. Anti-staphylococcal agents have been modified to inactivate penicillinase.
   *c. Broad-spectrum agents are effective against some gram-negative bacilli.
   d. Anti-pseudomonal agents are active against gram-negative cocci only.

[CL: KN]

Rationale: The broad-spectrum penicillins are active against most organisms sensitive to penicillin G and some gram-negative bacilli such as E coli.

3. An objective symptom of infection is the presence of:
   a. fatigue
   b. pain at the site
   *c. fever

d. malaise

[CL: CO]

Rationale: Fever is an objective (measurable) symptom of infection. Fatigue, malaise, and pain at the site are subjective.

4. Which of the following statements is correct regarding aminoglycoside antibiotics?
   a. High concentrations of penicillin enhance aminoglycoside activity.
   *b. Anaerobic bacteria are resistant to aminoglycoside therapy.
   c. Treatment of gram-negative sepsis is more successful with aminoglycosides alone.
   d. Aminoglycosides act by penetrating cell wall membranes.

   [CL: KN]

   Rationale: Anaerobic bacteria are resistant to aminoglycosides because oxygen is required for uptake of the antibiotic into the cell.

5. As a result of amphotericin B administration, the following electrolyte imbalance may be seen:
   a. hypermagnesemia
   b. hyponatremia
   c. hypercalcemia
   *d. hypokalemia

   [CL: KN]

   Rationale: Hypokalemia may occur in patients on amphotericin B therapy due to alteration in renal function. Additionally, hypomagnesemia may also occur.

CHAPTER 47: ANTI-INFLAMMATORY MEDICATIONS

Situation from Text

Situation 47-1

Marvin Ungerman, aged 50, has rheumatoid arthritis for which he is being treated through the health clinic.

1. Mr. Ungerman has been placed on drug therapy with ibuprofen (Motrin) 200 mg three times a day. The clinic nurse will provide the following information when teaching him about this drug:
   a. Wear a hat outdoors to reduce sun exposure.
   b. Expect water retention and weight gain.
   c. Use in conjunction with aspirin for relief of pain.
   *d. Take with food to reduce gastric irritation.

   [NP: IM, CL: AP]

   Rationale: A common effect of ibuprofen use is gastric irritation. If this occurs, the drug should be taken with food, milk, or an antacid.

2. When evaluating Mr. Ungerman on return visits to the clinic, the nurse will monitor the following with regard to ibuprofen therapy:
   a. potassim level
   *b. bleeding time
   c. T_3, T_4 levels
   d. urine amylase
   [NP: EV, CL: KN]

   Rationale: Nonsteroidal anti-inflammatory agents such as ibuprofen impair platelet aggregation and prolong bleeding time. Patients need to be evaluated on a routine basis for evidence of bleeding disorders.

3. Three months later, Mr. Ungerman continues to experience arthritic pain despite ibuprofen therapy. His physician plans to place him on gold therapy with gold sodium thiomalate (Myochrysine). Prior to therapy, Mr. Ungerman will be assessed for the following contraindication to its use:
   a. aspirin allergy
   b. peptic ulcer disease
   c. narrow angle glaucoma
   *d. congestive heart failure

   [NP: AS, CL: CO]

   Rationale: Contraindications of gold sodium therapy include patients with congestive heart disease, since gold deposits can worsen the condition.

4. In order to administer gold sodium thiomalate correctly to Mr. Ungerman, the nurse will plan to:
   *a. agitate the vial to ensure uniform suspension
   b. keep the patient NPO before giving
   c. use any subcutaneous site for injection
   d. keep medication cool for injection

   [NP: PL, CL: KN]

   Rationale: The bottle of gold sodium thiomalate should be agitated by rolling the vial between hands to warm the solution and ensure uniform suspension.

5. The nurse will teach Mr. Ungerman about adverse side effects of gold therapy, which include:
   a. seizures

b. angina
*c. rashes
d. hypertension

[NP: IM, CL: CO]

Rationale: The most common adverse side effects occur as a result of gold deposits in the skin, causing rashes, pruritis, and pigment changes.

6. Which of the following statements by Mr. Ungeran indicates successful patient teaching?
a. "The medication should be used only if it is a dark yellow."
b. "Getting direct sunlight will help relieve side effects."
*c. "It may take 6 to 8 weeks for benefits to be felt."
d. "It is best to walk for 30 minutes after the gold injection."

[NP: EV, CL: AN]

Rationale: Gold sodium thiomalate is slow acting and 6 to 8 weeks may be required before benefits will be noticed.

<u>**Additional Situation Not Presented in Text**</u>

Hashem Sajid is seen in the physician's office with complaints of exquisite pain in his left knee. The area is red and swollen. An initial diagnosis of gouty arthritis is made.

1. Mr. Sajid is to begin colchicine .5 mg po orally. The nurse will anticipate the following dosage schedule:
a. hourly until pain is resolved
*b. hourly during the acute phase
c. every two hours as maintenance dosage
d. every four hours during the acute phase

[NP: PL, CL: CO]

Ratoinale: Colchinsine is given orally in doses of .5 mg to 1.2 mg every hour during the acute phase of gout until pain is resolved or a total of 4 mg in 24 hours is reached.

2. During the acute phase of gouty arthritis, the nurse will instruct Mr. Sajid to report the following side effect of cholchinsine:
a. confusion
*b. diarrhea
c. hair loss
d. tinnitis

[NP: IM, CL: AP]

Rationale: Gastrointestinal symptoms, such as diarrhea, should be reported during the acute phase and may indicate a need to alter the dosage of colchicine.

3. Symptoms of gouty arthritis subside, and Mr. Sajid will begin maintenance therapy with allopurinol 300 mg po orally twice daily. It will be important for him to:
*a. increase fluid inake
b. take on an empty stomach
c. reduce physical activity
d. avoid exposure to sunlight

[NP: IM, CL: CO]

Rationale: Increasing oral intake to at least 3000 cc per day reduces the formation of uric acid stones in the kidney.

4. The nurse will provide diet teaching for Mr. Sajid in order to control acute gout attacks. The foods which he should avoid include:
   a. dairy products
   b. fiber and grains
   *c. organ meats
   d. citrus fruits

   [NP: IM, CL: AP]

   Rationale: Organ meats are high in purine and could precipitate an acute gout attack.

5. Should Mr. Sajid require an analgesic, which of the following would be most appropriate?
   a. codeine
   b. ibuprofen
   c. aspirin
   *d. acetaminophen

   [NP: PL, CL: CO]

   Rationale: Patients taking allopurinol should not take aspirin or aspirin-containing products due to the tendency for platelet alteration and potential for bleeding. Acetaminophen is recommended if an analgesic is necessary.

6. When evaluating Mr. Sajid for successful therapy, the best clinical indicator would be:
   a. serum phosphorous and calcium
   b. white blood cell count
   *c. serum uric acid levels
   d. eosinophil count

   [NP: EV, CL: AP]

   Rationale: It will be important to monitor uric acid levels and red blood cell counts on a routine basis in order to evaluate and alter drug therapy:

<u>Review Questions from Text</u>

1. The prostaglandins have a diversity of action which includes:
   a. vasoconstriction
   b. decreased cardiac output
   *c. increased capillary permeability
   d. platelet aggregation

   [CL: KN]

   Rationale: The prostaglandins, produced and released under certain conditions, have actions which include increased capillary permeability, vasodilation, increased cardiac output, and inhibition of platelet aggregation.

2. Prostaglandins have the following effect on the stomach lining:
   a. stimulation of gastric secretions
   b. inhibition of mucous production
   c. histamine release
   *d. stabilization of gastric mucosa

   [CL: KN]

   Rationale: The release of prostaglandins inhibits gastric acid secretion and stabilizes the gastric mucosa.

3. Misoprostol (cytotec) is contraindicated in the following patient condition:
   *a. pregnancy
   b. gastric ulcers

c. glaucoma
d. diabetes mellitus

[CL: CO]

Rationale: Misoprostol produces uterine contractions which may endanger pregnancy.

4. Short-term anti-inflammatory medications are used for:
 a. one to two months only
 b. a temporary cure
 *c. pain relief
 d. minimal side effects

[CL: CO]

Rationale: Anti-inflammatory medications developed for short-term use provide pain relief and should be administered for only one to four weeks. Severe side effects can develop as a result of short-term therapy.

5. Which statement is correct regarding substances that play a role in inflammation?
 a. Bradykinins cause profound vasoconstriction.
 *b. Histamines encourage migration of phagocytic cells.
 c. Protease builds up collagenous connective tissue.
 d. Hydrolases cause bronchospasm in the lung.

[CL: KN]

Rationale: Histamines encourage phagocytic cells in the blood stream to migrate to the place of injury. The phagocytic cells then attempt to engulf foreign particles present, releasing proteases and hydrolases in the process.

6. Salicylates are thought to relieve arthritic pain by:
 a. enhancing platelet aggregation
 b. releasing neurological blockers
 c. stimulating bradykinin synthesis
 *d. inhibiting prostaglandin synthesis

[CL: KN]

Rationale: Salicylates act to relieve the pain associated with arthritis by inhibiting prostaglandin synthesis.

7. The nonsteroid anti-inflammatory drugs:
 *a. are administered cautiously to patients with renal disease
 b. do not cross the placental barrier and are safe for pregnant women
 c. are used as a substitute for patients allergic to aspirin
 d. are slowly absorbed from the gastrointestinal tract

[CL: CO]

Rationale: Nonsteroidal anti-inflammatory agents decrease glomerular filtration rate and decrease renal blood flow; therefore, they should be used cautiously in patients with renal disease.

8. Nonsteroid anti-inflammatory drugs which are used for short-term therapy only include:
 a. piroxicam
 b. fenoprofen
 *c. phenylbutazone
 d. ibuprofen

[CL: KN]

Rationale: Phenylbutazone (Butazolidin) has many adverse side effects and is used only for short-term therapy.

9. While the exact mechanism of action is not known for D-penicillamine (Cuprimine), it is effectively used to treat:
   a. gouty arthritis
   *b. rheumatoid arthritis
   c. gastric ulcers
   d. resistant acne vulgaris

   [CL: KN]

   Rationale: D-penicillamin (Cuprimine) is a nonsteroidal anti-inflammatory agent which is used to treat rheumatoid arthritis. It is thought to have immunosuppressive activity.

10. An adverse side effect of meclofenamate sodium (Meclomen) is:
   *a. diarrhea
   b. hair loss
   c. peripheral neuritis
   d. chrysiasis

   [CL: KN]

   Rationale: Meclofenamate sodium, a salicylate-like medication, has been known to cause diarrhea which can be severe in some cases.

Additional Review Questions Not Presented in Text

1. Most of the nonsteroid anti-inflammatory drugs act by:
   a. reducing production of T-cells and B-cells
   *b. inhibiting the enzyme cyclo-oxygenase
   c. stimulating chemotaxis of inflamed cells
   d. increasing release of superoxide radicals

   [CL: KN]

   Rationale: By inhibiting the enzyme cyclo-oxygenase, the nonsteroid anti-inflammatory drugs block the synthesis of prostaglandins. The prostaglandins are potent vasodilators and increase the inflammatory process.

2. The joint pain associated with gout is caused by:
   *a. urate crystals deposited in synovial fluid
   b. purine deposits on ligaments of long bones
   c. prostaglandin synthesis in the central nervous system
   d. histamine release cells in the tissue surrounding the joint

   [CL: KN]

   Rationale: Gout, a metabolic disorder of purine metabolism, is associated with pain and swelling in the joints, resulting from urate crystals deposited in synovial fluid.

3. Which of the following drugs are commonly given together?
   a. D-penicillamine and corticosteroids
   b. ibuprofen and aspirin
   *c. indomethacin and antacids
   d. allopurinol and Vitamin C

   [CL: CO]

   Rationale: Due to the effect of indomethacin on gastric mucosa, it is often given with antacids to reduce gastric upset.

4. Antigout agents, known as the uricosurics, include probenecid and sulfinpyrazone. These agents act by:

a. increasing the activity of leukocytes and synovial cells
b. stimulating the breakdown of purine in the liver
*c. inhibiting the tubular reabsorption of uric acid
d. inhibiting the conversion of xanthine to uric acid

[CL: KN]

Rationale: Uricosurics act to reduce symptoms associated with gout by inhibiting the tubular reabsorption of uric acid.

5. Which of the following statements is correct regarding non-steroidal anti-inflammatory drugs and their interactions with other agents?
*a. Increased bleeding may occur with anticoagulants.
b. Increased anti-inflammatory effects occur with aspirin.
c. Decreased ulcerogenic effects occur with corticosteroids.
d. Increased antihypertensive effects occur with captopril.

[CL: CO]

Rationale: The concomitant administration of nonsteroidal anti-inflammatory drugs and anticoagulants results in increased bleeding.

CHAPTER 48: THE PRINCIPLES OF ANTINEOPLASTIC CHEMOTHERAPY

Review Questions from Text

1. In comparing malignant and benign neoplasms, malignant neoplasms are characterized by:
   a. slow, controlled growth
   b. new growth
   c. encapsulation
   *d. ability to metastasize

   [CL: CO]

   Rationale: Malignant tumors or neoplasms differ from benign tumors in that they have the ability to invade surrounding tissue and metastasize.

2. During the S phase of cell division, the following activities take place:
   a. resting state
   *b. DNA synthesis
   c. specialized protein synthesis
   d. cell mitosis

   [CL: KN]

   Rationale: During the S phase, actual DNA synthesis occurs, taking from 10 to 20 hours to double the DNA complement.

3. According to the Stem Cell Theory:
   a. all of the cells in a primary tumor are thought to be of clonal origin
   b. the stem cell population has limited ability to reproduce
   c. all members of a stem cell population are involved in cell division at the same time
   *d. the primary tumor arises from a clonogenic population

   [CL: KN]

   Rationale: According to the Stem Cell Theory, only a small cell population has the potential to reproduce the entire tissue from its genetic storehouse.

4. The first chemotherapeutic agent, found in 1919, was:
   *a. nitrogen mustard
   b. hydroxyurea
   c. dacarbazine
   d. adriamycin

   [CL: KN]

   Rationale: In 1919 it was discovered that nitrogen mustard had leukopenic activity. Administration of chemotherapy began around 50 years ago.

5. Which of the following statements is <u>correct</u> regarding adjuvant chemotherapy?
   a. This treatment manages primary tumor growth.
   *b. It is the use of agents to destroy micrometastasis.
   c. This group of agents is used to treat overt metastasis.
   d. It is the use of drugs to stimulate viral oncogenes.

   [CL: KN]

   Rationale: Adjuvant chemotherapy is the administration of chemotherapy for the purpose of destroying micrometastasis and preventing the development of secondary tumors following the removal of the primary tumor.

6. Cell cycle-specific agents affect the cell during:
   a. the entire cell cycle
   b. mitotic division only
   *c. one phase of the cell cycle
   d. resting phase only

   [CL: KN]

   Rationale: Cell cycle-specific chemotherapeutic agents are designed to affect the cell during a specific phase of the cell life cycle.

7. An example of a cell cycle-nonspecific chemotherapeutic agent is:
   *a. cisplatin
   b. bleomycin
   c. vincristine
   d. fluoracil

   [CL: KN]

   Rationale: Cisplatin is an example of an alkylating or cell cycle-nonspecific agent used to treat disseminated carcinomas of the breast, ovaries, testes, and lungs.

8. Historically, chemotherapy was used as:
   a. primary treatment for malignant disease
   b. specific agents for particlar primary tumors
   *c. treatment of hematologic and metastatic tumors
   d. management of side effects of tumor growth

   [CL: KN]

   Rationale: Historically, chemotherapy was not considered first-line treatment for malignant disease. The major use of these agents was for treatment of hematologic and metastatic tumors.

9. Which of the following statements is <u>true</u> regarding the history of antineoplastic agents?
   a. The use of chemotherapy dates back to the Egyptians' use of opium.
   b. The first antimetabolic agents were introduced in the 1970s.
   *c. The drug Mustargen was first given to patients in 1942.
   d. Introduction of the antibiotics occured during the 1930s.

   [CL: KN]

   Rationale: Mechlorethamine (Mustargen) was first administered to patients in 1942.

10. Cytotoxic drugs are generally more effective:
   a. against resting cells
   b. when tumor burden is high
   c. when there is greater organ impairment
   *d. against dividing cells

   [CL: KN]

   Rationale: Chemotherapeutic agents are generally more effective against dividing cells than against resting cells.

<u>Additional Review Questions Not Presented in Text</u>

1. Cell cycle-nonspecific antineoplastic agents:
   a. are effective against small tumors where the growth fraction is high
   b. are referred to as "schedule dependent" when given in multiple repeated fractions
   c. work by causing a biochemical blockade at a specific phase of the cell cycle
   *d. are dose dependent and are administered in a bolus fashion

[CL: CO]

Rationale: Antineoplastic cell cycle-nonspecific agents are dose dependent rather than schedule dependent. The degree of cell kill is directly proportional to the amount of drug given.

2. Which statement correctly describes a basic principle of antineoplastic chemotherapy?
*a. To achieve total cell kill, drugs are administered in combination or in sequences.
b. The presence of a single clonogenic malignant cell yields insufficient offspring to affect the host.
c. There is a significant contribution of host immune mechanisms in augmenting chemotherapy.
d. A specific dose of a specific chemotherapeutic agent destroys a specific number of cells.

[CL: CO]

Rationale: The best way to achieve total cell kill is to administer chemotherapeutic agents in combination or in sequences. This approach is a way of dealing with residual tumor cells after only one agent has been administered.

3. The term "growth fraction" refers to the:
a. number of neoplastic cells lost from the tumor mass
b. fraction of cells in mitosis at a given time
*c. number of tumor cells involved in cell division
d. time required for a tumor population to double itself

[CL: KN]

Rationale: The term "growth fraction" (GF) refers to the overall number of proliferating neoplastic cells or tumor cells involved in cell division. This is a crucial factor in the effectiveness of drug therapy.

4. In reference to cell resistance to chemotherapy, Type I resistance occurs when:
a. tumor cells are temporarily resistant
*b. permanently resistant tumor cells cannot be affected by the drug
c. tumor cells receive less than adequate drug exposure due to local conditions
d. antibodies are produced by the tumor cell

[CL: KN]

Rationale: Type I resistance to chemotherapy occurs when permanently resistant tumor cells cannot be affected by the drug at all.

CHAPTER 49: ANTINEOPLASTIC CHEMOTHERAPY

Situations from Text

Situation 49-1

Hannah Berry is a 52-year-old with disseminated breast cancer. She has been admitted to the oncology unit for chemotherapy.

1. Prior to administration of fluorouracil (5FU) to Ms. Berry, the nurse will check the following lab data:
   a. sodium and potassium
   b. sedimentation rate and sodium
   *c. white blood cell count and platelets
   d. liver enzymes and amylase

   [NP: AS, C: AP]

   Rationale: Because of side effects of bone marrow depression, patients receiving fluorouracil should be assessed prior to treatment for a WBC of less than 3,500/mm^3 or platelets below 100,000/mm^3.

2. Ms. Berry begins a three-day course of intravenous fluorouracil. The nurse will plan to include the following intervention:
   a. restrict fluid intake
   *b. perform frequent oral care
   c. limit meat extracts
   d. monitor thyroid studies

   [NP: PL, CL: CO]

   Rationale: Stomatitis is a frequent effect of fluorouracil therapy; therefore, frequent oral care limits the occurrence and severity of this side effect.

3. When the nurse teaches Ms. Berry about drug therapy, the following information will be included:
   a. Eliminate foods high in tyramine.
   *b. Report dark, tarry stools.
   c. Avoid antiemetics.
   d. Eat foods high in fiber.

   [NP: IM, CL: CO]

   Rationale: Side effects of fluorouracil include gastrointestinal ulcers. Patients should be taught to be aware of and report evidence of GI bleeding, such as dark, tarry stools.

4. After successful administration of fluorouracil, Ms. Berry is to be discharged home on cyclophosphanide (Cytoxan) orally. Discharge teaching will include:
   a. taking Cytoxan with meals
   b. doubling doses if one is missed
   c. taking Cytoxan at bedtime
   *d. drinking plenty of fluids

   [NP: IM, CL: AP]

   Rationale: Bladder toxicity is related to Cytoxan therapy, especially on long-term oral use. Drinking plenty of fluids reduces the risk of developing related complications.

5. The nurse will monitor the following lab value on a routine basis while Ms. Berry is on Cytoxan:
   *a. liver enzymes

b. uric acid levels
c. calcium
d. potassium

[NP: EV, CL: AP]

Rationale: Liver dysfunction may be noted in patients taking Cytoxan. Liver enzymes should be monitored closely.

6. Which of the following statements by Ms. Berry indicates the need for further patient teaching?
   a. "I may lose my hair due to this chemotherapy."
   b. "Soft toothbrushes will reduce bleeding gums."
   *c. "Red urine means that I am getting rid of the medicine."
   d. "I should weigh myself and report unexpected weight gain."

[NP: EV, CL: AN]

Rationale: Red urine is an indication of severe hematuria and should be reported immediately. This is a sign of hemorrhagic cystitis and is related to Cytoxan therapy. Sudden weight gain may indicate retention of water resulting from syndrome of inappropriate antidiuretic hormone (SIADH), also related to Cytoxan therapy.

Situation 49-2

Randolph Alvin, aged 49, continues to receive chemotherapy for multiple meyloma. Medication therapy includes doxorubicin and carmustine. He is being cared for on the Medical Oncology Unit.

1. While Mr. Alvin is receiving doxorubicin (Adriamycin) via peripheral intravenous infusion, the nurse will monitor:
   *a. 12 lead ECGs
   b. uric acid levels
   c. potassium levels
   d. abdominal films

[NP: AS, CL: AP]

Rationale: Cardiac toxicity has been related to Adriamycin use. The ECG should be monitored for changes on a routine basis.

2. Mr. Alvin complains of burning and swelling at the IV site through which Adriamycin is infusing. The nurse's best action would be to discontinue the IV and:
   a. place not packs over the site for at least 24 hours
   b. medicate with morphine sulfate as needed for pain
   c. elevate the extremity and apply pressure at the site
   *d. inject sodium bicarbonate subcutaneously at the site

[NP: IM, CL: AP]

Rationale: If extravasation of Adriamycin is suspected, the specific antidote is 3-5 ml of 7-8.5% sodium bicarbonate injected subcutaneously at the site. Ice packs may also be used intermittently for 18 to 24 hours.

3. In addition, Mr. Alvin is to receive carmustine (BCNU) via slow infusion for two days. The nurse will expect to give the following along with this agent:
   a. antigout medication
   b. leucovorin rescue
   *c. antiemetics
   d. Vitamin B_{12}

[NP: PL, CL: CO]

Rationale: Nausea and vomiting are acute toxic effects of BCNU and occur approximately 6 hours after beginning the infusion. Antiemetics should be given along with the chemotherapy.

4. When evaluating Mr. Alvin for bone marrow depression related to BCNU therapy, the nurse will do so:
   a. 2 days after the dose
   *b. 3-6 weeks after the dose
   c. 1-2 weeks after the dose
   d. 1 month after the dose

   [NP: EV, CL: KN]

   Rationale: Bone marrow depression related to BCNU therapy occurs approximately 3-6 weeks after administration.

5. Two weeks after discharge from the hospital, Mr. Alvin is readmitted with symptoms related to hypercalcemia. He is to be treated with mithramycin (Mithracin) via intravenous infusion. The nurse will monitor Mr. Alvin for acute toxic signs of this drug, which include:
   *a. facial flushing and epistaxis
   b. confusion and stomatitis
   c. purple bands in nail beds
   d. breast tenderness

   [NP: IM, CL: AP]

   Rationale: A unique toxic effect of mithramycin is a hemorrhagic syndrome causing facial flushing, epistaxis, and/or hematemesis.

6. With regard to mithramycin therapy, the nurse selects the nursing diagnostic category Potential for Injury for Mr. Alvin. This nursing diagnosis is related to:
   a. seizures
   *b. bleeding tendencies
   c. psychotic reactions
   d. ataxia

   [NP: AN, C: AN]

   Rationale: Mithramycin causes bone marrow depression (especially thrombocytopenia), and patients are at risk for bleeding.

<u>**Additional Situation Not Presented in TExt**</u>

Sam Heller is a 23-year-old newly diagnosed with testicular cancer. He is scheduled to undergo chemotherapy after recovery from surgery.

1. Mr. Heller is to begin receiving bleomycin (Blenoxane) intravenously once a week for 4 weeks. The nurse will assess him for potential side effects, which include:
   *a. fever
   b. esophagitis
   c. thrombocytopenia
   d. confusion

   [NP: IM, CL: AP]

   Rationale: Fever is a common adverse effect related to bleomycin therapy. Fever generally occurs only on the first day of therapy.

2. The cumulative dosage of bleomycin will be limited to less than 400 units because of the potential for:
   a. cardiotoxicity
   b. neurotoxicity
   *c. pulmonary fibrosis

d. bone marrow depression

[NP: AN, CL: CO]

Rationale: Pulmonary fibrosis is a dose-related complication seen with cumulative doses of bleomycin greater than 400 units.

3. Psychological support for Mr. Heller would include the following nursing intervention:
   a. informing him that he will never be able to father children
   *b. using an honest approach when describing usual side effects of chemotherapy
   c. maintaining an attitude of control and power in order to provide a secure environment
   d. encouraging him to feel depressed about his devastating disease and chemotherapy

[NP: IM, CL: CO]

Rationale: Patients are most likely to comply with therapy if they understand the adverse effects of chemotherapeutic medications and what effects may be expected. An honest approach facilitates trust in the caregiver and allays fear.

4. In addition to bleomycin, Mr. Heller will receive vincristine intravenously weekly. The nurse will monitor him for:
   a. hypoglycemia
   b. hypercalcemia
   c. hirsutism
   *d. tingling of the extremities

[NP: AS, CL: AP]

Rationale: Paresthesias are common adverse effects of vincristine therapy.

5. When planning nursing care for Mr. Heller, the following nursing action should be included:
   a. Restrict fluids during treatment.
   b. Limit dosage of acetaminophen.
   *c. Observe for IV drug infiltration.
   d. Place patient in isolation.

[NP: PL, CL: CO]

Rationale: Vincristine is corrosive to tissues, causing cellulitis, phlebitis, and necrosis if infiltrated into subcutaneous tissues.

6. For discharge teaching, the nurse will include the following information about his chemotherapy:
   a. All chemotherapy causes hair loss.
   b. Normally, red urine will be seen related to vincristine.
   *c. Stool softeners may prevent constipation related to vincristine.
   d. A high protein diet is best tolerated on chemotherapy.

[NP: IM, CL: AP]

Rationale: Paralytic ileus and constipation are related to vincristine therapy; stool softeners may be given prophylactically.

Review Questions from Text

1. Which of the following is the mot accurate means of dose calculation for chemotherapeutic agents?
   *a. body surface area
   b. body weight
   c. age
   d. total body fat

[CL: KN]

Rationale: The most accurate means of calculating dosages for all antineoplastic drugs is by using body surface area.

2. Guidelines for the preparation of chemotherapeutic agents include utilizing:
   a. patient care units for mixing agents
   b. oral pipetting of certain agents only
   c. disposal of waste in the standard manner
   *d. face mask and protective clothing for the preparer

[CL: KN]

Rationale: When mixing chemotherapeutic agents, the preparer should wear a face mask and protective clothing to guard against airborne particles or aerosolization of the drug.

3. In general, alkalizing agents act by:
   a. substituting an enzyme in protein metabolism
   *b. inactivating the cell replication process
   c. forming electrophilic bonds in the cytosine of DNA
   d. affecting cells in the GO (resting) phase

[CL: CO]

Rationale: Alkylating agents are derived from sulfur mustard gases and form electrophilic bonds with the guanine in DNA, thereby inactivating the cell replication process.

4. The alkylating agent cyclophosphamide (Cytoxan):
   a. requires a one-step metabolic activation
   b. crosses the blood-brain barrier
   c. increases activity when given with corticosteroids
   *d. acts on both normal and abnormal cells

[CL: KN]

Rationale: Cyclophosphamide is not a tumor-specific antimetabolite and is capable of cross-linking DNA in many normal cells as well as abnormal cells.

5. Which of the following agents would be most useful against primary brain tumors?
   a. melphalan
   b. cyclophosphamide
   *c. carmustine
   d. cisplatin

[CL: CO]

Rationale: As an alkylating nitrosourea, carmustine is useful against primary and metastatic brain tumors because it is lipid soluble and crosses the blood-brain barrier.

6. As a group, the antimetabolites act as antineoplastic agents by:
   *a. interfering with the pathways of dividing cells
   b. exerting the greatest effect on GI phase
   c. cross-linking RNA replication
   d. producing toxic coenzymes

[CL: CO]

Rationale: Antimetabolites interfere with the metabolic pathways of dividing cells by their similarity to vitamins, coenzymes, or normal cell intermediary products.

7. The toxic effects of methotrexate on normal cells can be reduced by the administration of:
   a. levorphanol
   b. cytarabine
   *c. leucovorin
   d. allopurinol

   [CL: KN]

   Rationale: Methotrexate is a folic acid antagonist which affects normal as well as malignant cell growth. In order to reduce potentially fatal toxic effects, leucovorin is administered to "rescue" the normal cells. Leucovorin provides a form of folic acid which can only be used by normal cells.

8. Antineoplastic agents which act by inhibiting pyrimidine synthesis include:
   a. hydroxyurea
   b. thioguanine
   c. cisplatin
   *d. fluorouracil

   [CL: KN]

   Rationale: The antimetabolite fluorouracil (5-FU) works by inhibiting pyrimidine synthesis and, thereby, altering DNA synthesis.

9. For patients on thioguanine therapy, it will be important to monitor the following level:
   a. calcium
   *b. uric acid
   c. sodium
   d. potassium

   [CL: CO]

   Rationale: Thioguanine is a purine antagonist, resulting in increased purine and uric acid levels. Secondary gouty arthritis is associated with abnormally high uric acid levels.

10. The following is <u>correct</u> with regard to the vinca alkaloids:
   a. cell cycle-nonspecific
   *b. derivative of the periwinkle plant
   c. similar in antitumor spectrum
   d. effective in oral doses

   [CL: KN]

   Rationale: The vinca alkaloids are derivative of the periwinkle plant and are cell cycle-specific.

<u>Addtional Review Questions Not Presented in Text</u>

1. A unique adverse effect of the anthracyclines (doxorubicin and daunorubicin) is:
   a. photosensitivity
   *b. cardiotoxicity
   c. psychosis
   d. neurotoxicity

   [CL: KN]

   Rationale: Patients treated with either of the anthracyclines may develop a dose-dependent cardiomyopathy similar to congestive heart failure.

2. The main advantage of using hormones as antineoplastic therapy is that they have:
   *a. minimal bone marrow depression

b. cell cycle-specific action
c. few adverse side effects
d. a specific mode of action

[CL: KN]

Rationale: The major advantage of the use of hormones in the treatment of certain neoplasms is that they do not cause bone marrow depression.

3. The antineoplastic agent L-Asparaginase (Elspar) is:
a. used as a last resort in the treatment of testicular tumors
b. toxic to gastrointestinal mucosa and hair folicles
c. active only in the mitotic phase of cell division
*d. represents the first enzyme to be used to treat cancer

[CL: KN]
Rationale: Asparaginase is unique in the field of cancer treatment in that it is the first enzyme to be successful in the treatment of cancer. This agent is primarily used in the treatment of acute lymphoblastic leukemia.

4. A nursing implication for patients receiving the radioactive isotope sodium idodide (^{131}I) would be to:
a. collect all urine excreted in 12 hours
b. maintain isolation for one month
*c. monitor for swelling or sensations of fullness in the neck
d. give thyroid hormone along with the isotope

[CL: CO]

Rationale: The adverse reactions of sodium radioiodine for the treatment of thyroid cancer are mild, but patients may complain of fullness or swelling in the neck.

5. Estramustine phosphate (Emeyt) is used primarily for treatment of:
a. metastatic breast cancer
b. disseminated liver cancer
*c. prostatic carcinoma
d. primary lymphoma

[CL: KN]

Rationale: Estramustine is a combination of nitrogen mustard and a derivative of estradiol which is particularly effective against metastatic prostate cancer in patients resistant to estrogen.

CHAPTER 50: IMMUNOTHERAPY AND BIOLOGICAL RESPONSE MODIFIERS

Situation from Text

Situation 50-1

Carl Pazos is a 33-year-old recently diagnosed with AIDS. He is being treated through a public health clinic specializing in immune altered patients.

1. Mr. Pazos is to begin therapy with Zidovudine (AZT) 250 mg orally. The nurse will anticipate the following dosage schedule:
 a. every 8 hours
 b. twice a day
 *c. every 4 hours
 d. four times a day

 [NP: PL, CL: KN]

 Rationale: Because of the short half-life of AZT, the drug must be taken every 4 hours around the clock in order to achieve therapeutic drug levels.

2. The nurse will teach Mr. Pazos about the side effects to be expected with AZT, including:
 a. photosensitivity
 b. alopecia
 c. fever and chills
 *d. nausea

 [NP: IM, CL: CO]

 Rationale: Common side effects of AZT therapy include nausea, anorexia, and severe headaches.

3. Upon his return visits to the clinic, the nurse will evaluate Mr. Pazos' response to AZT therapy. Which of the following lab values would be especially important to note?
 *a. complete blood count (CBC)
 b. creatinine and BUN
 c. calcium and phosphorus
 d. potassium and magnesium

 [NP: EV, C: CO]

 Rationale: Severe bone marrow depression is an acute toxic effect of AZT therapy. The CBC should be evaluated routinely and, if patient becomes severly anemic, therapy may need to be altered.

4. Should Mr. Pazos experience severe headaches, he would be instructed to:
 a. take indomethacin
 *b. contact the physician
 c. take acetaminophen
 d. drink extra fluids

 [NP: IM, CL: AP]

 Rationale: Drugs such as indomethacin and acetaminophen may increase the toxic effects of AZT. Patients should be taught to contact the physician before using any medications.

5. While providing care for Mr. Pazos after six months of AZT therapy, the nurse will be mindful of which of the following?
 a. respiratory protection
 *b. AIDS transmission precautions

c. isolation precautions
d. no precautions necessary

[NP: PL, CL: AP]

Rationale: AIDS patients on AZT are still able to transmit the virus to others; therefore, appropriate precautions need to be observed.

6. Additional assessment of Mr. Pazos which should be employed on a routine basis would be to:
 a. expect patient to be depressed and withdrawn
 b. observe for serious systemic side effects
*c. check mucous membranes and skin for areas of breakdown
 d. monitor cardiac rhythm prior to drug administration.

[NP: AS, C: AP]

Rationale: An intact integument is the best first line of defense against invading organisms, particularly in patients susceptible to infection.

__Additional Situation Not Presented in Text__

Patricia Hightower is a 64-year-old who has undergone successful heart transplant surgery. She is being cared for in the Surgical Intensive Care Unit.

1. On the third postoperative day, Mrs. Hightower is to start cyclosporine (Sandimmune) intravenously. Which of the following data should be noted prior to therapy with this agent?
 a. serum amylase
*b. creatinine and BUN
 c. LDH and CPK
 d. T_3T_4 levels

[NP: AS, CL: CO]

Rationale: Due to the nephrotoxic effects of cyclosporin, the creatinine and BUN should be noted for the baseline and monitored throughout treatment.

2. Which of the following findings would the nurse report promptly after assessing Mrs. Hightower?
 a. evidence of hair loss
 b. heart rate of 100 pbpm
 c. urine output of 40 cc/hr
*d. drainage from incision

[NP: AS, CL: AP]

Rationale: Due to the immunosuppressive nature of cyclosporin, any evidence of infection should be reported immediately.

3. After three days of intravenous therapy with cyclosporin, Mrs. Hightower is to start oral dosage. The nurse will administer oral cyclosporin:
*a. on an empty stomach
 b. with meals
 c. with an antacid
 d. prior to bedtime

[NP: IM, CL: CO]

Rationale: Food delays absorption of cyclosporin, and it is best administered before meals.

4. When planning specific nursing care for Mrs. Hightower related to cyclosporin therapy, the nurse will include:

a. weighing patient once a week
b. limiting mobility
c. maintaining isolation
*d. performing oral care

[NP: PL, CL: AP]

Rationale: Gum hyperplasia is a side effect of cyclosporin therapy. The nurse not only provides frequent oral care, she/he should teach the patient regarding its importance.

5. The nurse will monitor Mrs. Hightower for side effects related to cyclosporin therapy, which include:
a. nausea
b. alopecia
*c. tremors
d. palpitations

[NP: IM, CL: KN]

Rationale: Tremors are often seen as adverse effects of cyclosporin therapy.

6. Which of the following statements by Mrs. Hightower indicates a need for further teaching?
a. "I should stay away from people with colds or flu."
b. "It will be important for me to maintain a nutritional diet."
*c. "For a fever, I should take aspirin and call the doctor."
d. "It would be best to refrain from alcoholic beverages."

[NP: EV, CL: AN]

Rationale: Aspirin and aspirin-containing products may compound immunosuppression and should not be taken along with cyclospirin therapy.

Review Questions from Text

1. T-cells play the following role in the immune response:
a. producing antibody-like proteins
*b. assisting B-cells in antibody synthesis
c. producing specific antibodies
d. inhibiting the humoral response

[C: KN]

Rationale: T-cells assist the B-cells in the synthesis of antibodies. This is a "helper" role only as they do not produce antibodies or antibody-like proteins.

2. In humans, B-cells mature in the:
a. immature thymus gland
b. liver and pancreas
c. epiphysis of long bones
*d. Peyer's patches in the intestines

[CL: KN]

Rationale: B-cells mature in bursa-equivalent areas located in Peyer's patches in the intestines.

3. One method by which tumor cells escape detection by the host organism is by:
a. stimulating a strong host immune response
b. initiating an early host response
*c. blocking factors which cover the antigenic sites on cancer cells
d. mechanical obstruction of tumor cells by area leukocytes

[CL: CO]

Rationale: The presence of blocking factors or antibodies by tumor cells can inhibit the ability of the host organism to recognize the tumor cells as foreign.

4. Passive nonspecific immunotherapy occurs when:
*a. serum from healthy individuals is injected into cancer patients
b. serum from patients in remission is injected into patients with active disease
c. immunosuppressive substances from cancer patients are removed
d. live immunocompetent lymphocytes are transferred to cancer patients

[CL: CO]

Rationale: Passive nonspecific immunotherapy is the injection of serum from healthy individuals into cancer patients.

5. Host defenses play a role in retarding tumor growth, spread, or recovery from disease as evidenced by the following example:
a. Spontaneous tumor regression occurs in patients with large tumor burdens.
*b. Cancers heavily infiltrated by lymphocytes have a better prognosis.
c. Weak cell-mediated immune response to chemotherapy shows a better prognosis.
d. Appearance of metastatic disease occurs in all patients in 15 to 30 years.

[CL: CO]

Rationale: Patients with lymphocyte-predominant breast tumors have a well-documented improved prognosis over patients without lymphocytic infiltration.

6. The function of lymphokines is to activate:
a. tumor-specific antibodies
b. B-cells
*c. macrophages
d. killer T-cells

[CL: CO]

Rationale: When T-cells are sensitized by foreign antigens, soluble factors called lymphokines are released. An example is migration inhabitory factor (MIF), which activates and draws tissue macrophages to the tumor cell site.

7. A goal of cancer immunotherapy is to:
a. produce remission as a single agent in cancer therapy
b. promote tumor-nonspecific immunity
*c. stimulate immunocompetence in cancer patients
d. bypass side effects of traditional chemotherapy

[CL: KN]

Rationale: One of the basic goals in cancer immunotherapy is to promote and stimulate immunocompetence by active or passive methods.

8. Immunorestorative immunotherapy is utilized to:
a. replace the patient's immune system
*b. augment the patient's immune response
c. bypass the patient's effector cell response
d. prevent overstimulation of the immune response

[CL: KN]

Rationale: Immunorestorative immunotherapy uses substances such as interferon to augment the patient's own immune system.

9. When preparing a BCG injection, the following precaution must be taken:
   a. Prepare skin well with alcohol prep.
   *b. Protect the vaccine from light when stored.
   c. Use any diluent for reconstitution
   d. Store in a dry warm area after reconstitution.

   [CL: KN]

   Rationale: The vaccine BCG should be protected from light and kept in refrigeration to retain potency.

10. Adverse effects of interferon therapy include:
   *a. flu-like symptoms
   b. seizures
   c. peripheral neuritis
   d. alopecia

   [CL: KN]

   Rationale: Commonly seen side effects of interferon therapy include flu-like symptoms, such as fever, chills, myalgia, fatigue, and/or headache.

<u>**Additional Review Questions Not Presented in Text**</u>

1. The following patient criterion is used when considering eligibility for immunotherapy:
   *a. small tumor burden
   b. severely immunosuppressed
   c. negative skin patch testing
   d. progression beyond Stage III

   [CL: CO]

   Rationale: Patients who have had tumor reduction procedures will benefit from immunotherapy, due to small tumor burden.

2. Active nonspecific immunotherapy is the stimulation of the immune response by:
   a. administration of antibodies from normal individuals
   b. injection of the tumor cell and its products
   *c. administration of attenuated live bacteria or their products
   d. transplantation of normal bone marrow

   [CL: KN]

   Rationale: Active nonspecific immunotherapy is achieved by administration of live attenuated bacteria or their products, such as the bacillus Calmette-Guerin (BCG) vaccine.

3. The most successful combination of interferon therapy involves:
   a. alpha and beta interferon
   b. alpha and BCG vaccine
   c. beta and BCG vaccine
   *d. gamma and beta interferon

   [CL: CO]

   Rationale: Alpha and beta interferons share the same receptor on their cells and when given together compete for the same receptors. Since gamma interferon has a different receptor, it is given with either beta or alpha interferon for enhanced therapeutic effect.

4. Initial studies of tumor necrosis factor (TNF) have shown that therapeutic actions include:

a. single agent effectiveness against cancer
b. stimulated Killer T-cell and B-cell activity
c. counteracting adverse side effects of interferon therapy
*d. stimulating macrophase mediated antitumor activity

[CL: CO]

Rationale: While the exact role of TNF has not been determined, it has been shown to stimulate macrophage mediated antitumor activity. TNF therapy appears to be best utilized in combination therapy rather than as a singlw antitumor agent.

5. The use of antithymocytic globulin (Atgam) is to:
a. stimulate T-cells and B-cells
*b. reduce thymus-dependent lymphocytes
c. recruit circulating macrophages
d. prevent weight loss in cancer patients

[CL: KN]

Rationale: Atgam is an immunosuppressive drug which reduces the number of T-lymphocytes. Atgam is limited to renal allograft rejection.

CHAPTER 51: OVERVIEW OF ANATOMY AND PHYSIOLOGY OF THE GASTROINTESTINAL SYSTEM

Review Questions from Text

1. The pyloric glands produce:
   *a. mucus
   b. ptyalin
   c. hydrochloric acid
   d. pepsin

   [CL: KN]

   Rationale: The pyloric glands produce mucus with protects the gastric mucosa.

2. The hormone which regulates the rate of gastric emptying is:
   a. gastrin
   b. pepsinogin
   *c. enterogastrone
   d. trypsin

   [CL: KN]

   Rationale: Enterogastrone, a hormone produced in the small intestine, helps to regulate gastric emptying.

3. Which statement is <u>correct</u> concerning the gastrointestinal system?
   a. The esophagus is 2.5 cm long.
   b. The ileum is part of the large intestine.
   *c. The large intestine is approximately 1.5 meters long.
   d. The duodenum is considered a part of the stomach.

   [CL: KN]

   Rationale: The large intestine is composed of the cecum, colon, and rectum and is about 1.5 meters long.

4. The primary function of villikinin is to:
   *a. allow the villi to absorb more nutrients
   b. stimulate peristaltic activity in the large intestine
   c. inhibit the entrance of chyme into the small intestine
   d. stimulate the production of musuc from the villi

   [CL: CO]

   Rationale: Villikinin is a hormone secreted by the intestinal wall which allows the villi to absorb increased nutrients through active transport and passive diffusion.

5. Approximately 2000 ml of alkaline secretions are secreted daily by:
   a. Brunner's glands
   b. goblet cells
   c. oxyntic cells
   *d. crypts of Lieberkuhn

   [CL: KN]

   Rationale: The crypts of Lieberkuhn are small glands located along the surface of the small intestine. These glands secrete approximately 2000 ml of alkaline secretions daily. The secretions contain special enzyme which enable final digestion of food before absorption.

6. Digestion within the small intestine is dependent on:

a. peptidases for splitting neutral fats into fatty acids
b. lipase for splitting peptides into amino acids
c. lactase for splitting starch into disaccharides
*d. bacteria for splitting food by-products

[CL: KN]

Rationale: Bacterial action in the small intestine helps in splitting food by-products.

7. Which statement is correct concerning nervous system control of the alimentary canal?
a. The parasympathetic nervous system decreases gastric secretion.
*b. The sympathetic nervous system slows or stops GI tract function.
c. The parasympathetic nervous system decreases intestinal motility.
d. The sympathetic nervous system increases intestinal mucus production.

[CL: KN]

Rationale: The effect of the sympathetic nervous system on the gastrointestinal system results in slowing or cessation of function.

8. The liver performs the following functions except:
a. producing bile from old defective red blood cells
b. playing a role in varbohydrate, fat, and protein metabolism
*c. synthesizing Vitamins A, D, and B_{12}
d. synthesizing cholesterol and clotting factors

[CL: CO]

Rationale: The liver stores, rather than synthesizes, Vitamins A, D, and B_{12}. The liver performs more than 500 individual functions.

9. As an endocrine gland, the pancreas secretes:
a. trypsin inhibitor
b. sodium bicarbonate
*c. glucogen
d. chymotrypsin

[CL: KN]

Rationale: The pancreas produces insulin and glucogon as an endocrine function. Chymotrypsin is released as an exocrine function.

10. The primary role of cytochrome P-450, released by the liver, is to:
a. stimulate steroid release as a stress response
*b. deactivate and detoxify medications and other substances
c. produce fibrinogen, prothrombin, and factor V
d. deaminate amino acids, forming urea

[CL: KN]

Rationale: Cytochrome P-450 is a substance produced in the liver which plays a vital role in drug biotransformation.

Additional Review Questions Not Presented in Text

1. The stimulus for contraction of the gallbladder is:
a. alkaline chyme in the small intestine
b. fat-soluble vitamins in the small intestine
c. acid chyme in the stomach
*d. fatty foods in the chyme

[CL: KN]

Rationale: Normal contraction of the gallbladder is stimulated by the presence of acid chyme in the duodenum or fatty foods in the chyme.

2. Which of the following have the greatest inhibition of gastric emptying?
 a. carbohydrates
 *b. fats
 c. proteins
 d. ethyl alcohol

[CL: CO]

Rationale: Fats delay gastric emptying for as long as 3 hours. Alcohol, on the other hand, is quickly absorbed through the epithelial wall of the stomach.

3. Intrinsic factor is produced by:
 a. villi in the small intestine
 b. Kupffer cells in the liver
 *c. parietal cells in the stomach
 d. goblet cells in the duodenum

[CL: CO]

Rationale: Intrinsic factor, essential for B_{12} absorption, is produced by parietal cells in the stomach.

4. Which stage of digestion occurs in response to the sight, taste, or smell of food?
 a. mediary
 b. gastric
 *c. cephalic
 d. voluntary

[CL: KN]

Rationale: The cephalic digestive phase begins when the stomach secretes gastric juices in response to the sight, smell, or taste of food.

5. The normal pH of gastric secretions is:
 *a. 1.0-3.5
 b. 4.5-6.0
 c. 7.8-8.0
 d. 8.0-8.3

[CL: KN]

Rationale: Gastric secretions have a pH range of 1.0-3.5, while small intestinal secretions range 7.8-8.0.

CHAPTER 52: MEDICATIONS TO TREAT GASTRIC HYPERACTIVITY

Situation from Text

Situation 52-1

Artie Simon is a 24-year-old who is on the telemetry unit following a motor vehicle accident during which he suffered a head injury. He has a tracheostomy, nasogastric tube, and a central line.

1. Mr. Simon is receiving cimetidine (Tagamet) 300 mg IVPB every 6 hours to reduce the risk of gastric ulcer formation. The nurse will avoid rapid intravenous infusion due to the potential for:
   a. hyperthermia
   b. hypertension
   *c. bradycardia
   d. seizures

   [NP: PL, CL: AP]

   Rationale: During rapid intravenous infusion of cimetidine, patients may develop bradycardia and cardiac arrest.

2. The nurse will monitor Mr. Simon for which of the following side effects related to cimetidine therapy?
   a. tetany
   *b. abdominal pain
   c. visual disturbances
   d. cough

   [NP: IM, C: AP]

   Rationale: Patients on cimetidine therapy may experience gastrointestinal side effects such as nausea, diarrhea, and/or abdominal pain.

3. Mr. Simon also receives aluminum hydroxide (Amphojel) 30 cc via nasogastric tube every 4 hours. The nurse will plan to check him for:
   a. hypersensitivity reaction
   b. oral thrush
   c. milk-alkali syndrome
   *d. constipation

   [NP: PL, CL: CO]

   Rationale: Patients taking aluminum products commonly experience constipation due to the combination of aluminum and bile salts.

4. Mr. Simon is receiving continuous tube feeding. Assessment reveals abdominal distention. He is to begin metoclopramide (Reglan). The nurse is aware of the following contraindication to its use:
   *a. bowel obstruction
   b. glaucoma
   c. cardiovascular disease
   d. pulmonary fibrosis

   [NP: AN, CL: CO]

   Rationale: The stimulation of bowel mobility may be dangerous in the case of bowel obstruction, perforation, or hemorrhage.

5. When administering metoclopramide, the nurse will monitor Mr. Simon for the following adverse effects:
   a. nausea and vomiting
   b. photosensitivity reactions
   *c. restlessness

d. tachycardia

[NP: IM, CL: AP]

Rationale: There is a high incidence of central nervous system effects related to metoclopramide therapy. These include restlessness, drowsiness, and extrapyramidal and parkinsonism-like reactions.

6. An appropriate outcome for Mr. Simon would be:
 a. gastric residual >150 cc
 *b. stools negative for occult blood
 c. at least 3 formed stools per day
 d. evidence of tube feeding around trach site

[NP: EV, CL: AP]

Rationale: Patients on drugs to prevent hyperacidity will be evaluated in terms of evidence of gastric bleeding or irritation. An outcome of successful treatment would be stool specimens negative for occult blood.

Additional Situation Not Presented in Text

Dessie Hildebrand is a 48-year-old tax accountant who has recently been diagnosed with peptic ulcer disease. She is to begin medical treatment and to be discharged with medications.

1. Mrs. Hildebrand is started on sucralfate (Carafate) 1 gm 4 times a day. A potential nursing diagnostic category pertaining to this patient would be:
 *a. Alteration in Bowel Elimination: constipation
 b. Potential for Injury: bleeding
 c. Noncompliance
 d. Decreased Cardiac Output

[NP: AN, CL: AN]

Rationale: A frequent adverse effect of sucralfate is constipation.

2. The nurse will plan to administer the sucralfate to Mrs. Hildebrand at the following site:
 a. with meals
 b. with an antacid
 *c. one hour before meals
 d. after each meal

[NP: PL, CL: AP}

Rationale: Sucralfate is best administered orally one hour before meals and at bedtime for optimum protection againt gastric acidity.

3. Mrs. Hildebrand is scheduled to receive ranitidine (Zantac) 50 mg po at bedtime. The nurse will inform the patient of the following common side effect related to this medication:
 a. fever and chills
 *b. headache
 c. tachycardia
 d. anxiety

[NP: IM, CL: KN]

Rationale: Few adverse side effects have been associated with ranitidine therapy; however, the most common effect reported is headache.

4. When evaluating Mrs. Hildebrand during routinely scheduled checkups, the nurse will note the following in relation to ranitidine therapy:
 *a. creatinine

b. red blood cell count
c. T_3, T_4 levels
d. potassium levels

[NP: EV, CL: CO]

Rationale: Ranitidine is excreted via the kidneys. Cautious administration is advised for patients with evidence of renal disease.

5. Gaviscon 30 cc po 4 times a day has been ordered for Mrs. Hildebrand. She will be instructed to report the following side effect related to its use:
 a. excessive bruising
 b. photosensitivity
 *c. diarrhea
 d. visual disturbances

[NP: IM, CL: CO]

Rationale: Antacids containing magnesium may cause diarrhea. If this occurs, the antacid should be switched to an aluminum-containing product.

6. When teaching Mrs. Hildebrand about taking antacids, the nurse will include the following information:
 a. Take antacids with all meals.
 b. Antacid tablets are equal to the liquid form.
 c. Antacids absorb the acid in the stomach.
 *d. Do not take other medications with antacids.

[NP: IM, CL: KN]

Rationale: Due to the possibility of drug interaction, antacids are best taken 1 to 2 hours before or after other medications.

<u>**Review Questions from Text**</u>

1. As a group, antacids act by:
 a. reducing gastric acid secretions
 b. absorbing gastric acid
 c. stimulating an alkaline secretion
 *d. raising the gastric pH

[CL: CO]
Rationale: Antacids interact with gastric secretions, neutralizing some of the hydrochloric acid secretion and increasing the gastric pH.

2. Sodium bicarbonate and calcium carbonate may be responsible for the development of milk-alkali syndrome, characterized by:
 a. hypocalcemia
 b. acidosis
 c. hypokalemia
 *d. hypercalcemia

[C: KN]

Rationale: Milk-alkali syndrome, caused by overuse of sodium bicarbonate and calcium carbonate, is characterized by hypercalcemia, alkalosis, and renal failure.

3. Anticholinergics, when administered with other agents:
 *a. relieve pain by inhibiting motility and secretions
 b. stimulate the release of acetylcholine at neuroeffector sites

c. stimulate gastric cells to produce pepsin and mucus
d. are indicated in the treatment of gastric ulcers

[CL: KN]

Rationale: Anticholinergics are used as adjuncts in the management of peptic ulcers. They relieve pain by inhibiting motility and secretions.

4. Which of the following statements is <u>correct</u> regarding antacids and drug interactions?
   a. Antacids increase the absorption of digitalis products.
   *b. Antacids decrease the absorption of tetracycline antibiotics.
   c. Aluminum products enhance the absorption of propranolol.
   d. Magnesium products increase the absorption of the phenothiazine.

   [CL: KN]

   Rationale: Antacids decrease the absorption of tetracycline antibiotics by binding with them to form complexes which are difficult to absorb.

5. When caring for a patient receiving an anticholinergic drug, a nursing action would be to:
   a. administer the drug with meals to enhance effectiveness
   b. observe the patient for symptoms of urinary retention
   *c. encourage the patient to avoid excessive heat
   d. prepare parenteral medications at least four hours before administering

   [CL: KN]

   Rationale: Anticholinergics suppress perspiration; therefore, patients should avoid excessive heat for they are at risk for heat stroke.

6. The belladonna alkaloids, such as balladonna and atropine, have the following characteristic:
   a. are slowly absorbed from the gastrointestinal tract
   *b. readily cross the blood-brain barrier
   c. depress the central nervous system in large doses
   d. stimulate the central nervous system in toxic doses

   [CL: KN]

   Rationale: The belladonna alkaloids are readily absorbed from the gastrointestinal tract and readily cross the blood-brain barrier.

7. Prolonged use of aluminum-containing antacids may cause hypophosphatemia, characterized by:
   a. increased appetite
   *b. muscle weakness
   c. irritability
   d. muscle rigidity

   [CL: KN]

   Rationale: When aluminum antacids bind with phosphate in the bowel, they produce hypophosphatemia with prolonged use. Symptoms of this adverse effect include muscle weakness, anorexia, and malaise.

8. In addition to their neutralizing ability, aluminum antacids have the following action:
   a. stimulation of peristalsis
   b. increased gastric muscle tone
   *c. delayed gastric emptying
   d. reduced number of parietal cells

   [CL: KN]

Rationale: Aluminum antacids relax gastric smooth muscles and delay gastric emptying in addition to their neutralizing action.

9. The Acid Neutralizing Capacity (ANC) is defined as the:
   *a. mEq of HCl required to keep an antacid suspension at a pH of 3.0 for 2 hours
   b. ability of the antacid to change the gastric pH to 5.0 and maintain for 2 hours
   c. mEq of HCl absorbed by an antacid within a 24-hour period in vitro
   d. amount of antacid required to neutralize 10 mEq of HCl to a pH of 4.0

   [CL: KN]

   Rationale: The Acid Neutralizing Capacity (ANC) is expressed as the mEq of hydrochloride required to keep an antacid suspension at pH 3.0 for 2 hours <u>in vitro</u>. A high ANC denotes an effective antacid.

Additional Review Questions Not Presented in Text

1. Cimetidine acts to reduce gastric irritation by:
   a. coating the stomach lining with an insoluble protective coating
   *b. blocking the action of histamine in the parietal cells
   c. stimulating the release of histamine which inhibits gastrin
   d. blocking the production of pepsinogen in the chief cells

   [CL: CO]

   Rationale: Cimetidine occupies the H_2 receptor sites in parietal cells and blocks stimulation by histamine. Histamine is associated with the secretion of gastrin and acetylcholine.

2. A nursing action associated with sucralfate (Carafate) includes which of the following?
   a. administer with meals
   b. crush if giving via n/g tube
   *c. give cimetidine 2 hours before or after
   d. give along with antacids

   [CL: KN]

   Rationale: Cimetidine, along with other drugs such as phenytoin and tetracycline, may bind with sucralfate in the stomach. To facilitate bioavailability of cimetidine, it should be given 2 hours before or after administration of sucralfate.

3. Mylanta is a combination antacid which contains the following ingredients:
   *a. aluminum hydroxide, magnesium, simethicone
   b. calcium carbonate, simethicone
   c. magnesium, simethicone
   d. calcium carbonate, aluminum hydroxide, magnesium

   [CL: KN]

   Rationale: Mylanta contains aluminum hydroxide magnesium, and simethicone. Such a combination may reduce gastric side effects.

4. A disadvantage related to calcium carbonate therapy is:
   a. high cost
   *b. acid-rebound
   c. secondary hypermagnesemia
   d. short duration of action

   [CL: KN]

   Rationale: Calcium carbonate is the only antacid which causes a rebound hyperacidity after neutralization of the gastric content.

CHAPTER 53: ANTIEMETIC AND EMETIC MEDICATIONS AND ANTIHISTAMINES

Situation from Text

Situation 53-1

Edgar Randazzo, aged 50 years, is receiving chemotherapy for cancer of the stomach. To reduce the nausea and vomiting related to the treatment, various antiemetics are being tried.

1. Mr. Randazzo is to receive prochlorperazine (Compazine) 10 mg IM 30 minutes before the scheduled chemotherapy. Prior to administration, the nurse will check the:
   a. pupillary response
   *b. blood pressure
   c. complete blood count
   d. age of patient

   [NP: AS, CL: AP]

   Rationale: Due to potential for hypotension and orthostatic hypotension, the patient's blood pressure should be assessed prior to administration of phenothiazines.

2. While Mr. Randazzo is on procholorperazine therapy, the nurse will provide the following intervention:
   a. restrict oral fluids
   b. encourage large meals
   *c. frequent oral care
   d. provide distractions

   [NP: IM, CL: AP]

   Rationale: An adverse side effect related to therapy with phenothiazines, such as prochlorperazine, is dry mouth. The nurse should provide frequent oral care to increase comfort.

3. The nurse will monitor Mr. Randazzo for side effects of prochlorperazine, which include:
   a. urinary frequency
   b. alopecia
   *c. blurred vision
   d. insomnia

   [NP: IM, CL: CO]

   Rationale: Many of the side effects related to prochlorperazine therapy involve neurological effects such as blurred vision and sedation.

4. For discharge home, Mr. Randazzo is given a prescription for diphenidol (Vontrol) po 50 mg q 4 hours prn nausea/vomiting. The nurse will instruct him about the following side effect related to this drug:
   *a. auditory hallucinations
   b. diarrhea
   c. abdominal pain
   d. photosensitivity

   [NP: IM, CL: AP]

   Rationale: Auditory and visual hallucinations have been reported with the use of diphenidol. The patient should report these side effects to the physician.

5. Which of the following statements by Mr. Randazzo indicates the need for further discharge teaching?
   a. "I should get up slowly from a lying position."
   *b. "It would be okay to have wine with my dinner."

c. "I should avoid drving a car while taking my medication."
d. "If I have difficulty voiding, I should call the doctor."

[NP: EV, CL: AN]

Rationale: Antiemetics may have an additive effect when taken with alcohol. Patients should be taught to avoid drinking alcohol when taking these medications.

6. When evaluating Mr. Randazzo for effectiveness of antiemetic therapy, the following outcome is important:
   a. mild hypotension
   b. central nervous system depression
   c. output greater than intake
   *d. acid-base balance

[NP: EV, CL: CO]

Rationale: Optimally patients on antiemetic therapy will not experience nausea or vomiting and will not demonstrate evidence of dehydration or acid-base imbalance.

<u>**Additional Situation Not Presented in Text**</u>

Yolanda Williams, age 2 years, is admitted to the emergency room by her parents after ingesting a poisonous substance.

1. Before giving Yolanda ipecac syrup, it will be <u>most</u> important for the nurse to assess:
   *a. exact substance ingested
   b. pulse rate and blood pressure
   c. degree of cooperativeness
   d. amount of substance ingested

[NP: AS, CL: AP]

Rationale: Before giving any emetic, the substance which was ingested must be known. Some agents, such as strong acid or alkali, can cause more damage if vomiting is induced.

2. The nurse administers ipecac syrup 15 cc po to Yolanda. In addition, the nurse will administer:
   a. a mild sedative
   b. an antacid
   *c. a glass of water
   d. 2 oz of milk

[NP: IM, CL: CO]

Rationale: At least 8 ounces of water should be administered along with ipecac syrup to increase volume in the stomach and facilitate vomiting.

3. An action by the nurse which may facilitate vomiting is:
   *a. bouncing the child
   b. rubbing the abdomen
   c. keeping the child supine
   d. preventing excessive movement

[NP: IM, CL: KN]

Rationale: The emetic effect can be enhanced by bouncing a child or walking an adult.

4. If Yolanda does not vomit within 20 to 30 minutes of a repeated dose of ipecac, the nurse will plan to:
   a. administer another emetic
   *b. prepare for gastric lavage

c. give additional oral fluids
d. start an IV

[NP: PL, CL: CO]

Rationale: If vomiting does not occur after the second dose of ipecac, the patient should be prepared for gastric lavage or given charcoal to absorb the ipecac. Ipecac may cause gastrointestinal bleeding if absorbed.

5. After Yolanda has a large emesis, the nurse will plan to:
   a. observe the child for one hour and discharge
   b. take vital signs and discharge with instructions
   *c. admit to the hospital for observation
   d. admit to the hospital for surgery

[NP: PL, CL: CO]

Rationale: Most patients who ingest poisonous toxins should be hospitalized for at least 24 hours for observation.

6. The nurse will teach Yolanda's parents about the following precautions:
   a. Give ipecac syrup if petroleum distillates are ingested.
   b. Utilize "universal antidotes" whenever possible.
   *c. Do not induce vomiting if child is unresponsive.
   d. Call the poison control center after giving ipecac syrup.

[NP: IM, CL: AP]

Rationale: There is increased risk of aspiration if vomiting is induced in patients with significant central nervous system depression or an absent gag reflex.

<u>Review Questions from Text</u>

1. As a group of drugs, antiemetics:
   a. are best administered after vomiting occurs
   *b. act either locally or centrally
   c. treat rather than prevent vomiting
   d. cause local irritation of gastric mucosa

[CL: KN]

Ratonale: Antiemetics act locally or centrally to relieve nausea and vomiting. They are used to prevent nausea and vomiting rather than to treat the cause.

2. An extrapyramidal side effect which may occur with administration of high doses of phenothiazine drugs is:
   *a. spasms of the tongue, face, neck, and back
   b. drowsiness
   c. nasal congestion
   d. rebound hypertension

[CL: CO]
Rationale: Extrapyramidal symptoms seen with high doses of phenothiazines include acute dystonia, which is characterized by spasms of the tongue, face, neck, and back.

3. Which of the following statements correctly describes scopolamine hydrobromide (Hyoscine)?
   a. It has a long duration of action.
   b. The drug is most effective for postoperative nausea.
   c. The drug can be used to treat urinary obstruction.
   *d. It produces blurred vision and a dry mouth.

[CL: KN]

Rationale: Scopolamine is an anticholinergic agent which is most effective in preventing motion sickness. Major side effects are blurred vision and dry mouth.

4. Antihistamines produce antiemetic effect by:
   a. enhancing the chemoreceptor trigger zone
   b. stimulating the vestibular portion of the eighth cranial nerve
   c. inhibiting local gastric irritation and secretions
   *d. reducing stimulation on the vomiting center

   [CL: KN]

   Rationale: Antihistamines inhibit the transmission of impulses along the vestibular portion of the eighth cranial nerve. They also act on the vomiting center to reduce stimulation.

5. An example of an antidopaminergic antiemetic is:
   a. diphenhydramine (Benadryl)
   b. benzquinamide (Emete-Con)
   *c. promethazine (Phenergan)
   d. cyclizine (Marezine)

   [CL: KN]

   Rationale: Antidopaminergics work by reducing sensitivity to dopamine stimulation in the chemoreceptor trigger zone in the vomiting center. An example of such an agent is promethazine (Phenergan).

6. Side effects related to phenothiazine use include akathisia, which is characterized by:
   a. expressionless face
   b. hysterical reaction seizures
   *c. a need to be in constant motion
   d. forgetfulness about current events

   [CL: KN]

   Rationale: Akathisia refers to motor restlessness and anxiety. Patients may pace back and forth or have continuous nonpurposeful movement of an extremity.

7. A nursing implication associated with the use of the Transderm-Scop system is:
   a. Apply the patch indefinitely for control of nausea.
   b. Place patch on the chest wall for best results.
   c. Apply after the antiemetic effect is needed.
   *d. Teach about the side effect of drowsiness.

   [CL: CO]

   Rationale: Patients using the Transderm-Scop system need to be cautioned about drowsiness, a common adverse effect. Patients using the patch should not operate heavy equipment.

8. In general, antiemetics are contraindicated in the following patient situation:
   a. glaucoma
   *b. pregnancy
   c. gastric ulcers
   d. metastatic cancer

   [CL: KN]

   Ratoinale: Due to possible teratogenic effects, antiemetics are contraindicated during pregnancy.

9. An example of a cannabinoid antiemetic is:
   *a. dronabinol (Marinol)

b. fluphenazine (Protixin)
c. diphenidol (Vontrol)
d. dimenhydrinate (Dramamine)

[CL: KN]

Rationale: Dronabinol (Marinol) is a cannabinoid which has the principal psychoactive substance found in cannabis sativa (marijuana). This controlled substance is indicated for persons receiving chemotherapy who have not responded to other antiemetics.

Additional Review Questions Not Presented in Text

1. Patients scheduled to receive buclizine hydrochloride should be assessed for an allergy to:
   a. acetaminophen
   *b. tartrazine
   c. iodine
   d. penicillin

   [CL: KN]

   Rationale: Buclizine contains tartrazine, which can cause an allergic reaction in persons sensitive to it.

2. An example of a locally acting antiemetic is:
   a. triflupromazine (Vesprin)
   *b. phosphorylated carbohydrate (Emetrol)
   c. meclizine (Bonine)
   d. nabilone (Cesamet)

   [CL: KN]

   Rationale: Phosphorylated carbohydrate solution (Emetrol) is a locally acting protective agent which relaxes gastrointestinal muscle spasms. This prevents as many afferent impulses from reaching the vomiting center.

3. When giving benzquinamide (Emete-Con) intravenously, the nurse should watch the patient closely for:
   a. vertigo
   b. depressed respirations
   c. hypotension
   *d. increased blood pressure

   [CL: KN]

   Rationale: When giving benzquinamide IV, adverse effects which may be seen include hypertension and transient dysrhythmias.

4. A nursing implication associated with apomorphine hydrochloride administration is:
   a. reverse effects with thorazine intramuscularly
   b. observe for restlessness and insomnia
   *c. observe for respiratory depression
   d. give by intravenous bolus

   [CL: CO]

   Rationale: Apomorphine hydrochloride is a mild narcotic which causes sedation and may depress the respiratory center.

CHAPTER 54: MEDICATIONS FOR COMMON DIGESTIVE PROBLEMS (DIGESTANTS AND INTESTINAL PREPARATIONS)

Situation from Text

Situation 54-1

Ida Vinnett is a 70-year-old who has been cared for in a nursing home since a massive stroke two years earlier.

1. According to the nurse's notes, Ms. Vinnett has not had a stool in four days. Prior to giving her a laxative, the nurse will check for evidence of:
   a. confusion
   *b. fecal impaction
   c. anxiety
   d. urinary incontinence

   [NP: AS, CL: AP]

   Rationale: Laxatives are contraindicated if there is evidence of abdominal obstruction or if the patient has a fecal impaction.

2. Ms. Vinnett is to receive bisacodyl (Dulcolax) orally. It is best to administer this drug with:
   *a. water
   b. milk
   c. an antacid
   d. food

   [NP: IM, CL: KN]

   Rationale: Bisacodyl is best taken with water. It should not be taken with an alkaline solution such as milk or an antacid because theenteric coating dissolves in the stomach, where the medication can cause severe cramping.

3. After bowel evacuation, Ms. Vinnett is to begin taking psyllium hydrophilic mucilloid (Metamucil) daily. The nurse will include the following intervention in her plan of care:
   *a. Administer at least 8 oz of fluid with medication.
   b. Mix medication with evening meal.
   c. Add all of the patient's medications to the Metamucil.
   d. Discontinue Metamucil if no bowel movement noted in four hours.

   [NP: IM, CL: AP]

   Rationale: Metamucil should be administered in juice or fluid and followed with at least 8 ounces of fluid to prevent intestinal impaction or obstruction.

4. Metamucil should be given with caution if Ms. Vinnett has:
   a. arthritis
   b. glaucoma
   c. hepatic dysfunction
   *d. diabetes mellitus

   [NP: IM, CL: AP]

   Rationale: Metamucil contains sugar, which can affect the blood glucose level in patients with diabetes mellitus.

5. The nurse will expect to see results of Metamucil:
   a. after one week
   *b. within 1 to 3 days
   c. after 2 weeks

d. within 12 hous

[NP: PL, CL: KN]

Rationale: Bulk-producing agents may take from 1 to 3 days to be effective.

6. Ms. Vinnett is to receive magnesium hydroxide (Milk of Magnesia) prn every evening. The nurse will assess for evidence of renal disease because this agent contains a high concentration of:
 a. purine
 b. iron
 c. potassium
 *d. sodium

[NP: AS, CL: AP]

Rationale: Because of its high concentration of sodium, magnesium hydroxide should be given cautiously to patients with renal disease.

Additional Situation Not Presented in Text

Spencer Suarez is a 62-year-old who is in the recovery phase after acute pancreatitis. He has just begun taking soft foods and is being cared for on the medical unit.

1. Mr. Suarez is to receive pancrelipase (Cotazym) 2 tabs orally with each meal. Prior to beginning this medication, the nurse will assess for the following allergy:
 a. iodine
 *b. pork protein
 c. beef protein
 d. penicillin

[NP: AS, CL: KN]

Rationale: Pancrelipase is contraindicated in patients who are allergic to pork protein.

2. The nurse will plan the following intervention for Mr. Suarez while on pancrelipase therapy:
 a. Give an antacid along with the drug at meals.
 *b. Hold milk products within 1 hour of taking the drug.
 c. Have patient chew capsules thoroughly.
 d. Give one tablet between meals.

[NP: PL, CL: CO]

Rationale: Patients should not take milk products or antacids within an hour of taking pancrelipase.

3. The nurse will encourage Mr. Suarez to eat the following diet while on pancrelipase:
 a. low protein and low fat
 b. high carbohydrate and high calorie
 *c. balanced fat, carbohydrate, and protein
 d. high fat and protein

[NP: IM, CL: KN]

Rationale: It is important for patients on pancreatic enzymes to eat a well-balanced diet, including protein, carbohydrates, and fats. A well-balanced diet helps to alleviate indigestion.

4. When evaluating Mr. Suarez's response to pancreatic therapy, evidence of the following indicates a need to alter the medication:
 *a. steatorrhea
 b. flatulence

c. abdominal cramping
d. excessive burping

[NP: EV, CL: AP]

Rationale: Steatorrhea (fatty stool) is an important finding in patients on pancreatic enzymes. If fatty stools are noted, the dosage of pancrelipase may need to be adjusted.

5. Mr. Suarez develops diarrhea secondary to antibiotic therapy. He is to receive diphenoxylate hydrochloride (Lomotil) 2 tabs orally prn each diarrhea stool. The following effect is related to this therapy:
 a. anxiety
 b. bradycardia
 *c. drowsiness
 d. urinary retention

[NP: AN, CL: KN]

Rationale: Diphenoxylate can cause sedation. Patients should avoid tasks which require alertness.

6. A nursing intervention which should be included in Mr. Suarez's care plan would be:
 a. Restrict oral fluids.
 b. Monitor for hypotension
 c. Keep NPO if evidence diarrhea.
 *d. Check bowel sounds every shift.

[NP: IM, CL: CO]

Rationale: Diphenoxylate can contribute to the development of paralytic ileus; therefore, the nurse should check bowel sounds at least every shift.

<u>**Review Questions from Text**</u>

1. The pancreatic replacement enzyme pancrelipase (Cotazym) is utilized in the following patient situation:
 a. pernicious anemia
 b. post gallbladder surgery
 *c. cystic fibrosis
 d. hypochlorhydria

[CL: KN]

Rationale: Pancrelipase is used for symptomatic treatment of malabsorption syndromes such as cystic fibrosis.

2. A nursing intervention associated with the administration of antidiarrheal absorbents is to:
 *a. hold other medications for 2 hours after administration
 b. give absorbents at least 3 times daily for soothing effect
 c. discontinue if a fruity odor is apparent in the stool
 d. administer absorbents sparingly due to risk of addiction

[CL: KN]

Rationale: Absorbents have a tendency to bind with drugs given concurrently, thereby inhibiting their absorption. It is best to separate absorbents and routine medications by at least 2 hours.

3. Which of the following statements is correct regarding diphenoxylate hydrochloride (Lomotil)?
 a. It should be given to patients with infectious diarrhea.
 b. The drug is used to control antibiotic-induced pseudomembranous colitis.
 c. Lomotil is classified as a class III drug.
 *d. It contains atropine, causing dry mouth and blurred vision.

[CL: KN]

Rationale: Lomotil contains a small amount of atropine, which can cause side effects such as dry mouth, blurred vision, nausea, and vomiting.

4. The primary agent in paregoric tincture which acts as an anti-diarrheal is:
   a. meperidine
   b. atropine
   *c. morphine
   d. belladonna

]CL: KN]

Rationale: Paregoric tincture contains 2 mg morphine per 5 ml and 45 percent alcohol. Morphine is very effective in treating diarrhea, but is not commonly used.

5. The intestinal flora modifiers such as lactobacillus acidophilus (Lactinex) have the following action:
   a. destroy diarrhea-producing bacteria in the gut
   *b. encourage the growth of normal intestinal flora
   c. build a protective layer of mucous along the gut wall
   d. replace antibiotics in treating certain causes of diarrhea

[CL: CO]

Rationale: Patients on antibiotic therapy often have diarrhea because the normal bacterial flora of the intestine are destroyed. Lactinex encourages the growth of normal intestinal flora and reduces gastrointestinal complications associated with antibiotic therapy.

6. The belladonna preparation Donnagel is contraindicated in the following condition:
   a. diabetes mellitus
   b. Parkinson's disease
   c. peptic ulcer disease
   *d. narrow-angle glaucoma

[CL: KN]

Rationale: Donnagel contains atropine and hyoscyamine sulfate. These medications are contraindicated inpatients with narrow-angle glaucoma.

7. Which of the following statements regarding castor oil is correct?
   a. It stimulates gastric emptying
   *b. This laxative inhibits water reabsorption from the intestinal lumen.
   c. Castor oil should be taken with meals for a cathartic effect.
   d. It is the drug of choice for patients with ulcerative colitis.

[CL: KN]

Rationale: Castor oil is a contact/stimulant laxative which directly stimulates small intestine smooth muscle and inhibits water and electrolyte reabsorption from the intestinal lumen.

8. Patients taking cascara sagrada with milk of magnesia should be alert to the following side effect:
   a. foul smelling urine
   b. fruity odor to the breath
   c. oily skin
   *d. reddish or yellow-brown urine

[CL: CO]

Rationale: Patients taking cascara may notice a change in urine color. The drug may tint acid urine a yellow-brown or alkaline urine a reddish color.

9. Which of the following agents stimulates Auerbach's Plexus to induce peristalsis?

*a. senna
b. calcium polycarbophil
c. loperamide
d. docusate calcium

[CL: KN]

Rationale: Senna, an anthraquinone derivative, is converted to active aglycones in the colon. The aglycones stimulate Auerbach's Plexus to induce peristalsis and bowel evacuation.

Additional Review Questions Not Presented in Text

1. The agent found in over-the-counter products such as Ex-Lax and Feen-A-Mint is:
   a. senna
   *b. phenolphthalein
   c. castor oil
   d. belladonna

   [CL: KN]

   Rationale: Phenolphthalein, a contact/stimulant laxative, is similar to bisacodyl in action. Because of its pleasant taste, it is used in products such as Ex-Lax and Feen-A-Mint.

2. The belladonna products are associated with the following action(s):
   *a. preventing spasms and cramping associated with diarrhea
   b. decreasing gastric and small bowel motility
   c. stimulating mucus secretion and protecting bowel lining
   d. depressing the opiate receptors which regulate intestinal motility

   [CL: KN]

   Rationale: Belladonna alkaloids prevent spasms and cramping which frequently accompany diarrhea. There is no evidence that this class of drugs actually exerts a selective effect on the bowel to control diarrhea.

3. Bulk-forming laxatives:
   a. produce harmful nutritional side effects
   *b. expand as water is absorbed into the fecal contents
   c. empty both the large and small intestines
   d. interfere with Vitamin A absorption

   [CL: CO]

   Rationale: Bulk-forming laxatives absorb water into the fecal contents and expand, adding bulk to the stool. The increased bulk stimulates peristalsis of the large intestine rather than the whole bowel.

4. Osmotic laxatives are associated with the following effect:
   a. has a long action time
   b. ruptures egg capsules of parasites
   *c. produces a liquid stool which cleanses the bowel
   d. causes a catharsis with an isotonic saline solution

   [CL: CO]

   Rationale: Osmotic laxatives are rapid acting and hypertonic, producing a liquid stool by diffusion of fluid into the bowel. They are often used to cleanse the bowel for diagnostic tests or to flush poisons or remove parasites.

CHAPTER 55: MEDICATIONS UTILIZED IN HEPATIC AND BILIARY DISEASE

Situation from Text

Situation 55-1

Albert Shinn is a 56-year-old with alcoholic cirrhosis. He is admitted to the telemetry unit for care. Mr. Shinn is lethargic and confused. His abdomen is distended and firm; pitting edema is noted of the lower extremities.

1. A nasogastric tube is inserted, and Mr. Shinn is to receive lactulose (Cephulac) via n/g tube every 4 hours. The nurse will anticipate the following effect of this drug:
   a. nausea and vomiting
   *b. frequent stools
   c. tremors and muscle spasms
   d. skin rash

   [NP: PL, CL: CO]

   Rationale: Lactulose is a synthetic derivative of the sugar lactose and is a nonosmotic cathartic which induces evacuation of the bowel.

2. When evaluating Mr. Shinn for the effectiveness of lactulose therapy, the nurse will check the following:
   a. complete blood count
   b. total serum protein
   *c. ammonia levels
   d. stools for occult blood

   [NP: EV, CL: AP]

   Rationale: The action of lactulose in the bowel is the conversion of ammonia to ammonium for evaluation in the stool. The reduction in the ammonia level alleviates some of the symptoms associated with hepatic failure.

3. Mr. Shinn is scheduled to receive neomycin for short-term management of acute cirrhosis. The nurse will expect to administer this medication via:
   a. subcutaneous injection
   b. intravenous administration
   c. intramuscular injection
   *d. nasogastric tube

   [NP: PL, CL: CO]

   Rationale: When treating hepatic encephalopathy, neomycin is given only orally or via the nasogastric tube. This agent acts directly in the colon to reduce the breakdown products of urea and protein. Only a very small percentage of neomycin is absorbed systemically.

4. While Mr. Shinn is on neomycin therapy, the nurse will check the daily lab work for elevation of:
   a. amylase
   *b. creatinine
   c. white blood cells
   d. T_3, T_4

   [NP: AS, CL: AP]

   Rationale: Patients with normal renal function excrete the small amount of meomycin which is absorbed systemically. If renal impairment is present, the drug may accumulate and cause further renal damage.

5. The nurse notes alteration in skin integrity related to the pruritus associated with hepatic dysfunction. Mr. Shinn is started on cholestyramine (Questran) via nasogastric tube. The nurse will anticipate reduced pruritus

within:
*a. 1 to 3 weeks
b. 2 to 4 days
c. 24 hours
d. 5 days

[NP: PL, CL: KN]

Rationale: The therapeutic effect of cholestyramine is not usually noted until 1 to 3 weeks after initiation of therapy.

6. During the acute phase of hepatic encephalopathy, the nurse will plan to eliminate the following from Mr. Shinn's diet:
*a. protein
b. sodium
c. potassium
d. fats

[NP: PL, CL: CO]

Rationale: The breakdown of protein further increases the buildup of urea and ammonia during the acute stage of encephalopathy. Protein is slowly added to the diet as the patient recovers.

Additional Situation Not Presented in Text

Grace Guisti is a 38-year-old healthcare worker in an active emergency room. She is scheduled to receive the hepatitis B vaccine (Heptavax B).

1. When assessing Ms. Guisti for contraindications to Heptavax B administration, the nurse will report evidence of:
a. peptic ulcer disease
b. immunosuppression
c. history of arthritis
*d. yeast allergy

[NP: AS, CL: AP]

Rationale: A hypersensitive reaction may occur in patients who are allergic to yeast, which is used to produce the recombinant vaccine.

2. The nurse will administer the vaccine via intramuscular injection into which of the following sites?
a. vastis lateralis
b. gluteus
*c. deltoid
d. ventral gluteal

[NP: IM, CL: KN]

Rationale: The preferred site for intramuscular injection of Heptavax B is the deltoid muscle in the adult.

3. The nurse will teach Ms. Guisti about possible adverse effects related to Heptavax B, which include:
a. cough
*b. low-grade fever
c. hallucinations
d. seizures

[NP: IM, CL: CO]

Rationale: A low-grade fever is common following the injection. The fever occurs during the first 48 hours.

4. The nurse will plan the following dosage schedule for Ms. Giusti:

*a. 3 injections--initial dose followed by additional doses at one and six months
b. 2 injections--six months apart
c. 3 injections--initial dose followed by additional doses at three and six months
d. 2 injections--one month apart followed by a booster yearly

[NP: PL, CL: CO]

Rationale: The Heptavax B is given in three doses. The initial dose is followed by additional doses at one and six months.

5. The best criterion for evaluating Ms. Giusti for success of the Heptavax B vaccine is:
a. absence of active disease
*b. presence of serum anti-HB
c. presence of serum HB antigens
d. elevation of IGM antibodies

[NP: EV, CL: KN]

Rationale: After completion of Heptavax B vaccine, the patient should be assessed for the presence of serum anti-HB to determine if the patient has immunity. Another dose may be necessary for adequate immunity.

6. Which of the following statements by Ms. Giusti indicates the need for further patient teaching about Heptavax B?
a. "I may notice some pain and redness at the injection site."
b. "It is very important to stay on schedule for the Heptavax injections."
c. "This injection does not protect me against Hepatitis A."
*d. "I could get the AIDS virus from this vaccine."

[NP: EV, CL: AN]

Rationale: The AIDS virus is not transmitted. However, the AIDS antibodies are transmitted, but are usually absent after 6 months.

Review Questions from Text

1. The antidotal therapy for acetaminophen overdose is:
a. naloxone (Narcan)
b. protamine sulfate
c. Vitamin K
*d. N-acetylcystein (Mucomyst)

[CL: KN]

Rationale: Mucomyst provides glutathione to the liver cells, preventing cell damage from the build-up of acetaminophen metabolites.

2. Which of the following drugs is an aldosterone antagonist, useful in the management of ascites?
*a. spironolactone (Aldactone)
b. furosemide (Lasix)
c. acetazolamide (Diamox)
d. ethacrynic acid (Edecrin)

[CL: KN]

Rationale: In hepatic disease, ascites develops because of several factors, one of which is increased aldosterone production. Fluid retention is further increased due to decreased aldosterone metabolism in the liver. Spironolactone (Aldactone) is an aldosterone antagonist which produces a helpful diuresis.

3. Symptoms related to Phase I of hepatic encephalopathy include:

a. coma and asterixis
b. stupor and abnormal sleep pattern
*c. agitation and personality change
d. lethargy and asterixis

[CL: KN]

Rationale: The symptoms related to Phase I of hepatic encephalopathy are personality changes, agitation, vacant stare, and difficulty performing calculations.

4. A side effect of Heptovax B (hepatitis B vaccine) is:
*a. pain and soreness at injection site
b. fever that may reach 103 degrees F
c. bleeding tendency
d. generalized pruritus

[CL: KN]

Rationale: The most common adverse effect of Heptavax B is pain and soreness at the injection site.

5. Which of the following agents improves protein tolerance in patients with advanced hepatic cirrhosis?
a. Vitamin K
b. furosemide (Lasix)
*c. lactulose (Cephulac)
d. folic acid

[CL: CO]

Rationale: Lactulose is effective in reducing ammonia levels in patients with encephalopathy and improving protein tolerance in patients with advanced cirrhosis.

Additional Review Questions Not Presented in Text

1. A major constituent of gallstones is:
a. potassium phosphate
b. sodium chloride
*c. cholesterol
d. iron

[CL: KN]

Rationale: The three substances which usually precipitate to form gallstones are cholesterol, calcium salt of bilirubin, and calcium carbonate.

2. Which of the following is correct regarding monoctanoin?
a. It is a naturally occurring bile salt.
*b. This agent is only effective when in contact with a gallstone.
c. Monoctanoin should be administered for at least 9 months.
d. It inhibits the intestinal absorption of bile salts.

[CL: KN]

Rationale: Monoctanoin is a semisynthetic esterified glycerol which is used to break down gallstones. It is only effective when in contact with the stone.

3. Adverse effects associated with chenodiol (Chenodeoxycholic acid) include:
a. muscle tremors
b. photosensitivity
*c. diarrhea

d. urinary retention

[CL: KN]

Rationale: Diarrhea is the most common side effect of chenodiol. Hepatatoxicity is also a possible effect resulting from the breakdown of chenodiol.

CHAPTER 56: ENTERAL AND PARENTERAL AGENTS

Review Questions from Text

1. Which of the following statements is correct regarding the process of metabolism?
   a. Anabolism is the breaking down of complex cellular materials.
   b. Catabolism is the synthesis of cellular materials for growth.
   *c. If food intake exceeds metabolic demands, anabolism occurs.
   d. If food intake is less than metabolic demands, weight is gained.

   [CL: KN]

   Rationale: Anabolism is the synthesis of cellular elements for the process of cellular growth, maintenance, and tissue repair. When food intake exceeds metabolic demands, anabolism occurs and weight gain results.

2. The hormone which favors catabolism is:
   a. insulin
   *b. epinephrine
   c. growth hormone
   d. testosterone

   [CL: KN]

   Rationale: Epinephrine acts to mobilize substrates to provide energy, resulting in catabolism. The action of epinephrine results in inhibition of protein and carbohydrate synthesis.

3. When nutrients are not supplied to the body in adequate amounts, the following process occurs:
   a. Glycogen stores are used last as the liver acts to increase blood glucose.
   *b. Fats are broken down to form fatty acids and ketone bodies.
   c. Visceral proteins are the major substrate for protein anabolism.
   d. As urinary nitrogen increases, a positive nitrogen balance develops.

   [CL: KN]

   Rationale: When nutrients are not supplied to the body in adequate amounts, as in starvation, the body begins to break down fats to fatty acids and ketone bodies for energy in order to spare protein.

4. The milk-based meal replacement formulas are:
   *a. used in patients with an intact digestive system
   b. low in protein and high in carbohydrate
   c. nutritionally incomplete but high in minerals
   d. used in patients with lactose intolerance

   [CL: CO]

   Rationale: Meal replacement formulas which are milk-based are nutritionally complete and used in patients with an intact digestive system. They are high in lactose and should not be used for patients who are lactose intolerant.

5. A general principle concerning the administration of commercial feeding formulas is that:
   a. hypo-osmolar formulas have a tendency to cause diarrhea
   b. protein content is 50 percent of the total calories
   *c. fats increase calories without increasing osmolarity
   d. most formulas provide 20 calories per ml when fixed full strength

   [CL: KN]

   Rationale: The fat content in most commercial formulas can be up to 47 percent of the total calories. Fats increase the calorie content without increasing osmolarity.

6. Parenteral fat emulsions (PFE) are contraindicated in patients with:
   a. peptic ulcer disease
   b. acute renal failure
   c. muscle wasting disease
   *d. acute pancreatitis

   [CL: KN]

   Rationale: PFE administration is contraindicated for patients with disturbances in fat metabolism, such as patients with acute pancreatitis associated with hyperlipemia.

7. During initial administration of a lipid emulsion, the nurse performs the following intervention:
   a. administers the emulsion at the rate 10 ml/minute for first 30 minutes
   *b. observes for signs of an allergic reaction
   c. uses an in-line filter for IV administration
   d. observes for tissue necrosis at administration site

   [CL: KN]

   Rationale: Adverse reactions to intravenous lipid emulsion can include allergic reactions, such as chills, fever, diaphoresis, chest pain, or back pain. Initial administration should begin at 1 ml/minute for the first 15 to 30 minutes.

8. When assessing the patient receiving enteral or parenteral feedings, the nurse is aware that:
   *a. thirst may be a sign of dehydration from hyperosmolar enteral feedings
   b. light, flaky, reddened skin may indicate impending hyperosmolar shock
   c. patients with food allergies can tolerate enteral feedings without reactions
   d. hyperosmolar-induced edema occurs as a result of fluid overload

   [CL: KN]

   Rationale: Thirst is one of the first signs of impending dehydration from administration of hyperosmolar enteral formulas.

9. A possible cause of respiratory distress during administration of continuous tube feeding is:
   a. the feeding tube may be in the duodenum
   b. the patient is allergic to the tube feeding formula
   *c. a distended stomach interferes with diaphragmatic excursion
   d. a small bore feeding tube may impede ventilations

   [CL: CO]

   Rationale: When tube feeding is administered too rapidly, the distended stomach may be pushed up against the diaphragm and interfere with adequate chest expansion. This may result in respiratory distress.

10. A nursing intervention for patients receiving central TPN would be to:
   *a. initiate the solution slowly at a rate of 40 ml/hour
   b. change the TPN solution every 48 hours
   c. change the TPN IV tubing every 48 hours
   d. hang Ringer's lactate if TPN is interrupted

   [CL: KN]

   Rationale: A TPN solution should be initiated slowly, usually at a rate of 40 to 50 ml/hour and increased over a 24-hour period to the desired rate. This allows for the body to adjust to utilization of the TPN products.

Additional Review Questions Not Presented in Text

1. A central total parenteral nutrition (TPN):

a. is a hypotonic solution
b. always contains vitamins and trace elements
*c. provides a nitrogen-to-calorie ratio of 1:150 to 1:200
d. contains 850 fat calories per liter

[CL: KN]

Rationale: Central TPN is hypertonic and has a nitrogen-to-calorie ratio of 1:150 to 1:200. Vitamins and minerals are added as needed to the TPN.

2. When evaluating the patient receiving parenteral nutrition, the following lab data must be checked routinely:
*a. liver enzymes
b. T_3, T_4 levels
c. urinary amylase
d. creatinine clearance

[CL: CO]

Rationale: Patients may demonstrate hepatic dysfunction due to TPN substrate intolerance. Hepatic dysfunction is assessed by routine liver enzyme studies.

3. Which of the following is a sign/symptom of a catabolic state?
a. decreased temperature
*b. tissue edema
c. decreased respirations
d. elastic skin turgor

[CL: KN]

Rationale: Tissue edema, increased body temperature, poor skin turgor, and increased respirations are all signs of a catabolic state.

4. Important information to teach families of patients who will receive tube feedings at home includes:
a. storing tube feeding at room temperature
b. giving 100 cc of feeding over a 15-minute period
c. stopping tube feeding if greater than 3 stools per day
*d. placing patient in a sitting position for feeding

[CL: CO]

Rationale: To reduce the risk of aspiration, the family and patient should be taught to administer tube feeding in an upright position.

5. When administering parenteral fat emulsion, the nurse knows to:
a. shake the bottle vigorously to disperse fat globules
b. discard any unused portion after 24 hours
c. store the emulsion in the refrigerator
*d. discard the solution if oil separation has occurred

[CL: KN]

Rationale: The lipid emulsion should not be used if there is evidence that the oil has separated out or if there is an inconsistent texture or color.

CHAPTER 57: VITAMINS AND MINERALS

Review Questions from Text

1. Which of the following minerals is considered to be a macro element (bulk essential)?
   a. iron
   b. zinc
   *c. calcium
   d. fluorine

   [CL: KN]

   Rationale: Five minerals are considered to be essential for maintaining health and are needed by the body daily. These are calcium, magnesium, sodium, potassium, and phosphorus.

2. A mineral has the following characteristic:
   a. All are electropositive.
   b. All are organic and non-essential.
   c. They are carried by hormones.
   *d. They act on target organs.

   [CL: KN]

   Rationale: Minerals are naturally occurring nonorganic solid substances which are carried via the blood to target organs.

3. An example of a fat soluble vitamin is:
   a. biotin
   b. niacin
   *c. Vitamin K
   d. Vitamin B_{12}

   [CL: KN]

   Rationale: Four fat-soluble vitamins are utilized by the body. They include Vitamins A, D, E, and K.

4. Toxic side effects of Vitamin K include:
   a. insomnia
   *b. alopecia
   c. tetany
   d. decreased intracranial pressure

   [CL: KN]

   Rationale: Toxic side effects of Vitamin A are numerous. Alopecia, skin changes, hepatic dysfunction, and diplopia have been reported.

5. Vitamin D is used in the treatment of:
   a. hypercalcemia
   *b. hypocalcemia
   c. hyperparathyroidism
   d. hypomagnesemia

   [CL: KN]

   Rationale: Vitamin D increases the absorption of calcium in the gut and the reabsorption of phosphorus by the renal tubules. This vitamin is used in the treatment of hypocalcemia.

6. A role of Vitamin E in the maintenance of a healthy state includes:

*a. inhibition of hemolysis of red blood cells
b. enhances Vitamin K utilization
c. stimulates prostaglandin production
d. inhibits steroid metabolism

[CL: CO]

Rationale: Vitamin E appears to retard the hemolysis of red blood cells and has been found to be therapeutic in the management of certain anemias.

7. The proper rate for intravenous administration of phytonadione (Aquamephyton) is:
   a. 15 mg/10 minutes
   b. 5 mg/1 minute
   *c. 1 mg/minute
   d. 10 mg/2 minutes

[CL: KN]

Rationale: Aquamephyton is a derivative identical to Vitamin K_1. It should be given slowly by intravenous administration, not to exceed 1 mg/minute. Severe reactions have been reported as the result of rapid IV infusion.

8. Which of the following groups of patients are most likely to develop thiamine deficiency?
   a. newborns
   b. teenagers
   c. pregnant women
   *d. alcoholics

[CL: KN]

Rationale: Alcoholics are most likely to develop thiamine deficiencies due to inadequate dietary intake during periods of heavy drinking.

9. Which of the following statements is <u>correct</u> regarding drug interactions with Vitamin B6 (pyridoxine)?
   *a. B_6 enhances the peripheral metabolism of levodopa.
   b. B_6 inhibits hepatic metabolism of phenobarbital.
   c. Isoniazid decreases the urinary excretion of B6.
   d. Penicillamine decreases the urinary excretion of B6.

[CL: KN]

Rationale: Pyridoxine enhances the peripheral metabolism of levodopa when taken in doses of greater than 5 mg daily. When Vitamin B_6 and levodopa are taken concurrently, the dosage of levodopa may need to be increased.

10. Which of the following drugs is associated with elevated copper levels?
   a. nitroglycerin agents
   *b. estrogens
   c. prostaglandins
   d. antibiotics

[CL: KN]

Rationale: Elevated copper levels may be produced by estrogen compounds, thyroid, or corticotropin.

Additional Review Questions Not Presented in Text

1. A food which should be included in the diet of patients with zinc deficiency is:
   a. oranges
   b. margarine
   *c. cheese

d. spinach

[CL: KN]

Rationale: Zinc can be found in all cheeses, organ meats, sunflower seeds, wheat germ, and yeast.

2. Which of the following statements is correct regarding Vitamin C?
   a. It is an endogenous water-soluble vitamin.
   b. Vitamin C produces an alkaline urine when taken in high doses.
   *c. Vitamin C is necessary for utilization of folic acid.
   d. Smoking cigarettes decreases the daily requirements for Vitamin C.

[CL: CO]

Rationale: Vitamin C is necessary for the conversion of folic acid to folinic acid. Vitamin C cannot be synthesized by the body and must be supplied exogenously.

3. The nurse should be aware of the following factors when administering vitamins and minerals:
   a. Mineral oil should be avoided in all patients taking the B vitamins.
   *b. Intravenous solutions with multivitamins added should be protected from light.
   c. Vitamin D is best given on an empty stomach to enhance absorption.
   d. The dosage of Vitamin K is determined by Ptt levels.

[CL: CO]

Rationale: Vitamin mixtures are light sensitive; therefore, IV solutions containing vitamins should be covered to prevent degradation of vitamin products.

4. Manganese is a mineral which:
   a. is well absorbed from the gastrointestinal tract
   *b. activates several important enzymes
   c. affects the sensitivity of tissues to insulin
   d. is excreted in the urine

[CL: KN]

Rationale: Manganese is considered an essential mineral because it is an activator of several enzymes, including liver argenase and serum alkaline phosphatase.

5. Vitamin C should be avoided in patients who are taking:
   *a. anticoagulants
   b. calcium agents
   c. penicillin antibiotics
   d. birth control pills

[CL: KN]

Rationale: Vitamin C may interfere with the therapeutic effects of anticoagulants such as heparin and warfarin.

CHAPTER 58: MAJOR BODY ELECTROLYTES

Review Questions from Text

1. Sodium (Na^+) acts in the body to:
   a. inhibit electrical impulses within the cell
   *b. maintain serum osmolarity
   c. maintain muscle contraction
   d. regulate intracellular osmolality

   [CL: KN]

   Rationale: As the major cation in the extracellular fluid, sodium maintains osmotic pressure and serum osmolarity.

2. Administration of potassium is contraindicated for patients taking the following medication:
   a. aspirin
   *b. spironolactone
   c. lithium
   d. tetracycline

   [CL: KN]

   Rationale: Potassium products should not be given concurrently with potassium-sparing diuretics, such as spironolactone.

3. A sign or symptom of hypokalemia is:
   *a. muscle weakness
   b. increased reflexes
   c. loud heart sounds
   d. ST elevation on the ECG

   [CL: KN]

   Rationale: Skeletal muscle weakness is a common symptom of hypokalemia. In addition, patients may exhibit decreased reflexes and ST depression on the ECG.

4. A nursing intervention associated with administration of sodium polystyrene sulfonate (Kayexalate) is to:
   a. observe the patient for hyponatremia.
   b. allow suspension to separate; do not stir
   *c. urge patient to retain rectally for 30 to 60 minutes
   d. mix powder with an oil base solution

   [CL: KN]

   Rationale: This suspension lowers potassium by exchanging it with sodium in the intestine. When administering agent rectally, the patient should retain the enema for 30 to 60 minutes for optimal action.

5. When administering intravenous or oral calcium products, the nurse will monitor the patient for hypercalcemia. A sign of this would be:
   a. tetany
   b. Trousseau's sign
   c. Chvostek's sign
   *d. lethargy

   [CL: KN]

   Rationale: Signs/symptoms associated with ypocalcemia include drowsiness and lethargy due to neurological hypofunction.

6. Intravenous magnesium administration is contraindicated in the following patient situation:
   *a. heart block
   b. ventricular tachycardia
   c. pregnancy
   d. constipation

   [CL: KN]

   Rationale: Magnesium slows conduction in the heart; therefore, intravenous administration is contraindicated in patients with heart block.

7. In an acidotic state, the following serum electrolyte level occurs:
   a. hypomagnesemia
   b. decreased calcium
   c. decreased potassium
   *d. increased calcium

   [CL: CO]

   Rationale: In acidosis there is more ionized or free calcium, and serum calcium levels increase.

8. Patients taking oral calcium should be taught to:
   a. decrease intake of phosphate-containing foods
   b. take calcium chloride with meals
   *c. avoid taking calcium with tetracycline antibiotics
   d. increase intake of spinach, rhubarb, and bran

   [CL: KN]

   Rationale: Calcium products bind with tetracycline and inhibits absorption. Patients should avoid taking calcium with tetracycline antibiotics.

9. An important action associated with phosphate (HPO_4^-) is:
   a. stabilization of neuromuscular function
   b. regulation of acid-base balance through chloride shift
   c. maintenance of resting membrane potential
   *d. promotion of the phagocytic action of white blood cells

   [CL: KN]

   Rationale: Phosphate promotes the phagocytic action of white blood cells as well as supplying essential metabolic processes, such as ATP production.

10. A patient with an electrolyte imbalance demonstrates a high peaked T wave on the ECG. Which electrolyte imbalance does this sign indicate?
   *a. hyperkalemia
   b. hyponatremia
   c. hypophosphatemia
   d. hypermagnesemia

   [CL: CO]

   Rationale: Hyperkalemia, potassium excess, can produce high peaked T waves on the ECG.

Additional Review Questions Not Presented in Text

1. While administering potassium products, the nurse will monitor the patient for:
   a. depression
   *b. changes in heart rate

c. itching
d. constipation

[CL: KN]

Rationale: Patients receiving potassium chloride or any potassium product should be monitored closely for changes in heart rate and rhythm.

2. When assessing patients for hypomagnesemia, the nurse will look for the following sign/symptom:
 a. hypertension
 b. bradycardia
 *c. facial twitching
 d. hypoactive reflexes

[CL: KN]

Rationale: The assessment findings of hypomagnesemia are related to neuromuscular irritability and include hyperactive reflexes, tetany, and facial twitching.

3. Patient teaching for potassium products should stress:
 a. taking two doses at a time if one dose is missed
 b. using salt substitutes ad lib
 *c. continuing potassium for as long as on diuretics
 d. chewing potassium thoroughly before swallowing

4. Which of the following foods has the highest potassium content?
 a. 1 medium banana
 b. 2 to 3 medium apricots
 c. 1 medium orange
 *d. 1/2 cup dried peaches

[CL: KN]

Rationale: Dried peaches contain 28 mEq of potassium per 1/2 cup.

5. A nursing responsibility related to intravenous calcium administration is to:
 *a. monitor infusion to avoid infiltration
 b. monitor the ECG for peaked P waves
 c. mix calcium products with bicarbonate
 d. draw a calcium level immediately after infusion

[CL: KN]

Rationale: When administering calcium preapration intravenously, the nurse should monitor the infusion to avoid infiltration. Calcium preparations cause tissue irritation with potential necrosis.

CHAPTER 59: OVERVIEW OF ANATOMY AND PHYSIOLOGY OF THE EYE AND EAR

Review Questions from Text

1. A structure of the middle layer of the eye is the:
   *a. ciliary body
   b. cornea
   c. sclera
   d. retina

   [CL: KN]

   Rationale: The vascular middle layer of the eye is composed of the ciliary body, iris, and choroid.

2. The inner layer of the eye is composed of:
   a. diaphragm with a circular opening
   b. muscles which increase visual circular opening
   *c. nerve cells that translate light waves to neural impulses
   d. a thick, opaque posterior covering which adjusts to light

   [CL: KN]

   Rationale: The retina, inner layer of the eye, is composed of several layers of nerve cells which translate light waves into neural impulses which are then transmitted via the optic nerve to the brain.

3. Which of the following statements is <u>correct</u> regarding the fovea centralis?
   a. It contains rods which allow for color vision.
   *b. Cones are densely concentrated in the fovea.
   c. The fovea is the area of the eye which adjusts to dim light.
   d. The fovea is composed of nerve cells which are motion detectors.

   [CL: KN]

   Rationale: The fovea centralis is composed of cone cells and is the portion of the retina where visual acuity is the greatest.

4. The refractory mechanism occurs through which <u>correct</u> sequence to focus light rays on the retina?
   a. lens, cornea, vitreous humor, aqueous humor
   b. aqueous humor, cornea, vitreous humor, lens
   *c. cornea, aqueous humor, lens, vitreous humor
   d. cornea, vitreous humor, lens, aqueous humor

   [CL: CO]

   Rationale: The image enters the eye through the cornea and aqueous humor. It is then transmitted through the lens and the vitreous humor to the retina.

5. In myopia, the image focuses:
   a. on the peripheral portion of the retina
   *b. in front of the retina
   c. at a point behind the retina
   d. on the macula area of the retina

   [CL: KN]

   Rationale: Myopia is the inability to see distant objects. In this condition, the image focuses in front of the retina.

6. Which of the following statements correctly describes the accommodation reflex?
   a. It protects the cornea from damage by turning the eye upward when forcibly opened.
   b. Accommodation causes the pupil to become smaller when light is flashed into the eye.
   *d. It allows the pupil to become smaller as the gaze shifts from a close to a distant object.

   [CL: KN]

   Rationale: The accommodation reflex allows the pupil to become smaller when the gaze shifts from a distant to a close object. This allows us to see printed material as well as large or distant objects.

7. The vestibule is a portion of the:
   a. ossicles of the ear
   b. outer ear
   c. middle ear
   *d. inner ear

   [CL: KN]

   Rationale: The vestibule is a portion of the inner ear that is involved with changes in posture and balance.

8. Hearing impulses originate in the:
   a. malleus
   *b. organ of Corti
   c. semicircular canals
   d. incus

   [CL: CO]

   Rationale: The cochlea is stimulated by sound vibrations and the cilia of the organ of Corti send impulses to the brain via the acoustic nerve.

9. The function of the external ear is to:
   a. separate the middle and inner ear
   b. merge with the inner ear
   *c. funnel sound through the auditory canal
   d. convert sound waves into vibrations

   [CL: CO]

   Rationale: The function of the inner ear, which is composed of the auricle and meatus, is to funnel sound through the auditory canal to the middle and inner ear.

10. Normal intraocular pressure is:
   *a. 12 to 25 mmHg
   b. 50 to 60 mmHg
   c. 2 to 10 mmHg
   d. 30 to 46 mmHg

   [CL: KN]

   Rationale: Normally, intraocular pressure is maintained at 12 to 25 mmHg. In conditions such as glaucoma, the intraocular pressure rises to 60 mmHg or more.

Additional Review Questions Not Presented in Text

1. Which of the following statements is correct regarding the aqueous humor?
   a. It is found in the posterior chamber of the eye.
   b. Aqueous humor is continually produced by the choroid plexus.
   c. It furnishes nutritional support to the iris and retina.
   *d. Aqueous humor maintains intraocular pressure in the eye.

[CL: KN]

Rationale: Aqueous humor fills the anterior chamber and is produced by the ciliary body. It maintains the shape of the chamber and helps to regulate intraocular pressure.

2. Eye movement is controlled by the:
 a. third, fourth, and fifth optic nerves
 b. second, third, and fourth cranial neves
 *c. third, fouth, and sixth cranial nerves
 d. first, third, and fifth optic nerves

[CL: KN]

Rationale: Eye movement is controlled by the oculomotor (tihrd), trochlear (fourth), and abducens (sixth) cranial nerves.

3. Impulses from the medial half of the right eye:
 *a. cross to the left occipital lobe
 b. travel to the right occipital lobe
 c. cross to the left parietal lobe
 d. travel to the right parietal lobe

[CL: CO]

Rationale: In the optic chaism, impulses from the medial half of the eye cross to the opposite side of the brain, to either the right or left occipital lobe.

4. The function of the eustachian tube is to:
 a. direct sound waves into the inner ear
 *b. equalize air pressure in the middle ear
 c. secrete lubrication for the auditory canal
 d. vibrate against the tympanic membrane

[CL: KN]

Rationale: The eustachian tube connects the middle ear with the nasopharynx. It serves to equalize air pressure within the middle ear.

CHAPTER 60: MEDICATIONS USED IN EYE DISORDERS

Situation from Text

Situation 60-1

Inis Cave is a 76-year-old recently diagnosed with open-angle glaucoma. She is being treated at a university eye center.

1. Ms. Cave is to begin treatment with pilocarpine .25% 2 gtts every 6 hours. The nurse will caution her about the most common side effects of this drug, which are:
   a. pruritis and weakness
   b. sweating and fever
   c. anxiety and tremors
   *d. burning and itching

   [NP: IM, CL: KN]

   Rationale: Adverse ophthalmic effects of pilocarpine which are most commonly reported are burning and itching.

2. When assessing Ms. Cave after administration of pilocarpine, the nurse will anticipate the following:
   a. asymmetrically shaped pupils
   *b. constricted pupils
   c. dilated pupils
   d. increased accommodation

   [NP: AS, CL: CO]

   Ratonale: Pilocarpine is a direct-acting cholinergic which will cause pupil constriction.

3. The nurse will teach Ms. Cave about taking eye drops at home. The following information will be included:
   a. A stinging sensation indicates that the drug is working.
   *b. Visual acuity will be reduced in dim light.
   c. Dryness of the mouth and throat is related to pilocarpine.
   d. Eyelids should be massaged after administration.

   [NP: IM, CL: KN]

   Rationale: Patients using pilocarpine will experience reduced visual acuity in dim light as a result of the miotic action on pupils and cilliary muscles.

4. After a month of therapy on pilocarpine, Ms. Cave is to switch to timolol maleate (Timoptic) .25% 1 gtt BID. Prior to administration of this agent, the nurse will check for a history of:
   a. peripheral neuropathy
   b. iodine allergy
   *c. asthma
   d. peptic ulcers

   [NP: AS, CL: AP]

   Rationale: Timolol is a non-cardioselective $beta_1$- and $beta_2$-blocker. Therefore, patients with bronchial asthma or COPD should not receive this agent.

5. The nurse will teach Ms. Cave the following schedule for beginning timolol therapy:
   a. Discontinue pilocarpine for three days, then begin timolol.
   b. Continue both agents for one week, then gradually stop pilocarpine.
   c. Continue pilocarpine and timolol for three days, then stop pilocarpine.
   *d. Discontinue pilocarpine on the second day of timolol therapy.

[NP: PL, CL: CO]

Rationale: When necessary to switch from one antiglaucoma agent to timolol, discontinue the first agent (pilocarpine) on the second day of timolol therapy.

6. The nurse will monitor Ms. Cave for the following in relation to timolol therapy:
   *a. blood pressure
   b. level of consciousness
   c. reflexes
   d. potassium level

   [NP: IM, CL: CO]

   Rationale: A side effect of timolol therapy is hypotension; therefore, the blood pressure should be monitored during initial therapy.

Additional Situation Not Presented in Text

Henry Rosenblum is a 40-year-old who presents to the eye clinic with complaints of severe eye irritation and redness.

1. Tetracaine hydrochloride is instilled in each eye in order to examine Mr. Rosenblum. The nurse will warn him of the following effect:
   a. itching
   b. warm, flushed face
   *c. stinging
   d. temporary blindness

   [NP: PL, CL: AP]

   Rationale: A temporary side effect of tetracaine is stinging or burning of the eyes.

2. A diagnosis of conjunctivitis is made, and cultures are obtained. Mr. Rosenblum is to administer neomycin sulfate (Myciguent) ointment 4 times per day. It will be important for the nurse to determine if he has a history of:
   a. glaucoma
   b. thromobphlebitis
   *c. allergic reactions
   d. drug abuse

   [NP: AS, CL: CO]

   Rationale: Before administration with neomycin sulfate, a thorough history is important in order to determine previous allergic reactions. Allergic reactions to neomycin are frequently reported.

3. The nurse will teach Mr. Rosenblum to administer the ointment at home. The following information is appropriate:
   a. Do not remove any extra ointment from the eye.
   b. Keep the ointment chilled in the refrigerator at all times.
   c. Place the ointment on the upper eyelid and blink repeatedly.
   *d. Discard the first 1/4 inch of a new tube of ointment before using.

   [NP: IM, CL: AP]

   Rationale: The first 1/4 inch of the tube of ophthalmic ointment should be discarded as it may be too dry.

4. In order to reduce the possibility of systemic effects related to neomycin, the nurse will instruct Mr. Rosenblum to:
   a. use the drug only at night

b. rinse the eye with water after instilling ointment
*c. press inside corner of eye for 1 to 2 minutes
d. place a warm moist towel over closed eyes

[NP: IM, CL: CO]

Rationale: Applying pressure to the lacrimal sac for 1 to 2 minutes following administration reduces systemic absorption of the ophthalmic agent.

5. When evaluating Mr. Rosenblum for possible systemic effects of neomycin, the nurse will note the following lab value:
*a. creatinine
b. hematocrit
c. T_3, T_4 levels
d. calcium

[NP: EV, CL: AN]

Rationale: Systemic effects of neomycin include nephrotoxicity as evidenced by increasing creatinine levels.

6. Which of the following statements by Mr. Rosenblum indicates the need for further patient teaching?
a. "My vision may be blurred after instilling the ointment."
*b. "It is best to heat the ointment before using."
c. "I should avoid driving or operating machinery after use."
d. "After instilling the ointment, I should close my eyes for 1 to 2 minutes."

[NP: EV, CL: AP]

Rationale: By warming the ointment in the hand for a few minutes, the ointment can be instilled more easily. Excessive heat would damage the eye tisue.

Review Questions from Text

1. Fluorescein sodium can be used in the eye to:
a. fit soft contacts
*b. test lacrimal patency
c. remove foreign bodies from the eye
d. stain the eye for 60 minutes

[CL:KN]

Rationale: Fluorescein sodium, a nontoxic water-soluble dye, stains denuded areas of the epithelium of the eye. The preparation can be used to test lacrimal patency, demonstrated by the appearance of dye in nasal secretions.

2. The antiviral medication idoxuridine (IDU) is administered:
*a. for 5 to 7 days after healing has occurred
b. concurrently with boric acid solution
c. in a liquid form only
d. systemically to treat herpes simplex virus

[CL: KN]

Rationale: Idoxuridine should be administered for 5 to 7 days after healing has occurred in order to prevent a recurrence of herpes.

3. Anti-infammatory eye medications, such as dexamethasone, are used primarily for:
a. treatment of fungal infections
b. management of acute infections
c. long-term treatment of glaucoma
*d. reduction of permanent scarring

[CL: KN]

Rationale: Anti-inflammatory medications are used to treat some nonpyrogenic inflammatory conditions of the eye. Their action reduces inflammation and permanent scarring.

4. The direct-acting cholinergic miotics reduce intraocular pressure by:
   a. relaxing the sphincter muscle of the iris
   b. inhibiting ciliary muscle spasm
   c. reducing production of aqueous humor
   *d. decreasing resistance to outflow of aqueous humor

   [CL: CO]

   Rationale: The direct-acting cholinergic miotics reduce intraocular pressure by constricting the pupil, causing spasms of the ciliary muscle, and decreasing the resistance to outflow of aqueous humor.

5. When teaching the patient about insertion of Ocusert (pilocarpine), the following information will be included:
   a. Insert early in the morning initially.
   *b. Gently rinse with tap water prior to insertion.
   c. Continue using eye insert if irritation occurs.
   d. Leave insert in place for 14 days.

   [CL: KN]

   Rationale: Ocusert is an eye insert which releases pilocarpine slowly into the eye for a period of about 1 week. The insert should be rinsed gently with tap water prior to insertion to prevent a large initial release of pilocarpine.

6. Which of the following agents are cholinesterase inhibitors used to treat open-angle glaucoma?
   a. methazolamie (Neptazane)
   b. carbachol (Isopto Carbachol)
   *c. physostigmine (Eserine)
   d. betaxolol (Betoptic)

   [CL: KN]

   Rationale: Physostigmine is a cholinesterase inhibitor which inhibits cholinesterase and enhances the effect of endogenous acetylcholine on the eye.

7. Caution is advised when administering beta-adrenergic blockers, such as timolol maleate (Timoptic), with the following medication:
   a. potassium chloride
   *b. digoxin
   c. aspirin
   d. iodine

   [CL: CO]

   Rationale: Concurrent use of beta blocker ophthalmic agents with digitalis products may have an additive slowing effect on the cardiac conduction system.

8. Acetazolamide (Diamox) is used to treat glaucomas due to which of the following actions?
   a. production of systemic alkalosis
   *b. interference with production of carbonic acid
   c. production of osmotic diuresis
   d. direct contraction of ciliary muscles

   [CL: CO]

   Rationale: Acetazolamide is a carbonic anhydrase inhibitor which interferes with production of carbonic acid.

This leads to systemic acidosis and reduced aqueous humor formation.

9. Alpha adrenergic ophthalmic agents have the following effect on the eye:
   a. contraction of the constrictor muscle of the iris
   b. complete relaxation of the ciliary muscle
   *c. contraction of the dilator muscle of the iris
   d. inhibition of parasympathetic effects on the pupil

   [CL: KN]

   Rationale: Alpha adrenergic agents contract the dilator muscle of the iris, causing dilation of the pupil. These agents have only a slight effect on the ciliary muscle.

10. Osmotic diuretics used to treat eye disorders are used cautiously in the following patient condition:
   a. peptic ulcer disease
   b. increased intracranial pressure
   c. open-angle glaucoma
   *d. congestive heart failure

   [CL: KN]

   Rationale: Osmotic diuretics are used to treat glaucoma in patients resistant to the effects of miotics or carbonic anhydrase. Osmotic agents are given cautiously to patients with congestive heart failure because the heart may not be able to handle the larger fluid volume produced by the pulling of fluid from the tissues.

Additional Review Questions Not Presented in Text

1. Sytemic effects of the cycloplegic agent atropine (Atropisol) include:
   *a. dry mouth and tachycardia
   b. burning and itching with urination
   c. drowsiness and hypotension
   d. severe flushing and fever

   [CL: KN]

   Rationale: Systemic effects of atropine ophthalmic agents include the anticholinergic symptoms of dry mouth and tachycardia.

2. Epinephrine (Epifrin) is useful in treating:
   a. resistant inflammation
   b. accommodative esotropia
   c. acute eye infections
   *d. glaucoma

   [CL: KN]

   Rationale: Epinephrine is a catechloamine which decreases aqueous humor production and is useful in treating glaucoma.

3. The antibiotic chloramphenicol (Chloromycetin) should be used with caution due to the potential for:
   a. acute angle closure
   *b. aplastic anemia
   c. systemic lupus
   d. resistant bacterial strains

   [CL: KN]

   Rationale: Intravenous chloramphenicol can be used to treat serious eye infections. Its use should be limited, however, due to the risk of development of aplastic anemia.

4. The cholinesterase inhibitors are contraindicated for patients with:
   *a. iritis
   b. open-angle glaucoma
   c. convergent strabismus
   d. tacycardia

   [CL: CO]

   Rationale: The cholinesterase inhibitors are contraindicated when there is evidence of an inflammatory disease of the iris or ciliary body. These agents increase contraction of the ciliary muscle and may worsen the condition.

5. Patients who are at risk for developing cataracts are those who are taking:
   a. acetaminophen
   b. aspirin
   c. ibuprofen
   *d. nifedipine

   [CL: KN]

   Rationale: Drugs such as steroids and nifedipine (Procardia) are related to an increased risk of cataract formation. Analgesics protect against cataract formation.

CHAPTER 61: MEDICATIONS USED IN EAR DISORDERS

Review Questions from Text

1. A solution which can be used to irrigate the ears is:
   a. 10 percent acetic acid
   b. full strength hydrogen peroxide
   c. 50 percent ethyl alcohol
   *d. Burow's solution

   [CL: KN]

   Rationale: The most frequently used irrigating solution for the ears is Burow's solution (aluminum acetate solution).

2. Which of the following is considered a first line drug for treating otitis media?
   a. cefaclor
   *b. ampicillin
   c. erythromycin
   d. Bactrim

   [CL: KN]

   Rationale: First line drugs which are effective in treating otitis media are amoxicillin (Amoxil) and ampicillin (Polycillin).

3. Antihistamine-decongestant products are utilized along with antibiotics to treat acute otitis media. They work by:
   *a. improving eustachian tube patency
   b. resolving infectious process
   c. direct dilation of auditory canal
   d. stimulating ciliary movement in the midle ear

   [CL: KN]

   Rationale: Antihistamine-decongestants are thought to improve eustachian tube patency and enhance drainage from the middle ear.

4. When performing a nursing assessment on the patient requiring ear medications, the nurse is aware that:
   a. over-the-counter medications are free of ototoxic effects
   b. patients with renal dysfunction are less prone to ototoxicity
   *c. aminoglycoside antibiotics may damage the eighth cranial nerve
   d. vestibular damage causes loss of high-frequency sound perception

   [CL: KN]

   Rationale: Aminoglycoside antibiotics may damage the eighth cranial nerve, causing irreversible hearing loss.

5. The agent of choice for patients with otitis media resulting from Hemophilus influenzae is:
   a. Novafed
   b. penicillin V
   *c. ampicillin
   d. penicilin G

   [CL: KN]

   Rationale: Penicillin G and penicillin V are not effective against Hemophilus influenzae. The agent of choice is ampicillin.

Additional Review Questions Not Presented in Text

1. The nurse instructs patients and families on proper administration of ear medications, which includes:
   a. pulling the auricle downward and slightly in for the adult
   b. inserting cotton plugs after administration
   c. tipping the head toward the affected side before instillation
   *d. applying gentle pressure on the tragus after instillation

   [CL: KN]

   Rationale: To adminster ear drops properly, pull the auricle upward and back (for the adult). Press gently on the tragus after instillation to help move medication down into the canal.

2. "Swimmer's ear" is usually due to:
   a. gram positive organisms
   *b. gram negative organisms
   c. viral infections
   d. fungal infections

   [CL: KN]

   Rationale: Swimmer's ear is usually due to Pseudomonas acruginosa or other gram negative organisms.

3. Which of the following agents can be used to soften and remove cerumen deposits?
   a. Augmentin
   b. Ornade
   *c. Debrox
   d. Aerosporin

   [CL: KN]

   Rationale: Carbamide peroxide (Debrox) is a cerumenolytic agent which softens wax deposits and promotes normal removal.

CHAPTER 62: ENZYMES

Situation from Text

Situation 62-1

Stuart Ellsworth is a 78-year-old who is being cared for in a nursing home after several months of hospitalization for a massive CVA. He has a Stage IV sacral decubitus ulcer, 4 inches in diameter.

1. Decubitus wound care for Mr. Ellsworth includes the use of collagenase (Santyl) twice a day with sterile dressing changes. The nurse will monitor the patient within the first 24 hours for:
   a. hypotension
   *b. fever
   c. bradycardia
   d. reduced pulses

   [NP: AS, CL: CO]

   Rationale: During the first 24 hours of collagenase treatment, a fever may occur due to the accumulation of leukocytes at the wound site. This can be reduced by frequent aspiration of wound exudate.

2. The nurse will report the following persistent side effect of collagenase:
   a. pink moist skin
   b. development of granular tissue
   c. increased excudate
   *d. itching and stinging

   [NP: EV, CL: KN]

   Rationale: Itching and stinging often occur with initial therapy with topically administered enzymes. These symptoms should subside. If itching and stinging continue, the physician should be notified.

3. Prior to application of collagenase, the wound should be prepared by washing it with:
   a. soap and water
   *b. hydrogen peroxide
   c. Burow's solution
   d. Betadine solution

   [NP: IM, CL: AP]

   Rationale: Hydrogen peroxide is compatible with collagenase and can be used to prepare and clean the wound prior to application. The hydrogen peroxide should be followed by sterile normal saline.

4. The nurse will plan the following outcome for Mr. Ellsworth relative to collagenase therapy:
   *a. wound debridement
   b. elimination of infection
   c. repair of connective tissue
   d. elimination of granulocytes

   [NP: PL, CL: CO]

   Rationale: The purpose of collagenase is to debride wounds for promotion of healing. Collagenase has no antibacterial properties.

5. The nurse will implement the following intervention when applying collagenase:
   a. Keep the skin pH at 5.
   b. Apply to injured as well as healthy tissue.
   c. Put a silver based ointment around wound.
   *d. Apply to injured tissue only.

[NP: IM, CL: KN]

Rationale: Collagenase should be applied to injured tissue only, because it can cause erythema of healthy tissue. The surrounding tissue can be protected by an agent such as zinc oxide ointment.

6. Which of the following nursing diagnostic categories applies to Mr. Ellsworth in relation to collagenase therapy?
   a. Decreased Cardiac Output
   b. Sleep Pattern Disturbance
   c. Noncompliance
   *d. Potential for Injury: Bleeding

   [NP: AN, CL: AP]

   Rationale: Collagenase can induce bleeding and hemorrhage and should be used cautiously if evidence of hemorrhage exists.

<u>**Additional Situation Not Presented in Text**</u>

Annie Petitbon is a 48-year-old recovering from surgery for a ruptured gall bladder. She has an open surgical wound which is being packed with saline-soaked gauze sponges.

1. To aid wound healing, Ms. Petitbon is to receive papain (Papase) 2 tabs orally q.i.d. Prior to administering this agent, the nurse will note an allergy to:
   *a. papaya
   b. iodine
   c. pork
   d. beef

   [NP: AS, CL: KN]

   Rationale: Patients allergic to papaya may be sensitive to papain, which is derived from papaya.

2. The following lab value should be assessed before beginning papain therapy for Ms. Petitbon:
   a. calcium
   b. T_3, T_4 levels
   c. amylase
   *d. bleeding time

   [NP: AS, CL: AP]

   Rationale: Papain is contraindicated in patients with blood dyscrasia, as papain can prolong bleeding time.

3. Papain ointment 10% is also applied to the surgical wound. The nurse will avoid the following solution for irrigation:
   a. antiseptic soap
   b. normal saline
   *c. hydrogen peroxide
   d. sterile water

   [NP: PL, CL: CO]

   Rationale: Hydrogen peroxide should not be used to irrigate wounds which are treated with papain ointment, because it inactivates the enzymes.

4. When teaching Ms. Petitbon about taking papain tablets, the nurse will include the following information:
   a. Take tablets with an antacid to reduce gastric iritation.
   b. If a dose is missed, take a double dose to catch up.
   *c. Check with the physician before taking any other medication.
   d. Do not apply papain to healthy tissue.

[NP: IM, CL: CO]

Rationale: Drug reactions can occur with enzyme administration. The patient should check with the physician before taking another medication.

5. The nurse will monitor Ms. Petitbon for a neurological side effect of papain, such as:
   a. confusion
   b. neuropathy
   c. seizures
   *d. dizziness

   [NP: IM, CL: KN]

   Rationale: An adverse neurological effect of papain is dizziness.

6. Ms. Petitbon will need to be on oral papain for at least:
   a. 2 days
   b. 24 hours
   *c. 5 days
   d. 3 days

   [NP: PL, CL: KN]

   Rationale: Oral papain should be given 4 times a day for at least 5 days.

Review Questions from Text

1. As a class of drugs, enzymes are:
   a. given intravenously to aid digestion
   *b. synthesized proteins from plants or animals
   c. known to be immunologically neutral
   d. altered by the reactions which they mediate

   [CL: CO]

   Rationale: Enzymes are proteins which are synthesized from plant and animal sources. Enzymes are catalysts for chemical reactions, but are not altered by the reaction.

2. Which of the following statements is correct regarding sutilains (Travase) therapy?
   a. This enzyme is active on viable tissue.
   b. Airtight, dry dressings are applied after sutilains.
   *c. The skin pH should be kept at a range of 6.0 to 6.8.
   d. The medication is discontinued if no improvement in 7 days.

   [CL: KN]

   Rationale: Sutilains functions best in a pH range of 6.0 to 6.8. This proteolytic enzyme is inactive on viable tissue. Loose, wet dressings should be placed on wound after sutilains is applied.

3. In order to prepare the skin for sutilains (Travase) therapy, the following should be used:
   a. soap and water
   *b. isotonic saline
   c. hexachlorophene
   d. iodine

   [CL: KN]

   Rationale: The skin should be cleansed with water on isotonic saline prior to applying sutilains. The use of iodine, hexachlorophene, or detergents decreases the effectiveness of sutilains.

4. Prior to administration of fibrinolysin and deoxyribonuclease (Elase), the nurse will assess for the following allergy:
   a. papaya
   b. iodine
   c. pork
   *d. beef

   [CL: CO]

   Rationale: Elase is a proteolytic and fibronlytic enzyme derived from bovine sources. Patients allergic to beef may exhibit allergic reactions to this enzyme.

5. The nurse will include the following information when teaching the patient about enzyme replacement therapy:
   a. Enteric-coated tablets are to be chewed, then followed by water.
   *b. Mild stinging may occur when tablets are absorbed buccally.
   c. Bowel movements should increase while on digestive enzymes.
   d. Store enzyme tablets in the refrigerator.

   [CL: KN]

   Rationale: When digestive enzymes are absorbed buccally, mild stinging may occur. This is usually relieved by removing the tablet.

<u>**Additional Review Questions Not Presented in Text**</u>

1. The nurse will teach patients who are on pancreatin to avoid taking it with:
   a. caffeine
   b. a large amount of fluids
   c. meals
   *d. antacids

   [CL: KN]

   Rationale: Antacids negate the effects of pancreatin, and they should not be taken concurrently.

2. A side effect for which the nurse should monitor with regard to chymopapain intradiskal administration is:
   a. photosensitivity
   b. difficulty voiding
   *c. back pain
   d. drowsinss

   [CL: KN]

   Rationale: A common side effect of intradiskal administration of chymopapain is back pain, stiffness, and soreness. The back pain may continue for several days after administration.

3. A nursing responsibility in administering enzyme medications is to:
   a. reconstitute powdered drugs 2 hours before administration
   b. shake vigorously when mixing agent
   c. store reconstituted enzyme for no longer than 48 hours
   *d. before giving, perform a subcutaneous skin test

   [CL: CO]

   Rationale: Before enzymes are administered, skin testing should be performed by giving a small amount subcutaneously. If a wheal or signs of allergic reaction are noted, the enzyme should not be used.

4. Hyaluronidase (Wydase) is used to:
   a. facilitate medication absorption of intramuscular injections
   *b. reduce tissue sloughing due to vasoconstrictor intravenous infusions

c. treat patients with herniated lumbar intervertebral disks
d. increase intraocular pressure during ophthalmic surgery

[CL: KN]

Rationale: Hyaluronidase is amucolytic enzyme which has been shown to reduce sloughing of tissue, which can occur due to infiltration of vasopressor agents.

5. Which of the following enzyme agents is often utilized in cataract surgery?
*a. chymotrypsin
b. chymopapain
c. pancrelipase
d. papain

[CL: KN]

Rationale: Chymotrypsin is often used in cataract surgery. It is instilled into the eye prior to surgery to soften the lens for easier removal.

CHAPTER 63: MEDICATIONS FOR COMMON SKIN DISORDERS

Situation from Text

Situation 63-1

Joe Terranova is a 17-year-old with moderate to severe acne. He is evaluated in a dermatology clinic for treatment.

1. After washing with an antibacterial soap, Joe is to apply a topical anti-acne agent with benzoyl peroxide. The nurse will instruct him to:
   a. leave on skin for 6 hours initially
   b. apply to oily areas and cover with a dressing
   c. apply to entire face overnight
   *d. leave on for 15 minutes initially

   [NP: IM, CL: KN]

   Rationale: Benzoyl peroxide is applied to the skin and left on for 15 minutes on the first evening. The length of time which benzyol peroxide is left on the skin increases gradually until it can be left on overnight.

2. The nurse will caution Joe about overuse of the benzoyl peroxide cream, which is evidenced by:
   a. dizziness
   *b. dry, cracking skin
   c. increased acne
   d. nausea, vomiting

   [NP: IM, CL: AP]

   Rationale: Side effects of acne products, such as extreme dryness of skin, are increased with overuse of these products.

3. After one month of treatment with topical agents, Joe has not demonstrated improvement of acne. He is to begin treatment with tretinoin (Retin-A). The nurse will instruct Joe in the proper use of this product by teaching the following:
   a. Apply a thick layer of tretinoin three times a day.
   b. Expect therapeutic results after one week.
   *c. Keep the ointment away from eyes, mouth, and mucous membranes.
   d. Increase sun exposure to aid the healing process.

   [NP: IM, CL: KN]

   Rationale: After applying tretinoin to affected skin areas once a day, the hand should be washed thoroughly. Irritation will result if the agent is in contact with delicate mucous membranes.

4. The nurse will check Joe for the following effect of tretinoin:
   a. elimination of wrinkles
   b. permanent pigment changes
   c. oiliness of skin
   *d. peeling skin

   [NP: EV, CL: AP]

   Rationale: Within 48 hours, the skin generally becomes red and begins to peel. Pigment changes may occur, but these are temporary.

5. In addition, Joe is to begin therapy with isotretinoin (Accutane). The nurse will instruct him to:
   a. increase sun exposure
   *b. eliminate alcohol from diet

c. take for the rest of his life
d. take on an empty stomach

[NP: IM, CL: KN]

Rationale: Alcohol intake should be eliminated during therapy with isotretinoin because of potentiation of adverse effects.

6. When evaluating Joe for adverse effects of isotretinoin, the nurse will note the following:
*a. increased triglycerides
b. decreased cholesterol
c. increased HDL
d. decreased CPK

[NP: EV, CL: CO]

Rationale: Approximately one-fourth of patients on isotretinoin demonstrate elevated triglyceride levels with potential for increased cholesterol.

Additional Situation Not Presented in Text

Kim Wong is a 38-year-old who presents to the Emergency Department with second and third degree burns resulting from hot oil.

1. A first aid remedy which would not be employed for Ms. Wong would be to:
a. rinse clothing over burn in cold tap water
b. rinse wound in cold tap water
*c. apply butter or salve to area
d. remove clothing around wound

[NP: IM, CL: AP]

Rationale: First aid treatment for burns involves rinsing the burn with cold tap water. Clothing should be cooled with cold tap water and/or removed.

2. When evaluating Ms. Wong's skin burns, the following is characteristic of third degree burns:
a. pain
b. moist, thick-walled vesicles
c. erythema
*d. open thin-walled vesicles

[NP: AS, CL: KN]

Rationale: Third degree burns are characterized by thin-walled vesicles which are open. Pain is not usually associated with third degree burns because nerve endings are destroyed.

3. After rinsing the burn with sterile saline, mafenide (Sulfamylon) is applied with a sterile gloved hand. Because of this drug's systemic effect, the nurse will observe the patient for:
a. hallucinations
*b. labored breathing
c. hypotension
d. bradycardia

[NP: EV, CL: AP]

Rationale: Mafenide is a carbonic anhydrase inhibitor which may cause metabolic acidosis. Compensatory hypeventilation occurs to maintain a balanced pH. Should respiratory dysfunction occur, the cream should be removed.

4. Ms. Wong is transferred to the burn unit for continued care. The nurse will plan the following intervention:

a. Remove mafenide at night.
*b. Check skin for signs of super infection.
c. Discontinue if burning is noted when first applied.
d. Do not wash burn unless contaminated.

[NP: PL, CL: KN]

Rationale: The burned areas should be assessed frequently for evidence of super infections, such as foul purulent drainage.

5. The nurse will monitor Ms. Wong for potential hematological effects of mafenide, which include:
*a. bone marrow depression
b. polycythemia
c. early cyanosis
d. increased clotting time

[NP: IM, CL: AP]

Rationale: Adverse effects of mafenide include bone marrow depression and hemolytic anemia.

6. Ms. Wong's dressings are moistened with silver nitrate. Because of potential adverse effects of this agent, the following should be noted regularly:
*a. potassium and sodium levels
b. T_3, T_4 levels
c. calcium and phosphorus levels
d. magnesium and potassium levels

[NP: EV, CL: AP]

Rationale: Silver nitrate may precipitate fluid and electrolyte disturbances; therefore, sodium and potassium levels should be evaluated routinely.

Review Questions from Text

1. In addition to blood vessels and nerves, the dermis layer of the skin contains:
*a. collagen and elastin
b. keratinized tissue and keratohyalin granules
c. keratinocytes and prickle cells
d. adipose and loose connective tissue

[CL: KN]

Rationale: The second main layer of skin is the dermis, which contains collagen and elastin in addition to a network of nerves and capillaries.

2. Which of the following is correct regarding emollients?
a. The suspension requires shaking before application.
b. They have a drying effect on the skin when the water evaporates.
*c. Emollients have fixed oils as a base preparation.
d. They are predominantly water in base.

[CL: KN]

Rationale: Emollients have fixed oils, such as olive, flax-seed, or cottonseed, as a base and are used to treat dry, cracked skin.

3. A common side effect of acyclovir (Zovirax) is:
a. photosensitivity
b. hives
*c. mild pain

d. pigment changes

[CL: KN]

Rationale: Mild pain and transient buring are the major side effects of acyclovir.

4. When corticosteroids are used on the skin, they have the following action:
   a. fibrinolytic
   *b. vasoconstriction
   c. vasodilation
   d. proteolytic

[CL: KN]

Rationale: Corticosteroids have vasoconstrictive actions when used topically. In addition, they are anti-inflammatory and antipruritic.

5. The following information should be included for patients treated with dermatologic agents:
   a. A thick film or medication is applied over dry areas.
   b. Do not use soap and water on affected skin.
   c. A large amount of medication is applied to moist areas.
   *d. Any scales or crusts are removed before applying the medication.

[CL: CO]

Rationale: The area to be treated is cleansed well with soap and water. Any scales or crusts are removed before applying the medication.

6. When evaluating the effectiveness of skin medications, the following is important:
   a. Acute skin lesions should subside in 3 to 4 days.
   *b. Skin lesions are often slow to improve and require frequent evaluation.
   c. Noncompliance is a problem due to ineffectiveness of treatment.
   d. Lesions which do not show improvement in 24 hours need to be evaluated.

[CL: KN]

Rationale: Treatment of skin lesions may take considerable time. Some skin conditions are slow to heal and must be evaluated frequently, usually on a daily basis.

7. When a patient who is receiving medications for a skin disorder develops a reaction, the nurse will plan to:
   a. discontinue medications one at a time
   *b. obtain a complete medication history
   c. assume the rash is due to the current medication(s)
   d. continue all medications and document all nursing care

[CL: CO]

Rationale: Reactions to medications may occur up to a year after discontinuing; therefore, a complete medication history should be obtained. Generally, the patient is taken off all medications, if possible, to discover the problem.

Additional Review Questions Not Presented in Text

1. A serious dermatological reaction to medication is the Stevens-Johnson syndrome, which is characterized by:
   *a. erythema multiforme of the oral and anogenital mucosa
   b. seborrheic dermatitis of the scalp, face, and trunk
   c. open blisters in the folds of the skin
   d. systemic exfoliative dermatitis with dry lesions on trunk and arms

[CL: KN]

Rationale: Stevens-Johnson syndrome is a serious form of erythema multiforme involving the oral and anogenital mucosa.

2. When treating and assessing patients with pediculus (lice), the nurse is aware that:
   a. they are easy to treat
   b. cloth and paper gowns provide adequate protection
   *c. lymph nodes may be enlarged as a result of inflammation
   d. itching should ease as soon as lice are removed

   [CL: KN]

   Rationale: Lymph nodes may be enlarged as a result of inflammation due to lice. Itching may persist after the lice are dead if the skin is already irritated from scratching.

3. A common adverse effect of topical steroids is:
   *a. skin atrophy
   b. moist, weeping skin
   c. striae
   d. hyperpigmentation

   [CL: KN]

   Rationale: A common adverse effect of topical steroids is skin atrophy. This effect is often associated with potent topical corticosteroids.

4. Which of the following agents is efective in treating warts and molluscum contagiosum?
   a. benzoin
   b. permethium
   c. mafenide
   *d. cantharidin

   [CL: KN]

   Ratioale: Cantharidin is a keratolytic used for its exfoliation affect on epidermal cells only. It is used in treating warts and molluscum contagiosum.

5. Skin appendages include which of the following:
   a. prickle cells
   b. stratum germinativum
   c. papillary layer
   *d. fingernails

   [CL: KN]

   Rationale: Fingernails and toenails are skin appendages which are modifications of the keratinized layer of the epidermis.

CHAPTER 64: VACCINES AND IMMUNIZATIONS

Situation from Text

Situation 64-1

Evelyn Perez, aged 21 years, has given birth to a healthy baby girl named Alisa. Mrs. Perez is being cared for on the postpartum unit.

1. Mrs. Perez is to receive Rho(d) Immune Globulin. The nurse is aware that:
   *a. the mother is Rh negative and daughter Rh positive
   b. the daughter is Rh negative and the mother Rh positive
   c. the daughter is Rh negative and the mother Rh negative
   d. the mother is Rh positive and the daughter is Rh positive

   [NP: AN, CL: CO]

   Rationale: The Rho(D) Immune Globulin (RhoGAM) is used to suppress the immune response in nonsensitized Rh negative women who receive Rh positive blood, as in the case of delivering an Rh positive baby.

2. The nurse will plan to administer the RhoGAM injection within how many hours of delivery?
   a. 8
   *b. 72
   c. 48
   d. 12

   [NP: PL, CL: KN]

   Rationale: Administration of RhoGAM should be within 72 hours of delivery.

3. Mrs. Perez is concerned about when Alisa should begin immunizations. The nurse will explain that the earliest age for beginning immunization is:
   a. 12 days
   b. 1 year
   c. 4 months
   *d. 2 months

   [NP: IM, CL: KN]

   Rationale: The recommende schedule for childhood immunizations should begin at 2 months of age.

4. When Mrs. Perez brings Alisa in to the Well Baby Clinic for immunization, which of the following findings would contraindicate immunization at this time?
   a. anemia
   b. malnutrition
   *c. active infection
   d. slowed development

   [NP: AS, CL: AP]

   Rationale: Evidence of an active infection, such as a high fever, is a contraindication to immunization.

5. After Alisa receives the Diptheria and Tetanus Toxoid and Pertussis (DPT) vaccine, the nurse will teach Mrs. Perez about potential side effects, which include:
   a. mild arthralgia and lymphadenitis
   b. abdominal pain and tremors
   *c. anorexia and fretfulness
   d. paralysis and hypertension

[NP: IM, CL: AP]

Rationale: Common adverse effects related to DPT vaccine include anorexia and fretfulnss, in addition to redness and pain at the site of injection.

6. When Alisa is 15 months old, the nurse will plan to administer the following:
   a. DPT and DPV
   b. DPT and TB test
   *c. DPT, OPV, and MMR
   d. TB test and OPV

   [NP: PL, CL: KN]

   Rationale: It is recommended that children at age 15 months receive DPT, poliovirus, and measles, mumps, and rubella vaccines.

<u>**Additional Situation Not Presented in Text**</u>

Adrian Bacon is a 34-year-old who is planning a sojourn to Asia for a year of travel and photography. He presents to the County Health Department for appropriate immunizations.

1. Mr. Bacon will need to receive a typhoid vaccine. The nurse will plan to administer this vaccine by the following route:
   a. oral
   *b. subcutaneous
   c. intramuscular
   d. intravenous

   [NP: PL, CL: KN]

   Rationale: Typhoid vaccine is administered subcutaneously in doses of 0.5 ml to 0.1 ml for adults.

2. After Mr. Bacon receives a Cholera Vaccine, the nurse will teach him about possible side effects, which include:
   *a. malaise, low grade fever
   b. bradycardia
   c. hypotension
   d. hallucinations

   [NP: IM, CL: AP]

   Rationale: Frequent side effects associated with the Cholera Vaccine include malaise, low grade fever, flushing, pain, redness, and swelling at site.

3. The nurse will inform Mr. Bacon that immunity from the Cholera Vaccine will last approximately:
   *a. 3 to 6 months
   b. one year
   c. 2 years
   d. 10 years

   [NP: IM, CL: KN]

   Rationale: Immunity from the Cholera Vaccine is brief, lasting from 3 to 6 months. If exposure continues to be a risk, then a booster is recommended.

4. Mr. Bacon should receive a tetanus toxoid if he has not had one in the last:
   a. 6 months
   b. 5 years
   *c. 10 years
   d. 2 years

[NP: PL, CL: KN]

Rationale: Tetanus toxoid should be repeated for persons at risk every 10 years.

5. Just prior to departure, Mr. Bacon will receive Immune Globin because of exposure to areas with high risk. This provides passive immunity for:
   a. herpes zoster
   b. rabies
   c. hepatitis B
   *d. hepatitis A

   [NP: AN, CL: KN]

   Rationale: Immune Globin will provide passive immunity to hepatitis A exposure.

6. If continued risk is present, the nurse will advise Mr. Bacon to repeat the Immune Globin within:
   a. two years
   *b. three months
   c. eight months
   d. one year

   [NP: IM, CL: KN]

   Rationale: Immune Globin provides passive immunity for 6 weeks to several months.

<u>**Review Questions from Text**</u>

1. An advantage of passive immunity is that it:
   a. stimulates the body to produce antibodies
   *b. provides immediate protection
   c. persists for an extended period
   d. treats diseases effectively

   [CL: CO]

   Rationale: Passive immunity provides immediate protection, but does not last for an extended period of time. Its effectiveness in treating disease is limited.

2. An example of a toxoid vaccine is:
   a. polio
   b. smallpox
   *c. diptheria
   d. hepatitis A

   [CL: KN]

   Rationale: Diptheria is a toxoid vaccine in which detoxified but antigenically active poisons are administered. Toxoids provide an excellent immunity.

3. Children should not receive the attenuated measles vaccine before 15 months because:
   *a. maternal antibodies destroy the attenuated virus before antibody production occurs
   b. the child's immune system is too young to respond with antibody production
   c. the attenuated virus is too strong and will produce an active form of the disease
   d. antibodies which are produced by a child less than 15 months are immature

   [CL: CO]

   Rationale: Children younger than 15 months have passive immunity acquired from the mother. If immunized earlier than 15 months, the maternal antibodies will destroy the attenuated virus before the child's active immunity is stimulated.

4. Before administration of measles vaccine, the nurse should assess for an allergy to:
   a. iodine
   b. yeast
   c. penicillin
   *d. neomycin

   [CL: KN]

   Rationale: Neomycin is utilized in the production of the attenuated virus for the measles vaccine. Persons allergic to neomycin may react hypersensitively.

5. A nursing intervention associated with immunizations is to:
   a. teach patients that unusual side effects are to be expected
   b. mix vaccines at least 6 hours before administration
   *c. change the needle before injecting the vaccine
   d. keep vaccines in a dry warm place for storage

   [CL: KN]

   Rationale: By changing the needle after the vaccine has been withdrawn from the vial, local tissue reaction to the injection can be reduced.

6. The pathological organism responsible for chickenpox is:
   a. poliovirus III
   *b. varicella-zoster
   c. Bordetella
   d. Mycobacterium

   [CL: KN]

   Rationale: Varicella-zoster virus is the infective organism responsible for chickenpox.

7. What is the time required for development of active immunity in response to a vaccine?
   a. 6 months
   b. 6 hours
   *c. 5 to 14 days
   d. 25 to 75 days

   [CL: KN]

   Rationale: Active immunity may take from 5 to 14 days to develop after primary immunization.

8. The recommended time for Hemophilus influenza vaccine (Hib) is at:
   *a. 18 to 24 months
   b. 4 to 6 years
   c. 3 years
   d. 8 to 12 months

   [CL: KN]

   Rationale: The child who is high risk should be vaccinated for Hib if between the ages of 18 and 23 months. Otherwise, the initial vaccination should be given at 24 months.

9. Drug interactions associated with the Bacillus Calmette-Guerin (BCG) vaccine include:
   a. Immunosuppressive drugs enhance BCG response.
   b. BCG may inactivate aminoglycosides.
   *c. Active TB treatment drugs inactivate BCG.
   d. BCG facilitates theophylline excretion.

   [CL: KN]

Rationale: If active TB treatment drugs are given along with BCG, they will cause the vaccine to be ineffective.

Additional Review Questions Not Presented in Text

1. A possible serious adverse effect associated with pneumococcal vaccine (Polyvalent) is:
   a. lymphadenitis
   b. serum sickness
   c. Sudden Infant Death Syndrome
   *d. Guillain-Barre Syndrome

   [CL: KN]

   Rationale: Guillain-Barre Syndrome has been associated with patients receiving the pneumococcal vaccine or the hepatitis B vaccine.

2. Which of the following statements is correct regarding rabies immune globulin (RIB)?
   a. It is obtained from the plasma of hyperimmunized chicken donors.
   b. RIB should be administered 6 days after the rabies vaccine.
   *c. Half of the dose is administered into the wound, the other half intramuscularly.
   d. There are no known adverse effects associated with RIB.

   [CL: KN]

   Rationale: RIB is obtained from human donors. After a bite from an infected animal, half of the dose is given into the wound, while the other half is given intramuscularly.

3. The type of immunity which is achieved through mother to infant via breast milk is known as:
   a. passive immunity--artificially acquired
   *b. passive immunity--naturally acquired
   c. active immunity--naturally acquired
   d. active immunity--artificially acquired

   [CL: KN]

   Rationale: The mother transfers her antibodies to the infant via breast milk (or the placenta). This type of immunity is passive--naturally acquired.

4. Which of the following cells is responsible for producing antibodies in a sensitized host?
   a. macrophages
   b. T cells
   c. bursa cells
   *c. plasma cells

   [CL: KN]

   Rationale: When the plasma cells are stimulated to produce antibodies to a specific antigen, they will continue to do so for the lifetime of the cell.

CHAPTER 65: EMERGENCY SITUATIONS

Review Questions from Text

1. A nursing action for drug therapy in the acute care setting is to:
   a. administer drugs intramuscularly if the patient is hypotensive
   *b. administer drugs intravenously to patients with severe cardiac failure
   c. monitor cholesterol levels because many acidic drugs are bound to fat
   d. give drugs such as protamine sulfate over 2 minutes intravenously

   [CL: CO]

   Rationale: The intravenous route for medications is preferable for the patient with heart failure.

2. Drugs which may be given endotracheally in an emergency situation include:
   *a. epinephrine
   b. bretylium
   c. sodium bicarbonate
   d. dopamine

   [CL: KN]

   Rationale: If an IV access is not available, drugs such as epinephrine, atropine, and lidocaine can be administered endotracheally.

3. Which of the following emergency drugs is contraindicated in congestive heart failure?
   *a. beta blockers
   b. cardiac glycosides
   c. diuretics
   d. vasodilators

   [CL: CO]

   Rationale: Beta blockers block sympathetic response to increased fluid volume, worsening congestive heart failure.

4. Patients in pulmonary edema will demonstrate the following sign/symptom:
   a. thick, yellow sputum
   b. abdominal pain
   *c. severe dyspnea
   d. poor skin turgor

   [CL: KN]

   Ratoinale: Assessment findings related to pulmonary edema are severe dyspnea, pink frothy sputum, rales, hypertension, and tachycardia.

5. The following agent may be ordered for the patient in cardiogenic shock:
   a. propranolol
   *b. dobutamine
   c. atropine
   d. sodium bicarbonate

   [CL: KN]

   Rationale: Dobutamin (Dobutrex) is a positive inotropic agent which improves cardiac output and performance.

6. The drug of choice for the patient exhibiting status epilepticus is:
   *a. diazepam

b. epinephrine
c. propranolol
d. furosemide

[CL: KN]

Rationale: For the control of seizures in status epilepticus, diazepam (Valium) should be given slowly intravenously.

7. The patient with elevated T_3, T_4, and T_7 values with symptoms such as fever, tachycardia, tremor, and restlessness should receive the following agent:
a. diazepam
b. phenobarbital
*c. propylthiouracil
d. paraldehyde

[CL: KN]

Rationale: The patient is exhibiting signs and symptoms of thyroid storm. Propylthiouracil is a drug which can be used in this situation because it blocks the release of thyroid hormone.

8. In any emergency situation, the nurse's first priority is to:
*a. maintain a patent airway
b. take blood pressure and pulse
c. assist with placement of a central line
d. assess orientation

[CL: CO]

Rationale: A patent airway must be maintained and is a top priority for the nurse in an emergency situation.

9. A nursing assessment finding in the patient experiencing acute adrenal insufficiency is:
a. hypertension
b. Kussmaul respirations
c. pink, frothy sputum
*d. dehydration

[CL: KN]

Rationale: Patients in acute adrenal insufficiency exhibit signs of dehydration, hypotension, weakness, and abdominal pain.

10. The drug of choice in the event of cholinergic crisis is:
a. lidocaine
b. epinephrine
*c. atropine
d. digitalis

[CL: KN]

Rationale: Atropine sulfate produces an anticholinegic response to block release of acetylcholine and improve the patient's condition.

Additional Review Questions Not Presented in Text

1. A patient receiving an intravenous dose of naloxone (Narcan) too rapidly may experience:
*a. nausea and vomiting
b. dry skin and bradycardia
c. hypotension and insomnia

d. ventricular dysrhythmias and apnea

[CL: KN]

Rationale: Patients who receive naloxone too rapidly (IV) may experience nausea, vomiting, sweating, and/or tachycardia.

2. When administering nitroglycerine intravenously for unstable angina, the nurse will watch for the following side effect:
   a. hypertension
   *b. headache
   c. restlessness
   d. sedation

   [CL: KN]

   Rationale: Headache, hypotension, and flushing are common side effects associated with intravenous nitroglycerine.

3. The physician orders a "renal dose" dopamine infusion for the patient in cardiogenic shock. Which of the following ranges is appropriate:
   a. 15 to 20 mcg/kg/minute
   b. 0.5 to 1.5 mcg/kg/minute
   *c. 2 to 5 mcg/kg/minute
   d. 10 to 15 mcg/kg/minute

   [CL: CO]

   Rationale: In the range of 2 to 5 mcg/kg/minute, dopaminergic receptors are stimulated by dopamine. This increases glomerular filtration rate and urine output.

4. An example of a Group I drug which may cause liver damage in healthy individuals is:
   a. morphine
   *b. acetaminophen
   c. prednisone
   d. phenylbutazone

   [CL: KN]

   Rationale: Acetaminophen (Tylenol) is an example of a Group I drug which should not be used in patients with liver disease.

5. Assessment findings in patients in insulin shock include:
   *a. diaphoresis and headache
   b. anxiety and acetone odor to breath
   c. flushed dry skin and Kussmaul respirations
   d. dehydration and hypothermia

   [CL: KN]

   Rationale: Signs and symptoms related to insulin shock include diaphoresis, weakness, nervousness, headache, and unconciousness.

CHAPTER 66: MISCELLANEOUS AND ORPHAN DRUGS

Review Questions from Text

1. A nursing intervention associated with administration of dimercaprol (Bal in Oil) is to:
   a. maintain patient in supine position
   b. keep patient awake
   c. avoid excessive hydration
   *d. maintain urine alkalinization

   [CL: KN]

   Rationale: Dimercaprol is the antidote for arsenic, gold, and/or mercury toxicity by promoting urinary excretion. In order to protect the kidneys, the urine is kept alkaline.

2. The use of sclerosing agents such as sodium tetradecyl sulfate (Sotradecol) and morrhuate sodium is contraindicated in patients with:
   a. hyperparathyroidism
   *b. asthma
   c. myasthenia gravis
   d. G-6PD deficiency

   [CL: KN]

   Rationale: Sotradecol and morrhuate can cause asthmatic symptoms as an adverse effect; therefore, they are contraindicated in patients with the disease.

3. Patient teaching related to nicotine gum (Nicorette) includes the following information:
   a. Continue Nicorette gum for 6 months before tapering.
   b. Smoking cigarettes along with Nicorette is allowed in the first week.
   *c. Chew gum slowly and intermittently for 30 minutes.
   d. Chew each piece of gum for 2 hours before discarding.

   [CL: KN]

   Rationale: In order to ensure even buccal absorption of nicotine, the gum should be chewed slowly and intermittently for 30 minutes.

4. Side effects which are related to therapy with Antihemophilic A factor include:
   a. increased salivation and abdominal pain
   *b. chest tightness and wheezing
   c. hymphadenopathy and alopecia
   d. nausea and constipation

   [CL: KN]

   Rationale: Adverse effects of Antihemophilic A factor include chest tightness, wheezing, and other signs of allergic response.

5. A nursing intervention which should be planned for patients using minoxidil is to:
   a. wash scalp with strong soap
   b. discontinue if no results in one month
   c. restrict oral fluids
   *d. assess blood pressure regularly

   [CL: CO]

   Rationale: Changes in blood pressure may occur in patients using minoxidil for male pattern baldness; therefore, monitoring blood pressure regularly is important.

Additional Review Questions Not Presented in Text

1. Patients taking $Alpha_1$ proteinase inhibitor are at risk for development of:
   a. asthma
   *b. hepatitis B
   c. myasthenia gravis
   d. adrenal tumor

   [CL: KN]

   Rationale: Due to the potential risk of hepatitis B, patients should be vaccinated prior to taking $Alpha_1$ proteinase inhibitor. This preparation is obtained from pooled plasma.

2. Teaching information for the patient taking Beta-carotene (Max-Caro) should include:
   a. taking the medication on an empty stomach
   b. discontinuing medication if skin turns yellow
   *c. opening capsules and mixing with juice before taking
   d. getting at least 6 hours of sun exposure per day

   [CL: KN]

   Rationale: Beta-carotene capsules may be opened and mixed with juice. This Vitamin A precursor is best taken with meals.

3. An agent which is used to counteract the effects of organophosphate pesticide poisoning is:
   *a. pralidoxime chloride
   b. cellulose sodium phosphate
   c. edetate calcium disodium
   d. amiodarone

   [CL: KN]

   Rationale: Pralidoxime reactivates cholinesterase outside the central nervous system. This effect acts to reverse the anticholinesterase action of organophosphate pesticide poisoning.